CW00741997

SHORT LOAN

This

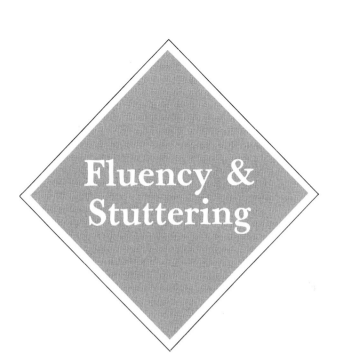

Fluency &
Stuttering

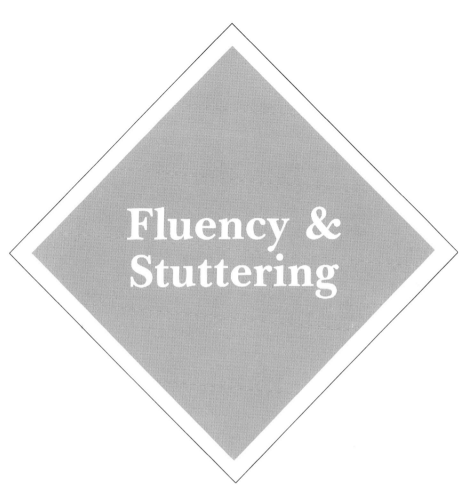

Fluency & Stuttering

C. Woodruff Starkweather
Temple University

PRENTICE-HALL, INC., Englewood Cliffs, New Jersey 07632

Library of Congress Cataloging-in-Publication Data

Starkweather, C. Woodruff.
  Fluency and stuttering.

  Includes bibliographies and index.
  1. Stuttering. I. Title
RC424.S69 1987   616.85'54   86-30556
ISBN 0-13-322462-7

Cover design: Wanda Lubelska
Manufacturing buyer: Harry P. Baisley

This book can be made available to businesses, industry,
organizations, associations, and mail order catalogers at
substantial discounts when ordered in quantity. For more
information, contact:

> Prentice-Hall, Inc.
> Special Sales Department
> College Division
> Englewood Cliffs, N.J. 07632
> (201) 592-2863

Printed in the United States of America

10 9 8 7 6 5 4 3 2 1

ISBN 0-13-322462-7   01

Prentice-Hall International (UK) Limited, *London*
Prentice-Hall of Australia Pty. Limited, *Sydney*
Prentice-Hall Canada Inc., *Toronto*
Prentice-Hall Hispanoamericana, S.A., *Mexico*
Prentice-Hall of India Private Limited, *New Delhi*
Prentice-Hall of Japan, Inc., *Tokyo*
Prentice-Hall of Southeast Asia Pte. Ltd., *Singapore*
Editora Prentice-Hall do Brasil, Ltda., *Rio de Janeiro*

To Aly

Remembering Anchor Bay,
La Lutece,
and Heart's Ease

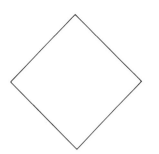

Contents

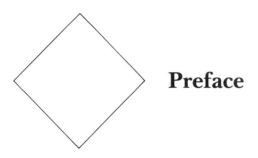# Preface

This book was written in response to several needs. A number of books on stuttering are already available for graduate students, clinicians, and researchers, and some provide extensive reviews of the literature. Others present a particular view of the disorder or provide some other useful contribution. However, even the most comprehensive books give only the skimpiest coverage to the topic of normal fluency. I have long believed that in stuttering, as in other speech and language disorders, an adequate understanding of the disorder could be derived only from an adequate understanding of the normal behavior that the disorder impairs. So in this book I have tried to cover the topic of normal fluency as fully as possible. Indeed, there is more detail in the first part of the book, where normal fluency is dealt with, than in later sections. This is done intentionally to respond to the need for information in this particular area.

I also believed that few of the books on stuttering dealt squarely with the matter of theory construction. There is a current belief in our field that the construction of theory is somehow deleterious, and it is true that there have been a number of abuses in the past—theories that were little more than speculation and personal opinion. But good theory construction—the fitting of one small piece of information to another so as to provide a more complete picture of the whole—is, in my view, a valuable contribution to any discipline. It has been valuable in the history of the other sciences, and there is no reason why it should not be in ours. I also believe that everyone reading an article based on an experiment constructs theory as a natural response to the new information the article provides. Theory construction is, in other words, inescapable—a reflexive reaction of the thinking mind. But because theory construction has had a bad reputation in our field, this reflexive response is suppressed. It occurs, but it is not made public. So I have tried in this book to do more than just describe the small pieces of information, the results of experimental research and clinical observations. I have tried also to show how each of these stones can be fitted with other stones to produce some kind of coherent edifice. There is a bonus in describing not only the information but what can be done with it. The bonus is that students learn not only the information but how to use it, and this is a valuable skill for the practicing clinician. New information is developing at a rapid rate, and we do our students a disservice if all we teach them are the current facts. We also need to show them how to apply the facts they will read about in the future so that they may continue to develop as professionals.

Finally, I believed that there was a gap in the books available on stuttering. A few provided extensive coverage of nearly everything written on the subject. And there were some that covered certain aspects of stuttering or a certain point of view about it. But missing was a book that covered just the important research and covered it at a level of detail so that the material could be included in the usual one-semester course. And so I made a selection of the ideas that I thought were important. But I recognized that the process by which I decided what was important needed also to be made public, so I have described in the Introduction the criteria that I used in selecting information to include.

In the end, this book is an attempt to discover and describe what we really know about stuttering and normal fluency—not what we think we know or what we would like to know, but what we really know. Such a goal is, of course, unreachable, but perhaps something valuable is achieved in the attempt to reach it.

CWS

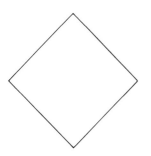

Acknowledgments

A textbook is constructed from information that has been discovered, analyzed, and disseminated by others. My ideas, the most recently laid course of stonework, rest on information quarried by others, and there will be many more placed on mine, and so on. So I want to acknowledge with gratitude the many speech, language, and hearing scientists whose efforts produced the information I have used in constructing this book. In the laboratories of our discipline, the small details of research are chiseled out with care, usually after everyone else has gone home to dinner. Speech, language, and hearing scientists usually expend this effort with little expectation of monetary reward. They are rewarded instead by an indescribable sensation—the "eureka" feeling. It is the feeling one has during a close encounter with a small nugget of information, cut from a larger vein of truth. It is from many of these small facts that really important ideas are built—theory that explains and clinical techniques that work. These small bits of truth are the stones in the foundation of our discipline. I salute the stonecutters.

I am, as always, thankful for the enlightened dedication of Charles Van Riper, who showed so many of us a trail through the woods to a bright clearing.

I am grateful to my family and to my colleagues at Temple University who had to deal with so many things that I failed to do because the better part of my mind was working on the problems of this book. Writing a book is, if nothing else, a wonderful excuse.

I am also grateful to a number of specific individuals who responded to my earliest request for reactions to the proposal for this book or who discussed it with me while I was writing it: Marty Adams, Stanley Ainsworth, Oliver Bloodstein, Dick Curlee, Dick Boehmler, Gloria Borden, Gene Brutten, Ed Conture, Jan Costello, Pearl Gordon, Dale Gronhovd, Steve Hood, Bill Leith, Hal Luper, Fred Murray, Maryann Peins, Bill Perkins, Dave Prins, Joe Sheehan, Hal Starbuck, Ken St. Louis, Mike Webster, Dean Williams, and Marcel Wingate. Their encouragement and assistance was important.

I have learned a great deal about stuttering from my clients, and am grateful to those who, in the midst of their misery, were willing to explain something to me. Thanks also to those students of Speech 545 who had the courage to discuss theoretical ideas. I am particularly grateful to students who worked on specific research projects: Janet Adler, Sharon Franklin, Judy Head, Paula Hirschman, Eddie Hoffman, Terrie Holland, Donna Hutt, Houri Kaloustian, Peggy Kline, Aly Lent, Jay Lucker, Mindy Myers, Sue Pfeuffer, Irwin Ronson, Arnold Shapiro, Terese Smigo, and Marylin Tassiello. I owe a lot to present and former Ph.D. students with whom so many ideas were discussed—Barbara Amster, Joy Armson, Barbara Corradi, and Meryl Wall—and postdoctoral Fellows Hannah Bell and Suzi Meyers, who contributed much work and thought. I owe more than I can say to the tireless energy, clear insight, and unshakable good will of my colleague Sheryl Gottwald. Most particularly, I am grateful to Hugo Gregory and Barry Guitar, whose detailed comments were helpful in revising the book.

Fluency &
Stuttering

Introduction

TOPICS COVERED IN THIS CHAPTER

♦ *The author's beliefs about:*
The importance of genetic/environmental interaction
The role of conditioning and learning in human behavior
The nature of stimuli that control fluency

♦ *The author's reasons for choosing information to include in the book*

♦ *Some common pitfalls of research*

♦ *Definitions of key terms:*
Speech
Language
Fluency
Disfluency
Stuttering

This introduction will describe the premises, assumptions, definitions, criteria, and beliefs that have been used in selecting information for the main body of the book and in commenting on it. It is important to understand that the ideas expressed in this introduction are axioms that I accepted and believed from the beginning. It is important because in this book I am going to try to separate fact from theory more clearly than they are usually separated, and my reasons for including some ideas and excluding others are not facts but beliefs.

BELIEFS ABOUT HUMAN BEHAVIOR

I have several beliefs about human behavior which are premises or axioms. These a priori assumptions form a background against which my evaluations of research and my conclusions about the nature of stuttering should be evaluated. First and foremost among these premises is my belief that human behavior is determined by an interaction between genetic factors and learning. We are all born with certain inherent capacities which constrain how much our behavior can be further changed by learning. Genetic influences provide physiological limits of strength, endurance, speed of movement, coordination, and sensory acuity. Because of these limitations, there are some things we will never be able to learn to do.

Genes also determine an organism's predilection to attend to certain types of stimuli and to respond in certain patterns of behavior. As well, they determine maturational patterns, causing some individuals to mature more quickly or for certain traits to develop before others. These genetic proclivities for patterns of behavior or maturation are partly universal and partly individual.

For example, as human beings we are all strongly predisposed, I believe, to respond to social stimuli. As a result, this secondary social reinforcement is often more important than a primary reinforcement, such as food. Hence the desire some individuals have to refrain from eating so that they will become more attractive. People are important sources of influence, perhaps the most important source of influence. To a certain extent, this is universally true. But some individuals react more strongly than do others to this influence. They are deeply affected by outside opinions. Other individuals, although still powerfully affected by outside opinions, are much more self-contained. Their own self-evaluations carry more weight with them than do the evaluations of others. We don't know for a fact whether or not these proclivities are genetically determined, but they might be.

In either event, such a proclivity never stands alone; it is always modified by the individual's exposure to the environment. All behavior, I believe, results from such genetic constraints and proclivities interacting with behavioral patterns that are learned as a result of exposure to the environment, primarily the social environment. This is another way of saying that the old question of nature vs. nurture is a "bad" question—a question with no answer. Everything we do results from a combination of our basic nature, genetically determined, and the results of our nurturing by the environment, primarily the social environment, in which we live.

Genetic alterations enable a species to track relatively slow changes in the environment, such as changes in the climate or prevailing sources of food. Genetic change can take place rapidly or slowly. Changes in body shape or size take place slowly, but sometimes a species adapts to an environmental shift as a result of a genetically determined alteration in behavior, and these adaptations occur more rapidly. But even the most rapidly changing genes, those that control social behavior (Wilson, 1978),[1] occur too slowly to cope with the fastest environmental changes. For these extremely rapid changes, individuals change by learning new patterns of behavior. Learning is consequently the individual's, not the species', way of adapting to life's moody whims.

I believe that we can best come to understand learning in humans through social learning theory (Bandura, 1969). In 1983, I presented a model based on social learning theory and adapted to speech and language behavior (Starkweather, 1983). The idea of this model was that a number of different conditioning processes may describe behavior change in speech and language. Furthermore, these processes function in humans primarily through social interaction and cognitive processes. Humans are social animals, and social stimuli are important to them. Fluency is no exception. As one dimension of speech and language behavior, fluency is also, I be-

---

[1]Wilson estimates that genes controlling social behavior in animals may alter the animal's behavior significantly in as few as ten generations.

lieve, capable of changing and of being changed by a variety of learning processes, for example, classical and instrumental conditioning, vicarious conditioning, and avoidance conditioning.

In most behavioral accounts, it is helpful to explore the form of the behavior one is interested in, and the form, or forms, of fluency will be examined in this book so that it will be clear what fluency looks and sounds like. Then, as a second step in understanding fluency as behavior, the stimuli that precede and follow it will be examined. These stimuli, the antecedents and consequences of fluency, are presumed (occasionally observed) to control fluency.

This examination will be influenced by my belief in the social learning theory model. In this model, the stimuli that control fluency are expected to consist largely of social and self-evaluative stimuli, although other sources of stimuli will not be overlooked. In other words, humans are motivated largely by the opinions and social interest of others and by their opinion of themselves. The antecedent stimuli are consequently the social circumstances, and this of course includes communicative (e.g., linguistic) events, which precede and presumably control variations in fluency. The consequential stimuli are the environmental changes that occur as a result of variations in fluency, but because the most important aspects of the human environment are (1) the internal environment (self-awareness) and (2) the social evaluations of others, the environmental consequences of any behavior are social, communicative, linguistic, and self-evaluative, for the most part.

Because the internal environment plays such an important role in this model, the antecedents and consequences of a behavior are often not directly observable. Antecedent stimuli must often be inferred from the circumstances under which a variation in the behavior occurs, and consequential stimuli must often be inferred from the apparent intentions of the person performing the behavior. This is a broader and more inferential behavioral model than is common, but I think that it is a model better suited to the development of understanding of speech and language behavior. Interested readers should consult my book, *Speech and Language: Principles and Processes of Behavior Change,* for a full description and application of this model to speech and language behavior.

CONSIDERATIONS IN DECIDING TO INCLUDE INFORMATION

It is no easy matter to decide whether a reported finding is an actual fact. The goal of research is to produce information that is true, and the truth of it should not be lessened by time or distance. Science seeks general and durable information (Agnew and Pyke, 1978).

Often this goal is not reached. Many "facts" are restricted to particular situations, groups of subjects, or periods. It is also often the case that a researcher will carry out an experiment but overlook some small detail so that an alternative explanation for the results is possible. Typically the alternative is really very unlikely and the experimenter's conclusion is most probably correct, but one cannot be certain. For all these reasons it is better to think of the truth of information not as an absolute value but as a relative value. In actuality, something is either a fact or not, but a close look at research literature makes it clear that a reported finding may be a fact or it may not. It is up to the reader to decide. If another experimenter has reported the same finding, that of course makes it more likely that the finding is factual.

But there are some other problems. Unfortunately, there are several built-in biases *against* truth in experimental research. These built-in biases result from the creative urge that motivates scientists to try to produce information. Anyone who has carried out a successful experiment which has increased understanding in an important area knows what a thrill it is. Your hair stands on end. Your palms sweat. Laboratories are sweaty, tremulous places, noisy with the sounds of discovery. It is exciting and fulfilling at the same time. And there are rewards for good research. There are rarely financial rewards, but the researcher may be rewarded by the admiration and approval of colleagues. The discovery is associated with the researcher's name. These are powerful motivations, and they tend to produce errors in research. The scientist wants so badly to find out something meaningful that errors of research design, mathematical mistakes, and alternative explanations of the results are simply overlooked in the heat of the moment. The Western system of science has developed a number of safeguards against these built-in biases. The major ones are prepublication reviews by peers and an insistence that experimental results be replicated before they are accepted as facts, and it is preferred that the replications be done by a different experimenter. But despite these safeguards, many questionable results are reported. For these reasons, one must evaluate each experiment and decide on the probability that the result represents fact or not.

In this book, each research result has been assessed in several ways. But it would be a mistake to call these criteria. I have not tried to create an algorithm for inclusion or exclusion, for deciding between fact and fancy. Although it is possible to develop such an algorithm (Andrews et al., 1983), doing so would be somewhat presumptuous. Some ideas are extremely compelling. They have explanatory power or they seem to fit well with other ideas. One wants to include them even if their empirical basis is questionable. So validity is not the only criterion for inclusion. But in deciding on validity in this book, I have considered a number of things. These are the number of subjects, replication, the logic of the experiment, soundness of the method, and limitations to the generalization of the results. Let us look at these considerations in more detail.

N—The Number of Subjects

An experiment that has been done with a small number (N) of subjects, even if the results are statistically significant, is less likely to be true for other people than an experiment that has produced significant results with a larger number of subjects. It may be a limited fact, true for a few. Unfortunately, in my view, there has been a trend recently in speech and hearing science for experiments to be reported with very small N's. One reason for this is the economic necessity of publishing, which makes researchers want to report their results as quickly as possible. This floods the journals with papers, which require time to process, which slows down the time of publication, which makes researchers all the more eager to get the work into print. It is a vicious cycle in more than one sense because the end result is the publication of many "facts" that are of questionable validity.

There are other reasons for the trend toward small N's. Sidman (1960) proposed a research model in which single subjects were run one after the other. The idea was to continue running single subjects until the outcome of running the next subject was clearly predictable. If applied in the way Sidman intended, this model would have provided standards for scientific truth as rigorous as any. But Sidman's model was often incorrectly used to justify the use of only a few subjects. Psycholinguistic research added to the trend. The psycholinguists believed that any one competent speaker of a language "knew" the rules of the language, and there was little room for individual variation. Therefore grammatical rules that were applicable to all speakers could be discovered by tapping the competence of one speaker. This idea also promoted a trend toward small N's in speech and hearing science, even in experiments unrelated to linguistic knowledge.

Replication

Whether or not an experiment has been replicated and whether this replication is by the same or another experimenter are both important considerations. Results that have not been replicated are less likely to be factual than results that have been replicated by the experimenters themselves, and these in turn are less likely to be factual than results that have been replicated by some other experimenter in another laboratory. However, one failed replication doesn't mean very much by itself. It is usually necessary to go beyond the replication and show how the first experimenter erred.

Related to this last point is an error of research interpretation that is more widely made than any. This error is attributing theoretical relevance to a nonsignificant result. An experiment that fails to find significant results does not provide evidence against the hypothesis it was designed to test. As Carl Sagan has put it: "The absence of evidence is not evidence of absence" (Sagan, 1977, p. 7). Many reviews of the literature include nonsignificant results and discuss them as if they balanced the account against significant results. Instead, such nonsignificant results should simply be omitted. To provide evidence against a stated hypothesis, a contrary hypothesis needs to be developed and a statistically significant result in support of the contrary hypothesis must be found.

Logic of the Experiment

Every experiment is basically a logical statement, beginning from certain premises and coming to specific conclusions. It is helpful, in evaluating research, to think of the article as an argument. The researcher presents the argument for his results. He defends them. It is up to readers to provide the argument for the prosecution. In the heat of discovery, scientists can easily come to conclusions that are not fully warranted by their own observations.

The most typical way in which this happens is overlooking some alternative explanation for the results. The method of the experiment is supposed to reduce these alternative explanations or eliminate them entirely, but it is easy to overlook one or more possibilities and design an experiment that doesn't cover all bases. There are many other ways that the logic of the experiment can be flawed. The premises of an experiment can be untenable. Sometimes an experimenter will begin by defining a construct (concept) in a certain way, which leads logically to the conclusions, but the original definition may be too restrictive or it may depart from known reality in some other way. The premises on which the argument is based have to be premises that most readers are willing to accept. But most typically, experimenters go too far in their conclusion. Because research is a creative enterprise, experimenters are personally proud of the information they have produced. They want it to be as important as possible, and this motive makes them overinterpret the results, drawing conclusions that are too broad. Most experiments produce results that mean something, but not as much as the experimenter believes.

Soundness of the Method

Simple errors in the method may render the observations invalid or inadvertently influence the results. Subjects may have been chosen in a way that predisposes the results in a certain direction or limits the generality of the findings. The measurements may have been made in a way that was not reliably consistent, so that changes could have occurred because of some variable other than the one being observed. Or the measurements may have been carefully made but not quite on target, not fully valid in the way numerical value was assigned to the construct. The analysis of the data can also influence the results if not done carefully. Anyone can make a mistake, and it is far easier to overlook an error when the resulting "fact" supports the experimenter's beliefs than when it doesn't.

But the most common methodological flaw is the presence of the experimenter. When the experimenter is actually present while the subjects are being run, and if they can see or hear the experimenter's reactions as they perform the experimental task, their performance will be affected. Adair (1973) describes behavioral research as a sociological event, in which the subjects and the experimenter reciprocally influence each other. These social influences have a way of altering, in some cases of producing, the "results."

This happens because subjects have a natural curiosity about the experiment they are participating in. They try to understand what the purpose of the experiment is. They usually form an opinion about its purpose. Whether this opinion is right or wrong, it influences their behavior. Hearing the experimenter give directions or talking to the experimenter before the experiment can often give clues about its purpose. Even though these may be false clues, they can influence the subject's performance because most subjects want to help. They want to discover something almost as much as the experimenter does. A few subjects may have the opposite motivation. They may be hostile to the purpose of the experiment and want to sabotage it, and this influences their behavior also. All these effects are quite unpredictable and can be controlled only by not letting the experimenter and the subject have any more to do with each other than is absolutely necessary. Ideally, experiments should be carried out by an assistant who is unaware of its purpose. Sometimes the experiment can be run by a computer.

Limitations of Generalization

In some cases, the results of an experiment apply only to a certain portion of the population of interest. This limits the generality of the findings and reduces their status as facts. For example, many experiments on stuttering are done with adult, usually young adult, subjects. This happens because college students are readily available in large numbers to many researchers. This restricts generality, particularly with regard to stuttering because the disorder is age-dependent; it occurs much more commonly in young children than in older children and adults; and it may have different characteristics in children. Many "facts" about stuttering are facts only for adults. Most experimenters use subjects near where they work, and this may influence the generality of findings. We don't really know, but stuttering may not be distributed evenly around the world. Most subjects are volunteers, and this means that they are predisposed to respond in a certain way. Often, the subjects of an experiment on stuttering are in therapy, and their attitudes and beliefs about stuttering have been heavily influenced by the therapy they are receiving. These beliefs may affect their behavior extensively. Also, exposure to a particular therapy may give them clues as to the purpose of the experiment, and this may in turn affect their behavior, or even produce the results, which are then reported as "facts" about stutterers in general, when actually they are just facts about stutterers who are presently in one particular type of therapy. Many of these restrictions on the generality of research results are unavoidable, but readers must nevertheless be aware of them and wait for replications before concluding that reported results are valid.

It is necessary, I believe, for readers to know the bases on which I have included or excluded certain experiments in the chapters that follow. Doing so makes me uncomfortable, however, because it may imply, to some readers, that I consider my own research free of "mistakes" of the kind just described. That is not the case. No researcher is free of these problems, although all good researchers try to deal with them.

An analogy can be made with religion, which is another avenue to understanding the truth of the universe. Like original sin, threats to the validity of an experiment are always with us. We can only strive to attain the unattainable ideal, searching for those things we have done that we should not have done and those things we have left undone that we should have done, confessing to them in our conclusions with statements that qualify the results, and promising ourselves that we will try to do a better job in our future research.

DEFINITION OF TERMS

The way in which a word or phrase is used, the meaning it has for the person using it, is like a premise. It is something given, an axiom on which later argument may be based. Not a fact, but a presupposition, the definition of a term needs to be given before the term is used. This section provides the definitions for special technical terms that are used throughout the book.

Speech

The word *speech* is used in this book to refer to the motor and neuromotor behaviors of human sound production for the purpose of conveying information through language.

Language

Language refers to (1) the knowledge of syntactic, semantic, and pragmatic rules for conveying information and (2) the behaviors, other than speech production, that result when people use these rules.

Fluency

It is difficult to get a grip on the concept of fluency because the speech-language-hearing profession has had a very narrow view of it since the earliest days of the profession. The word *fluency* connotes facility in speech and language performance. People who are fluent are so skilled in the performance of speech and language behaviors that they do not need to expend much thought or energy to it. Sounds, words, and sentences fall easily from their mouths, without hesitation, and are strung together one after the other rapidly and with few pauses. It ought to be said, however, that it is quite normal to acquire this very high level of skill in speech and language. Most people reach this level. It is normal to be fluent. This is not true of other sequential behaviors. A musician who plays an instrument with the same level of skill that is normal for speech is a very talented and advanced musician. Most human beings become this talented in speech performance. This suggests that speech and language are very special types of behaviors, for which humans are innately able to acquire high levels of skill. That may indeed be true, but remember how much we practice at talking. We practice talking far more than any musician practices an instrument. In fact, most musicians probably talk more than they play.

There are many types of fluency and many ways of looking at it. Because of the interest our field has always had in stuttering, we have always focused on the fluency of speech production, because stuttering is (most likely) a disorder of speech production. But it will help to put things into perspective to think about the other types of fluency. First, there is no reason why we should not, as we always have, use the word *fluency* to refer to the normally high levels of skill humans achieve in using language, as distinguished from speech.

Fillmore (1979) has described three types of language fluency. Although he didn't use these terms, his three types corresponded rather closely to three of the four major components of language: syntax, semantics, and pragmatics. Fillmore believed that speakers who are *syntactically fluent* have the ability to encode highly complex sentences representing a wide variety of complex content-form relations. *Semantically fluent* speakers have large vocabularies, to which they have full and ready access. *Pragmatically fluent* speakers always know what to say under a wide variety of social circumstances. The fourth major component of language, phonology, was not described by Fillmore, but his list can be augmented to include *phonologically fluent* speakers, who would have the ability to pronounce correctly and accurately long strings of syllables in unfamiliar combinations. They would probably be good at dialects and at pronouncing foreign languages too.

The reason for mentioning language fluency is to make it clear that language fluency does not seem to be a part of the problem of stuttering. Adult speakers who stutter have not been shown to lack syntactic, semantic, pragmatic, or phonological knowledge or skill, although few tests of any of these propositions have ever been made. Even if stutterers do lack some of these skills, it is unlikely that language fluency is part of the problem of stuttering, although there is a relation between language and stuttering that will be described later. Stutterers do not have a disability of language fluency, they have a disability of speech fluency. This is true both of adults and of children, although in children, in whom both systems are developing, it may be that there is a closer relation between language fluency and speech fluency than there is in adults. This point will be discussed later.

Speech fluency refers to a normal level of skill in the production of speech. This normal level of skill may be recognized in several ways, which are similar to the ways in which skill in any motor behavior may be seen. Speakers are fluent in their speech production if they produce normally long strings of sounds at a normally rapid rate without pausing or hesitation, and with a normal absence of effort. Speech fluency, then, may be defined as the ability to talk with normal levels of continuity, rate, and effort.

A word should be said here about rhythm. Normally fluent speech has a characteristic rhythm and disfluent or stuttered speech lacks this rhythm. It may be, then, that speech rhythm is also a dimension of fluency. But one theoretical account (Martin, 1979) suggests that the rhythm of speech is more of a support structure for speech production than a part of the skill itself. This, also, will be discussed later.

Disfluency (Dysfluency or Nonfluency)

Disfluency, dysfluency, and *nonfluency* are all terms that have in the past been used to refer to breaks in the continuity of speech production. They are avoided in this book for two reasons. First, speech fluency, as defined above, consists of more than just continuity, but refers to effort and rate as well. *Di(y)sfluency* and *nonfluency* seem not adequately descriptive because they do not specify which dimension of fluency is disrupted. Second, fluency is on a continuum. Speech is more or less fluent. Words like *disfluency* and *nonfluency* suggest that speech is either fluent or it is not. To replace these terms, I suggest the word *discontinuity*. This means specifically a break in the continuity of speech production, regardless of effort or rate. Discontinuities would always slow rate and would of course require some effort, but some discontinuities would slow rate more than others or be more effortful than others, and this distinction is clinically very important. It seems both accurate and useful to keep the dimensions of fluency separated in the words that are used to describe it.

Stuttering

It is always very difficult to define stuttering. There have been many attempts. I am particularly reluctant to do this because one of my purposes is to present facts before reaching theoretical conclusions. Yet a definition of stuttering implies that conclusions have been reached. Still, it is necessary to delimit the topic and make clear what is being referred to by the term. In this book the word *stuttering* will be used to describe a clinical entity, a disorder that can be reliably recognized by clinicians. Some of its primary symptoms are

1. An abnormally high frequency and abnormally long durations of sound, syllable, and word repetitions
2. An abnormally high frequency and abnormally long durations of sound prolongations and pauses

Another important symptom is abnormal amounts of effort in the production of speech, usually evident acoustically and physiologically by struggle, forcing, and tension in the vocal tract, occasionally by abnormally large amounts of cognitive activity related to speech production and in some stutterers, usually those who have experienced certain forms of therapy, by abnormally slow speech. It should be clearly understood that in this book speech that is continuous but abnormally slow is not considered fluent speech.

Other possible symptoms are the avoidance of sounds, words, situations, and listeners that the stutterer comes to believe are difficult; higher than normal levels of anxiety in response to speech and social situations; and a host of coping behaviors and mechanisms that are or have in the past been helpful to the stutterer in his struggles to talk. These symptoms might be summarized by noting that stuttering is a disorder in which the person knows what he wants to say but takes an abnormally long time to say it. The extra time is occupied by the characteristic behaviors described above.

REFERENCES

ADAIR, J., *The Human Subject: The Social Psychology of the Psychological Experiment*. Boston: Little, Brown, 1973.

AGNEW, N. McK., and PYKE, S., *The Science Game*, 2nd ed. Englewood Cliffs, N.J.: Prentice-Hall, 1978.

ANDREWS, G., CRAIG, A., FEYER, A-M., HODDINOTT, S., HOWIE, P., and NEILSON, M., Stuttering: a review of research findings and theories circa 1982, *Journal of Speech and Hearing Disorders*, 48 (1983) 226–46.

BANDURA, A., *Behavior Modification*. New York: Holt, Rinehart & Winston, 1969.

FILLMORE, C. J., On Fluency, in *Individual Differences in Language Ability and Language Behavior*. New York: Academic Press, 1979.

MARTIN, J., Rhythmic (hierarchical) versus serial structure in speech and other behavior, *Psychological Review*, 79 (1979), 487–509.

SAGAN, C., *The Dragons of Eden: Speculations on the Evolution of Human Intelligence*. New York: Random House, 1977.

SIDMAN, M., *Tactics of Scientific Research: Evaluating Experimental Data in Psychology*. New York: Basic Books, 1960.

STARKWEATHER, C. W., Speech fluency and its development in normal children, in *Speech and*

Language: Advances in Basic Research and Practice (vol. 4), ed. N. Lass. New York: Academic Press, 1981.

STARKWEATHER, C. W., *Speech and Language: Principles and Processes of Behavior Change.* Englewood Cliffs, N.J.: Prentice-Hall, 1983.

WILSON, E. O., *Sociobiology: The New Synthesis.* Cambridge, Mass.: Cambridge University Press, 1978.

The Dimensions
of Fluent Speech

INTRODUCTION

Writers attempting a description of stuttering have not included material on normal fluency, even though a substantial scientific literature on the rate, rhythm, and timing of normal adult speech has long existed. The development of fluency in children, a topic with a more obvious relevance to stuttering, has also been slighted, although the reason for this omission is easier to find. The early influence of Wendell Johnson's theory[1] of stuttering development led to a strong emphasis on the idea that discontinuities in preschool children, regardless of the form they took, were normal behavior. Descriptions of children's fluency development referred only to the frequency and type of discontinuities. But it is not just the continuity of speech that signals fluency. The rate of speech, the length of utterances, consistency in the duration of elements, and the overall quantity of speech are also signs of the facility with which speech is produced. With increased age, these signs show developmental change, signaling the growth of fluency in children. They talk more. They become able to talk in longer utterances, to speak more quickly, smoothly, and easily. And their speech timing improves.

It is important for the practicing clinician to know about these developmental changes, for the assessment of stuttering should be made—as the assessment of other speech and language disorders is made—by comparing the client's fluency with the level of fluency that would be expected for a normal person of the same age. This means that the clinician should know how easily nonstuttering children of various ages are usually able to

---

[1]Johnson (1961) believed that stuttering began to develop when parents, or other significant listeners, reacted emotionally to the normal disfluencies of a child. The child acquired the emotional reaction and began to struggle not to be disfluent.

talk, how to measure the variables that signal fluency in children, and how to compare a client's given level of fluency in any of its dimensions with the norms. The purpose of this first part is therefore to describe normal fluency—that is, the ease with which speech is produced—in adults and children.

Premises

Before discussing either the facts or the theory of fluent speech, it is necessary to determine the limits of the discussion. Not all facts are relevant. The relevancy of information depends on a number of premises. These premises are derived from several sources. One such source is the meaning of the word *fluency* (see Chapter 1). The boundaries of a discussion of fluency are also determined by the historical interests of at least three disciplines: speech-language pathology, psycholinguistics, and speech science. A few additional premises are derived from some commonplace observations that can be regarded as axiomatic.

I take it as given that fluency is a multidimensional behavior. That is, it involves a number of different behavioral variables, each of which is an aspect of fluency. Although I take this as a premise, there are some excellent reasons, based on empirical evidence, for doing so (Starkweather, 1981). The dimensions of fluency, it has been suggested, are the continuity or smoothness of speech, the rate of speech, and the effort a speaker makes in producing speech (Starkweather, 1981), but these are very broad categories, each of which consists of several variables. Also, a fourth category, the rhythmic structure of speech, should perhaps be added (Starkweather, 1982). It should be noted that of these four dimensions, continuity, rate, and rhythm have traditionally been considered aspects of speech *timing*, and are discussed in the speech science literature under that heading. Effort has also been examined by speech scientists, and a case can be made that effort is the primary dimension of fluency (Starkweather, 1982), and that the timing variables are secondary, simply reflections of effort (see the discussion later in this chapter).

The first dimension of speech fluency to be discussed is continuity. Fluent speech is continuous: it flows along without hesitation or stoppage. The word *fluency*, derived from the Latin for *flowing*, connotes this quality, and our intuitive recognition of highly fluent speakers is based partly on the ease and grace with which they produce long utterances without stopping.

Pauses and hesitations are usually divided into filled and unfilled pauses. The unfilled pause is simply a silence that lasts longer than a given interval, typically around 250 msec (Goldman-Eisler, 1958). An interval of silence less than a quarter of a second long is likely to result from junc-turing (briefly pausing to signal an otherwise obscure word boundary, as in distinguishing *black bird* from *blackbird*) and may not be a true pause. For this reason, Goldman-Eisler excluded pauses shorter than 0.25 second.

Filled pauses are signaled by the utterance of neutral or meaningless sounds, such as "um," "uh," "ah," "er," and so on. It is important, however, to be very precise about what stops during a discontinuity. It is not the production of sounds or words. To illustrate this point, consider the following passage. It would be considered less than perfectly fluent even when produced with continuous voicing and continuously moving articulators.

> What I mean, what I mean is, that, uh, when you, you, go to the, uh, store because, uh, you, you want some, need some, uh food or supplies or something, and, and, uh, the storekee-, the man, clerk, who, who waits, well not waits, but serves, you know, gets some-, something for you is, well, if he, if he, well if he is sort of, well, stern, or you know angry or something, then, well, then, I find it, well, I find it difficult to talk.

Words flow in this passage. Sound is continuously produced. What is not flowing in this passage is information. It is, it must be, the failure of *information* to flow at some expected rate that causes us to label such productions as low in fluency. This is not an idea that has been subjected to empirical verification, but a premise. There are several ways it could be tested, however. First, as above, continuous production of meaningless sound or repetitive (noninformation-bearing) words could be presented to listeners to see how they rate its level of fluency. Second, listeners could be asked to judge the fluency with which two productions of the same passage were made by the same speaker but at different rates. Speech pathologists, trained to listen for discontinuity, might judge the two passages to be equally fluent, but laymen might judge the more rapidly produced passage to be more fluent. Third, samples of speech could be manipulated so as to be produced at different rates *and* with different levels of continuity. The extent to which fluency judgments were predicted by each of the two variables could be assessed. Fourth, passages that differed in the amount of information they contained could be produced at the same rate by the same speaker. It might be that the passage containing more information would be judged as more fluently produced even though it was produced at the same rate and with the same continuity.

Experiments like this would determine if the flow of information at some expected rate (and the actual rate could be empirically determined for speakers of different ages) is the major determiner of judgments of fluency. Such tests might provide an empirical basis for what seems evident—that it is the flow of information, not the flow of sound, that results in the ordinary listener's judgment of fluency. Breaks in voicing or in the movement of articulators are *signs* of reduced fluency, and of course it is not possible to talk fluently when such breaks are occurring, but the reason these breaks interfere with fluency is, I believe, because information does not flow rapidly enough when they are occurring.

Some pauses are used intentionally to convey information, and these would not be considered discontinuities, because the flow of information continues, including the pause. Other pauses may convey information about the structure of the utterance but not about its content (Van Lancker, Canter, and Terbeek, 1981). Most listeners would not consider these pauses as discontinuities. Discontinuities may contain information about the speaker, but they do not convey information about the content of the utterance.

There are two nearly identical ways of measuring speech continuity: (1) the frequency of pauses and hesitations in a speech sample of known length and (2) the number of syllables produced without pausing. These two measures are essentially reciprocal. The first is the number of pauses per syllable; the other is the number of syllables per pause. The duration of pauses is another variable of interest. There is probably general agreement that longer pauses are more disruptive of fluency than shorter ones. Pauses differ not only in their duration but in a number of other ways, and there are several schemes of categorization, some descriptive of the pauses themselves, others based on the functions that pauses are thought to have.

Pauses may vary in length and they may be either silent or filled with "um," "uh," or some other semantically empty sound. The distinction between filled and unfilled pauses has been made by McClay and Osgood (1959), Goldman-Eisler (1968), and others. Clarke (1971) distinguishes between conventional and idiosyncratic pauses. *Conventional pauses* are ones that a competent speaker makes for emphasis or to signal something linguistically important, while *idiosyncratic pauses* are an aspect of performance, reflecting hesitation or uncertainty over word choice, style, or syntax. "A speaker who knows what he is going to say uses conventional pauses only" (Clarke, 1971, p. 71).

Although this distinction is a useful one to which I will return, it is not always so obvious which pauses are conventional and which are idiosyncratic. Some pauses that appear to be idiosyncratic, that is, pauses which occur because speakers are formulating thoughts and language, may nonetheless serve conventional purposes and be a useful part of language. It is a mistake to think of them as errors. Nevertheless, when people are asked to read aloud, they show only conventional pauses, located at syntactic boundaries and usually accompanied by a breath. By contrast, when the same people were asked to speak spontaneously on a comparable topic, composing their language as they spoke, they used idiosyncratic pauses as well, which are not restricted to syntactic boundaries (Henderson, Goldman-Eisler, and Skarbek, 1965; Clarke, 1971). The relation between pauses and uncertainty has been found by several other researchers. Specifically, pauses occur more frequently in or before sentences that are syntactically more complex (Rochester and Gill, 1973; Cook, Smith, and Lalljee, 1974).

In addition to pauses and hesitations, other breaks in speech continuity—what have always been called "disfluencies"—are repetitions of sounds, syllables, words, and phrases, prolongations of sounds, parenthetical remarks, such as "you know," and false starts, as in "I'm going to, I've got to leave now." Breaks in continuity have aways been considered an aspect of fluency by speech-language pathologists. By this I mean that they have been recognized as momentary stoppages in the forward flow of speech. Breaks in speech continuity may also be accepted as an aspect of fluency on the grounds that the behavior that occurs during the breaks occupies time without contributing information. This is a commonplace observation, but it implies that a certain model of fluency is being used, specifically a model in which *fluency* is defined as the easy flow of information. That is not the only element of the model, but it is one element, and it should be noted that it is consistent with the general definition of speech fluency given in the preceding chapter.

If it is acceptable that the flow of information is an aspect of fluency, then it follows that the rate at which meaningful speech is produced is an aspect or dimension of fluency. It was noted earlier that the central concept of fluency had to do with effort, facile speech being fluent speech. It is commonly observed that behaviors performed with greater facility are performed more rapidly. This idea, plus the idea that we intuitively label as breaks in fluency those behaviors that occupy time without contributing information, make it evident that speech rate is an aspect of fluency. We should, although we have not done so, think of the slow speaker as less fluent than the rapid one. It is odd that we have not thought of the slow speaker as lacking fluency because we have probably always recognized the rapid speaker (assuming good intelligibility and an even rhythm) as more skilled and fluent than the speaker whose rate is simply average. A more precise delimitation of the relation between rate and fluency will be a theoretical conclusion derived from information to be presented later.

The facility with which speech is produced is the central idea of fluency, as defined in the preceding chapter, so it would have to be conceded that ease of speaking is a dimension, perhaps the most central dimension, of fluency. But the measurement of effort is problematic, and for this reason there is only a little direct evidence bearing on the effort with which speech is produced, and virtually none for children's speech.

Another dimension of fluency is rhythm. This idea too is acceptable as a premise on the grounds that when excessive effort is used to achieve speech, that is, when speech is produced less fluently, the behaviors of which the effort is composed momentarily stop or slow speech. Then when the means to forward flow are again found, speech production resumes at a pace that is at least normal. These interruptions of course give to speech a lurching quality and detract from its more typical rhythm which contains certain regularities, to be described later. It also seems intuitively acceptable that fluent, facile speakers produce speech with fewer stops and starts, that is, in a more rhythmic way.

The preceding discussion is simply to say that continuity, rate, effort, and rhythm are qualities of speech that should be addressed in any discussion of fluency. That they are aspects of fluency is accepted as a premise. The following description will consequently be limited to findings pertaining to those four elements.

CONTINUITY

Findings

1. Unfilled pauses occur on the average every 4.8 words when speakers were providing narrative descriptions and every 7.5 words when they were engaged in discussion (Goldman-Eisler, 1968). In both of these cases, the speech was perceived by listeners to be "continuous."

2. Half of "continuous" speech time is divided into phrases that are less than three words long, with pauses between each phrase (Goldman-Eisler, 1958; 1968).

3. Only 10 percent of speech time is composed of phrases that are ten words or longer (Goldman-Eisler, 1958; 1961).

4. Pauses are distributed in a predictable way throughout utterance. They are more likely to occur before content words, such as nouns, verbs, adverbs, and adjectives, than before function words, such as prepositions, articles, and conjunctions (McClay and Osgood, 1959).

5. Pauses tend to occur at clause boundaries or where a decision over word choice is likely to be made (Goldman-Eisler, 1968; Boomer, 1970; Rochester and Gill, 1973).

6. Filled pauses tend to occur before words that are relatively high in uncertainty (Cook, 1971).

7. Filled pauses tend to occur before longer and more complex sentences (Cook, Smith, and Lalljee, 1974).

8. Filled pauses are much more common at the beginnings of clauses than within clauses (Boomer, 1965; Cook, 1971; Hawkins, 1971).

9. When the duration of pauses within clauses is compared with the duration of pauses between clauses, the within-clause pause is found to be shorter by about 100 msec (Grosjean and Deschamps, 1979; Hawkins, 1971).

10. Adults pause more often when explaining than when describing (Goldman-Eisler, 1968).

11. When people read out loud, they pause less often, their pauses are synchronized with their breathing, and the pauses occur at major syntactic boundaries. When the same people speak spontaneously, they pause more often, and some of the pauses are located intraclausally and not synchronized with breathing (Henderson, Goldman-Eisler, and Skarbek, 1965; Clark, 1971).

12. Hesitations and pauses are more common in material that is syntactically more complex (Rochester and Gill, 1973; Cook, Smith, and Lalljee, 1974).

13. In adults descriptions produce fewer disfluencies than interpretations (Goldman-Eisler, 1962).

14. Speakers pause longer before content words than before function words (Boomer, 1965; McClay and Osgood, 1965).

15. When recordings of spoken material are transcribed, or when spoken material is repeated, subjects do not repeat idiosyncratic pauses, but they do repeat conventional pauses (Clark, 1971).

Another way of looking at the continuity of speech, instead of counting the frequency of breaks in continuity, is to measure the length of unbroken, continuous segments of utterance. This can be done by counting the number of syllables that occur between pauses. Malecot, Johnston, and Kizziar (1972) made surreptitious recordings of fifty upper-middle–class Parisian French speakers as they conversed with each other. From these recordings a number of measures of speech timing were made, one of which was the length of utterance in syllables.

16. For adults, the length of utterance is about 6 to 9 syllables, on the average, although a proportion of utterances are very short, 2 to 5 syllables, and some are very long, 10 to 50 syllables (Malecot, Johnston, and Kizziar, 1972).

17. The distribution of utterance length in adults is quite skewed (Malecot, Johnston, and Kizziar, 1972).

18. There is a significant difference between the sexes in utterance length, women tending to be more fluent than men in this way (Malecot, Johnston, and Kizziar, 1972).

19. Malecot and his associates also observed a relation between utterance length and the speaker's profession. People who used oral language in their profession, such as lawyers and professors, tended to produce very long utterances.

Theory

It seems evident that pauses, whether filled or unfilled, are a common feature of speech. Few people would guess that we pause on the average every 4.8 words. We seem not to hear pauses and think of speech as more continuous than it actually is. Our perception of speech seems to be more continuous than the reality of it. In much the same way as listeners tend not to hear misarticulations in the speech of people they are familiar with, the pause, filled or unfilled, is simply overlooked. Presumably this happens because we focus on the content of communication. We listen to the ideas, not to the means for conveying them, and any sound or variation that does not contribute to these ideas is filtered out by our perceptual mechanism. That is not to say that pauses never convey information, but the information they sometimes convey has to do with the process of communication or with the speaker's level of uncertainty, rarely with the content.

The fact that pauses occur with a high frequency and are nearly universal in human speech suggests that they may serve some purpose. Human communication has evolved so as to provide for the intense socialization of our species, and it is unlikely that such a frequently occurring behavior is simply an error or momentary lapse in the process. To illustrate this idea, it is useful to compare pauses with slips of the tongue (spoonerisms), such as: "I'm not as drunk as some thinkle peep I am." Although slips of the tongue evidence certain regularities which reveal information about the nature of communication (Fromklin, 1971), they seem to be failures of the speech production or linguistic processes. They occur rarely, and both the speaker and any listeners react noticeably to them, usually with laughter or a comment. By comparison, pauses occur frequently and are not overtly reacted to by listeners. These differences suggest that pauses, unlike slips of the tongue, seem likely to have evolved as a functional aspect of oral language. The nature of that function becomes more evident when the distribution of pauses in utterance is examined.

The findings on the distribution of pauses (findings 4 through 15) seem related. They suggest that the frequency of pauses increases as the speech act, particularly its content, becomes more complex. In each of these studies, the speech act that presumably involved more cognitive activity—explaining versus describing, formulating versus reading, syntactically complex versus syntactically simple, interpreting versus describing, content versus function words—produced a higher frequency of pauses. There has been a presumption, from the earliest days of research in this area, that the pauses were occasions on which language was being formulated, and although it seems likely that this is true for some pauses it may not be true for all pauses. Clark's (1971) data indicate that people pause less and their pauses are found in different locations when they read aloud. During reading, language formulation is at least reduced, although it would be going too far to say that there is no language formulation associated with reading aloud. So it seems reasonable to conclude that *some* of the language formulation pauses drop out during oral reading, but some may remain.

In support of the idea that the two types of pauses are different in kind, Clark notes that idiosyncratic pauses convey no information and tend to be overlooked, but this is not true of conventional pauses, which are retained in transcribed or repeated material. Clark concludes that the "conventional pauses are information-bearing elements of the sentences" (p. 74) and that the "conventional pauses seem to have evolved in the language mainly for the benefit of the listener, whereas idiosyncratic hesitations are the product only of an overburdened speaker and give no help to the listener." This idea might be profitably supplemented by noting that it is not just the *over*burdened speaker, but all speakers who produce idiosyncratic pauses. Presumably, the presence of idiosyncratic pauses may lighten the burden of any speaker. We shall see in a moment just how the pause may help to lighten the speaker's burden.

The nature of normally fluent speech is elucidated not just by the frequency of pauses, but also by a consideration of the reciprocal of this idea—the length of continuous utterance between pauses. Findings 16 through 19 bear on this topic. The average duration of utterances is far down toward the lower end of the distribution. This means that although on the average people produce utterances that are rather short, occasionally they produce utterances that are very long, up to 50 syllables. So, although it is normal (average) for speech to be discontinuous, it is possible for the continuity of speech to exceed the average.

THE RATE OF SPEECH

Findings

1. Adult speakers of English speak at an average rate of 5 to 6 syllables per second (Walker and Black, 1950).
2. Rates are only slightly different in other languages (Malecot, Johnston, and Kizziar, 1972; Osser and Peng, 1964).
3. The rate at which continuous (i.e., pauses excluded) syllables can be produced is a function of (1) speed of articulatory movement and (2) the degree of coarticulatory overlap (Gay, 1978; Starkweather, 1981).
4. When rate is measured in words per minute, most of the variation is attributable to the duration and frequency of pauses. When these pauses are excluded, the variability of speech rate is much reduced (Goldman-Eisler, 1958).
5. With rate held constant, the average variability of overall duration of an utterance is about 3 to 4 percent (Kozhevnikov and Chistovich, 1965; Allen, 1975).
6. Speech can be compressed up to 275 wpm mechanically with little loss of comprehension, but comprehension declines rapidly at higher speeds (Foulke, 1971).

7. When communication failure is induced experimentally, speakers tend to slow down the rate of speech (Longhurst and Siegel, 1973).
8. The length of utterance is correlated with the rate of speech, rate being faster in longer utterances (Malecot, Johnston, and Kizziar, 1972).

Theory

Adult speakers of English produce about 5 syllables per second during continuous conversational speech (Walker and Black, 1950; Miller, 1951). In French, the rate is only slightly faster at 5.73 syllables per second (Malecot, Johnston, and Kizziar, 1972). This last study is of interest because the recordings were made surreptitiously, which may be important. Intuitively, one suspects that subjects would try to speak more correctly if they knew they were being recorded. Speaking more correctly might lead to several types of changes, such as more carefully articulated speech, more carefully structured sentences, and perhaps a slower rate.

In addition to their primary finding, Malecot, Johnston, and Kizziar (1972) found that the speech rate of women is more variable and their utterances are longer than men's, although they did not find a significant sex difference in rate. Such differences do exist at certain younger ages (see later discussion), but apparently not in adults.

It is perhaps important, in trying to understand the nature of speech rate, to recall the *non*segmental nature of speech production. The speech gestures which result in a stream of changing sound are continuous. The articulators stop moving only occasionally, and then for brief moments, so there are changes in velocity. The tongue lurches from one place to the other, sometimes pausing in its flight for a few milliseconds before moving on. We may hear this continuously changing stream of sound as a series of individual segments, but segmentation is not present in the speech gestures and movements, breathstream flow, and vocalization that produce speech. So we produce continuously what we hear segmentally.

When the rate of speech is discussed, this distinction must be borne in mind. The duration of syllables or of specific sounds is an important consideration in the perception of speech. Each sound has a characteristic duration, and our recognition of the sound depends partly on this. The characteristic duration is, however, a relative one. When we talk more rapidly, all segments are shortened, and when speech is slowed by a situational demand, such as the need to communicate against a noisy background, or by a syntactic demand, such as the end of a clause, all segments are lengthened. So the duration of segments is determined by their inherent duration and by the overall rate at which speech is produced, that is, the speed with which the speech gestures are performed and the extent to which adjacent speech gestures are allowed to overlap temporally. Consequently, important information about speech rate is to be found in studies that measure the duration of speech segments.

Mackay (1974) compared a number of different types of syllables and found that when a syllable began with a consonant it was likely to be produced faster than a syllable that began with a vowel. This effect was substantial enough so that even syllables that were longer by several sounds were produced faster if they began with consonants. For example a simple syllable, consisting of a single vowel, such as /a/ is likely to be produced more slowly than a consonants plus vowel (CCCV) syllable such as /skra/.

Rate is faster in longer utterances than in shorter ones. This effect does not seem to be attributable to speakers' attempts to finish a clause before taking a breath. There is more of a rate decrease during short utterances than there is a rate increase during long ones, which implies that it is the amount of information in the utterance that affects rate (Malecot, Johnston, and Kizziar, 1972; Starkweather, 1981).

The lips can move diadochokinetically at about 6 syllables per second, as can the tonguetip, and the tongueback can move at about 5 syllables per second (Fletcher, 1972). Tiffany (1980) pointed out in a careful analysis that the maximum rate and the ordinary rate of speech are about the same; that is, people talk about as fast as they can. Why this should be so, if it is true that the diadochokinetic (DDK) and the ordinary rate are not correlated (Lass and Sandusky, 1971), is unclear. If the rate of speech, averaged across many speakers, is about the same as the maximum DDK rate, averaged across many speakers, it follows that speakers in general talk about as fast as they can. But if the correlation between maximum DDK rate and speech rate is low, it means that the generality is untrue for a few speakers. These people must have diadochokinetic rates that are higher than the average, yet they talk at a rate below the average.

There is, however, another possibility that should be considered. In the experiment by Lass and Sandusky, no correlation was found. This does not mean that there is no correlation between DDK and speech rate. It means only that such a correlation was not found in the particular sample studied. The absence of evidence for a phenomenon is not the same as evidence for the absence of a phenomenon. Other attempts to find such a correlation should be made, and we should refrain from concluding that none exists until many attempts have failed.

Reaction time (RT) is the amount of time that elapses between the occurrence of an external stimulus and the beginning of some movement, such as bilabial closure for /pa/. Netsell and Daniell (1974) found that RT for /pa/ was approximately 200 msec. If one speech gesture can be made in a fifth of a second, it follows (at least mathematically) that five gestures can be made in 1 second. A syllable, of course, can consist of more than one speech movement, but the mathematical correspondence is striking, and confirms the other facts suggesting that we produce speech with movements that are made at nearly maximum velocity.

Several conditions are known to alter speech rate. In whispering, for example, rate is slower (Brown and Brandt, 1971; Parnell, Amerman, and

Wells, 1977), and rate is slower when speaking in noisy conditions (Hanley and Steer, 1949; Winchester and Gibbons, 1958; Ringel and Steer, 1963). Longhurst and Siegel (1973) asked listeners to say "What?" at predetermined times. The speakers reacted to the signal that information was not flowing by slowing their speech rate.

THE DURATION OF SPEECH SEGMENTS

Findings

1. The duration of consonants and vowels varies according to their inherent duration, their position in the utterance, their position in the word, the immediately adjacent sounds, the length of the word, and the word's frequency of usage (both in the language and in the speaker) (Umeda, 1975; 1977).

2. The duration of sounds reflects a continual speeding up and slowing down of speech rate (Starkweather, 1981), and these alterations seem to give the listener an additional cue about the syntactic structure of the utterance (Van Lancker, Canter, and Terbeek, 1981).

3. Segments are lengthened at the beginnings and endings of syllables, words, and phrases (Fowler, 1977).

4. All segments in a stressed syllable are lengthened, consonants and vowels alike (Huggins, 1978).

5. When speakers say the same thing repeatedly, the duration of adjacent segments tends to be negatively correlated. That is, if a sound is a little longer than usual, an adjacent sound is likely to be shortened to compensate (Kozhevnikov and Chistovich, 1965).

6. Segment durations are affected by adjacent sounds as in clustering effects and the effects of a following voicing feature (Huggins, 1978).

7. Segment durations are affected by position in the syllable (a syllable initial consonant—/s/ in "my seat"—is 10 to 20 percent longer than a syllable-final consonant—/s/ in "mice eat" (Huggins, 1978).

8. Segment durations are affected by the length of a word, for example, the duration of the syllable /bɔrd/ becomes progressively shorter in "board," "boarder," "bordering," "borderingly," but each additional unstressed syllable has less of a shortening effect than the previously added one (the idea of incompressibility) (Huggins, 1978).

9. Segment durations are affected by the length of a sentence; the longer the sentence, the shorter each word in it—compare "Joe" in "Joe called" to "Joe" in "Joe took father's shoe bench out" (Huggins, 1978).

10. Segment durations are affected by the position of the segment in the sentence, segments toward the end (prepausal) being lengthened— compare "Joe called" to "Call Joe" (Huggins, 1978). Vowels located at

the ends of phrases and utterances are some 100 msec longer than comparable vowels in nonfinal positions (Klatt, 1975; 1976).

11. A similar phenomenon occurs within phrases, segments located toward the end of the phrase being lengthened—compare "Jane married John Kalinsky" to "Jane Kalinsky married John." "Jane" is longer in the first example because it is the last (and only) element in the noun phrase (Huggins, 1974; Klatt, 1975; Goldhor, 1976).

12. In adults, the place of articulation has small effects on the duration of preceding vowels, vowels before labials being about 10 to 15 msec shorter than vowels before dentals or velars (Smith, 1978).

13. Differences in duration that exceed 15 to 20 percent can probably be perceived (Huggins, 1972).

14. Speech rate is not linearly related to segment duration—when a sentence is spoken twice as fast, some segments are shortened more than others, specifically the vowels are shortened more than the consonants (Huggins, 1978).

15. In speeded speech "timing contrasts" are reduced (Weismer and Ingrisano, 1979). The utterance-final segments in speeded speech were affected differently by the increased rate than other segments.

Theory

Although it is intuitively comfortable to measure the rate of speech by counting the number of syllables produced in a period of time, there are other ways of doing it. A closer view of the speed with which speech is produced can be provided by measuring the duration of individual speech sounds as they are produced in continuous utterance. Naturally, each sound has its own characteristic duration, but this inherent, or canonic, duration varies according to a number of contextual effects. It is these contextual effects that are of interest because they tell us that the rate of speech is not constant during continuous utterance. Rather it speeds up and slows down in minor variations that are predictable and interesting.

Two studies done by Umeda (1975, 1977) are important. Both of these studies were extensive analyses of monologues produced by an individual speaker and are consequently not necessarily representative, although most of her findings have been confirmed by other experiments in which samples of subjects were tested. However, in these confirming studies, the speech was not spontaneous.

Stressed syllables are longer than unstressed ones (Umeda, 1975). This is obvious, but the extent of the effect should be appreciated. Unstressed syllables are shortened so much that there is virtually little variation among them and little opportunity for them to be shortened more. They are all uniformly short. Gay (1978) has shown that at fast speech rates unstressed vowels cannot be further shortened. The variations that Umeda found are for vowels in stressed syllables. It is evident that, in addition to raising pitch and loudness to signal stress, we also slow the rate of syllable production on the stressed syllables to give them added weight.

In 1953, House and Fairbanks measured the duration of vowels in various types of nonsense syllables, such as /pip/ and /fuf/. They found that vowels were shorter when surrounded by voiceless consonants than when surrounded by cognate voiced consonants. They also found that vowels surrounded by stops were shorter than vowels surrounded by nasals and fricatives and that bilabial and velar consonants shortened the vowels they surrounded more than labiodental or alveolar consonants. A close analysis of these results suggests that it is the duration of the surrounding consonants that produces the effect. A longer consonant, such as a nasal or fricative, makes the neighboring vowel longer too, and a shorter consonant makes the vowel shorter. Umeda confirmed these findings but was able to distinguish between the effect of the following consonant and the effect of the preceding consonant. She found that the entire effect was produced by the following consonant.

The duration of vowels is longer in words that convey more information. This fact is derived from three of Umeda's (1975) observations: (1) vowels are longer in content than in function words; (2) vowels are longer in words that occur less frequently in the language; and (3) vowels are shortened in words that are said repeatedly during a conversation. Each of these observations seems to relate the duration of vowels to the amount of information conveyed by the word the vowel is in. Content words convey more information than function words, so the first two of Umeda's observations seem clearly to be related to uncertainty or information load.

The third observation also seems related to uncertainty. When a word is repeatedly used in connection with a particular topic, it seems reasonable to suppose that its predictability would be increased, and its information load reduced. So it would seem that the duration of vowels varies according to the information load of the word the vowel is in. Because the duration of vowels is a direct reflection of the rate of speech, it follows that speech may speed up or slow down according to momentary changes in the load of information in the utterance. It has long been known that the load of information fluctuates from moment to moment, and at one time this fact was used in connection with the idea that language is a linear series of units, each conveying some quantity of information. That view has long since fallen to the wayside with increased awareness of the hierarchical structure of language.

However, it is still a fact that information load varies from moment to moment, although it should be recognized that one of the main causes of this variation is syntactic structure. As a result, in a sentence such as "God isn't dead, He's just looking for a parking place," the load of information is very high at the beginning, since there is no way (given no context) to predict what the first word of the sentence is. Once the first word is known, however, it only takes a relatively few guesses, usually fifteen to twenty in an undergraduate class in speech pathology, to guess that the next word is "isn't." The reason that "isn't" conveys so much less information is that information about the structure of the sentence is conveyed by the first word. Once a listener has heard the first word, the probability of the second word being "isn't" is increased.

All this is to make clear that the level of information flow is not constant, but increases and decreases throughout utterance according to the words used and the structure of the sentences they are used in. Most important for an understanding of rate is the role played by syntactic structure, for there is always a large jump in uncertainty at a major clause boundary. After one clause has ended and before another one has begun the uncertainty is high and the load of information carried by the first word of a clause is correspondingly large. Information load and uncertainty are intimately related, because the amount of information conveyed by a linguistic item is a direct function of the amount of uncertainty preceding the item and is reduced by its expression.

If one looks even more microscopically at the flow of information, it should be intuitively evident that uncertainty is also raised just before a word is spoken, but that most of the information contained in a word is located in the first part of it. Compare your ability to understand " __is _____ence _____trates __he _____iple" with your ability to understand "Th__ sent____ illus_____ th__ prin_____." Much more information is conveyed in the sentence that lacks the second halves of its words than is conveyed by the sentence that lacks the first halves of its words.

Vowels are lengthened at the ends of words and phrases (Oller, 1973) and at the ends of clauses (Umeda, 1975). Umeda (1975) and Oller (1973) both suggest that these lengthening effects at the ends of words, phrases, and clauses may serve a useful communicative purpose by signaling the listener that a word, phrase, or clause boundary is approaching. This would mean that the moment-to-moment fluctuations in the rate of speech are a source of information about the syntactic structure of utterance. Of course, there are other ways of signaling syntactic structure, but such redundancies are common in language.

An experiment by Van Lancker, Canter, and Terbeek (1981) tested the idea that variations in rate and timing within the utterance may be used to signal syntactic structure. The authors asked a normal native speaker of English to say certain idiomatic expressions, such as "He has kicked the bucket," or "She is at the end of her rope." In one condition the speaker was to try to convey the idiomatic meaning, but in the other condition, the speaker was to attempt to convey the literal meaning. For example, "She was at the end of her rope," might have been part of a story about mountain climbing. After having the speaker generate a large number of pairs of expressions in which one was intended to be taken literally and one was intended to be taken idiomatically, the experimenters performed a spectrographic analysis of the sentence pairs. They found clear differences between the two types of sentences. Sentences that were intended to be taken literally were systematically longer and the extra time they were given was inserted at syntactic boundaries.

Thus, when a speaker is asked to convey the literal meaning of an idiomatic expression, he inserts time at syntactic boundaries. This has the function of signaling to the listener that the syntactic structure of the sentence is to be attended to. "She (pause) was (pause) at the end (pause) of her (pause) rope." When the idiomatic meaning is intended, the structure of the sentence is less important because the sentence has a whole meaning unto itself, much like a lexical item.

The duration of consonants also varies with the level of uncertainty. Like vowels, consonants have an inherent duration. This inherent duration then increases or decreases according to the phonetic environment. As with vowels, the moment-to-moment fluctuations in uncertainty seem to dictate further variations in the duration of consonants, their duration lengthening before a pause and then shortening after a pause. Umeda (1977) observed that consonants lengthened before a pause but that they did not lengthen at grammatical boundaries that were not accompanied by pausing. This suggests that the rate of speech still slows at these less distinct grammatical boundaries, but not enough to allow for the lengthening of the consonants, which have less capacity for change.[1] Umeda (1977) found that consonants in VCV syllables, on the average, were shortened by 30 msec following a pause and lengthened by 11 msec before a pause, an average change of 41 msec.

The duration of consonants is also altered according to their position in words. The consonants that introduce stressed syllables are shorter by 10 msec, on the average, when the syllable is in mid-word position than when the syllable initiates the word. This finding has been confirmed by Oller (1973) and Klatt (1974) in studies built around sentence tasks. When the syllable is at the end of the word, its consonants are shorter than the consonants in word-initial syllables but not as short as the consonants in mid-word syllables. This is different from the effect for vowels, but because vowels, being longer, contribute more to the duration of syllables, the overall effect is for syllables to be longer at the ends of words and shorter at the beginnings. Rate changes at word boundaries, although not as much as at sentence and clause boundaries. It seems reasonable to describe these microscopic changes in the rate of speech as correlated with changes in the

---

[1]Most consonants are shorter than vowels to begin with and so cannot shorten much more. Some consonants, specifically those with plosive qualities, are made with rapid movements and brief bursts of sound, which cannot be lengthened without destroying the character of the sound.

level of uncertainty (or information load) of the utterance. Like vowels, consonants also vary with the length of the word, the frequency with which the word occurs in the language, and whether the word is a content or a function word. Umeda (1977) was able to compare the effect of word length with that of word frequency for the consonant /s/. She found that frequency of occurrence predicted /s/ duration but not word length when it was kept independent of word frequency.

Klatt (1974) found that consonants were shorter in words that contained more syllables. We seem to skip quickly over long words that do not convey additional information. But, of course, longer words tend to be used less frequently in the language and as a result often do convey more information. It is as if we adjust the rate of our speech to maintain a more or less constant rate of information flow, slowing down when information is high, at syntactic boundaries, when using uncommon words, but speeding up when the flow of information is slow for the number of syllables.

The variability of speech sound durations may reflect one of two processes. It may be, as Klatt (1974) has suggested, that durational variability reflects less care on the speaker's part. This interpretation may be correct, but it may also be true that variability increases at locations in the utterance when additional demands are placed on the speaker to adjust the rate of speech. The findings regarding the variability of consonant duration suggest that variability increases at locations where the rate of speech changes— clause, phrase, and word boundaries. Apparently, durational targets become more difficult to achieve when the speaker attempts to change rate, either to speed up or to slow down.

The duration of speech segments can be altered by manipulating the feedback the speaker receives. The acoustic signal can be recorded, delayed slightly (50 to 500 msec) and then played back to the speaker loudly enough so that he or she cannot hear the original signal, a condition known as delayed auditory feedback (DAF). Under this experimentally induced condition, the duration of segments is prolonged.

We know that the DAF effect is not just a general slowing of rate because not all segments are prolonged equally. Those that are longer to begin with are prolonged more than those that are shorter (Agnello, 1966). The prolongation of individual segments may be appreciated by imagining oneself in the role of a speaker receiving delayed auditory feedback. You are talking and having proceeded, say, halfway through the production of an /s/, are informed by the delayed signal that you are only a quarter of the way through. So you continue to produce /s/, waiting, as it were, to hear confirmation that you have made enough of it to end it and move on to the next sound. Eventually, after an additional few hundred milliseconds, you realize that the sound has lasted long enough, and you move on to the next sound anyway, even though the acoustic signal says not to. Obviously, two types of feedback are present here, the first source of information being the acoustic feedback, the second being a sense of speech timing.

Huggins (1978) presents a general model of speech timing, noting that the duration "of a unit at one level is consistently affected by the number of other units at the same level that fall within a single unit at the next higher level." Thus (1) segment duration is affected by the number of other segments within a syllable; (2) syllable duration is affected by the number of other syllables within a word; and (3) word duration is affected by the number of words in the phrase, clause, or sentence.

Huggins makes the point that if the duration of segments in the first word of a sentence is determined by the total number of words in the whole sentence, then the speaker must have planned the entire sentence before producing the first word. A more parsimonious explanation could be based on the idea that the rate of speech is determined by the anticipated flow of information. In the latter case, one would not need to have planned the entire utterance but only to have some notion, more or less precise, about the amount of information it would contain. This allows for some foreknowledge of what is going to be said, which of course is present, but does not require that the sentence be syntactically planned at the outset.

COARTICULATION

Premises

Speech sounds are produced by movements of the speech mechanism. It is conceptually convenient to think of these movements as speech gestures. A speech gesture may be defined as a group of movements with the same purpose. In adjusting the vocal tract from one position to the next, the purpose is to get from the preceding to the following position. Because phonemes are combined in many different ways, it is useful to think of the movements of such a transition as consisting of two speech gestures. One moves away from the preceding position and the other gesture moves toward the subsequent position. These two speech gestures are perfectly continuous, flowing one into the other without hesitation in normal speech. Also, they vary in their physical characteristics (precise location, velocity, and so on) from person to person, and within a given speaker they vary with alterations in speaking rate, context, fatigue state, and so on. What remains constant is their purpose in adjusting the vocal tract toward a position. The position may be one of several that will have the desired acoustic effect. Several movements are usually involved in each of these speech gestures because of the coordinated activities of the phonatory, respiratory, and articulatory mechanisms. For example, to say /pa/ requires two gestures, each consisting of a number of movements. Movements in the first gesture would include bilabial adduction and velar elevation, at least. The second gesture would involve jaw depression, bilabial abduction, tongue retraction, glottal adduction, and some other movements.

Coarticulation refers to the fact that adjacent speech gestures can influence and interfere with each other. For example, the /s/ in "seat" has an acoustically different quality from the /s/ in "sat" because, in "seat" the tongue has already moved forward to the /i/ position during the time that the /s/ sound is being produced. From the point of view of timing, this means that the gesture to move into /i/ begins before the gesture to move away from /s/. In fact the gesture to move into /i/ may occur at the same time as the gesture to move *into* /s/. As far as timing is concerned, coarticulation refers to the fact that adjacent gestures may overlap in time, a gesture for a subsequent sound beginning before a gesture for a preceding sound has been completed.

In this discussion, the word *coarticulation* will be used to refer to the *extent* of this overlap. Previously, some investigators have been interested primarily in whether coarticulation was present or not under certain circumstances. Other investigators have measured the extent to which adjacent gestures may overlap temporally, a phenomenon called "undershoot." When timing and rate are the focus of attention, I believe it is more useful to think of coarticulation in this latter way, as a variable; to be aware that adjacent speech gestures can overlap *more or less*. This approach is valuable because the extent of coarticulation (undershoot) is related to the rate of speech production (Gay, 1978), and because it changes with development (Kuehn and Tomblin, 1974).

Findings

1. Coarticulatory overlap extends to adjacent sounds, and it may extend beyond immediately adjacent sounds (Amerman, Daniloff, and Moll, 1970). In a VCV utterance, the production of the first vowel may be influenced by the second vowel, in spite of the presence of the intervening consonant (Ohman, 1966).

2. In a CVVN utterance, coarticulation of the nasal does not extend as far back when there is a word boundary between the two vowels as when the two vowels are in the same word (McClean, 1973).

3. When the rate of speech is increased by instructions to talk faster, the extent of coarticulation is greater (Gay and Hirose, 1973; Gay et al., 1974; Gay, 1978).

Theory

Gay and his colleagues at the Haskins Laboratories asked subjects to say the same phrase at fast and at slow speeds. As predicted, the vowels were shorter in duration when speech was faster, but they retained their full vowel color and identity. For the vowels to retain their identity, the tongue must reach the position appropriate for the vowel, but in speeded speech it has to get to this position in less time than at normal rates. There are two ways time could be saved. The speech gesture could begin at the same time as in slow speech but the tongue could move more rapidly from one position to the next, or the gesture could begin earlier. In the latter case, the actual velocity of movement would not have to change, and this would be desirable because an extremely fast transition into a vowel position might change the perception of the vowel. Really rapid transitions tend to sound like consonants. And indeed, Gay and his colleagues observed that the velocity of tongue movement during rapid speech was not much different than during slow speech. Instead, the gesture was begun earlier, so that the tongue could move at an appropriate velocity to the appropriate position but still do so in less time. So at fast rates of speech coarticulatory overlap is greater. It seems reasonable to conclude that coarticulation is not just a passive influence of adjacent sounds on each other, but an active strategy that can be used to produce sounds more rapidly. This is not to say that movements of greater velocity may not also occur for certain sounds, which do not depend for their perceptual character on the speed of transition.

McClean (1973) asked speakers to produce a sequence of sounds in which a consonant was followed by two vowels, which were followed by a nasal. In one condition, this sequence of sounds contained a word boundary between the two vowels, for example /miæn/ in "me and you." In the other condition, the same sound sequence did not contain a word boundary between the two vowels, for example /miæn/ in "meander." McClean observed that the presence of a word boundary between the two vowels delayed the onset of the velar depression for /n/. Consequently, it could be said that the word boundary decreased the extent of coarticulatory overlapping. This is consistent with the observations that Umeda (1975; 1977) and others have made with regard to the duration of speech sounds. Both coarticulation and speech sound durations are a function of the rate of speech, which slows momentarily at word boundaries.

There are, logically, only two ways to change the rate of speech. One is to move the speech mechanism more rapidly and the other is to adjust the timing of speech gestures. Coarticulation is one important adjustment of this type. Another is reducing the duration of steady-state portions of vowels and continuants, and still another is to reduce the duration of pauses. There are consequently three different ways of changing timing to increase speech rate without changing the actual velocity of speech movements. This is important if, as Tiffany's (1980) and my own (1980) analyses suggest, humans talk at a rate that is close to the limits of their speed of movement. If the articulators are already moving at maximum, or nearly at maximum velocity, alterations in coarticulation may be a more available strategy for adjusting the rate of speech from moment to moment to signal the grammatical and lexical structure of the utterance.

There is a trade-off kind of relationship between rate of movement and coarticulation. Because we seem to talk very rapidly, close to our limits of movement speed, the availability of another way to increase rate may be an important consideration. When circumstances call for us to talk more quickly than our capacity for rapid movement will allow, we can still achieve the required speed by increasing coarticulatory overlap. A price is paid, however, because increased coarticulatory overlap moves speech production in the direction of decreased intelligibility, and highly coarticulated speech is slurred and hard to understand. This may be what happens in the speech of inebriated people. The alcoholic daze reduces reaction time and movement speed. The person attempts to compensate with further coarticulation and slurred speech results. Of course, it is also likely that articulatory precision is diminished by drunkenness, which would contribute to unintelligibility.

It is interesting to observe the relations between coarticulation as an aspect of speech rate and fluency in normal speakers. Coarticulation is also related to stuttering (see pp. 00) in that stutterers, early in the development of the disorder, seem to substitute the schwa (unstressed) vowel for full vowel color in stuttered syllables. The analysis in this section suggests the possibility that what appears to be schwa substitution in stuttering is actually a shortened version of the vowel motivated by a desire to hurry through stuttered syllables.

EFFORT

Premises

The effort that goes into speech production is an important aspect of fluency. It is characteristic of fluent speech that it is produced effortlessly. I take this to be a premise, not a fact or a theoretical position based on fact, because I know of no empirical way to establish a standard by which to determine what is considered a greater or smaller amount of effort. Nevertheless, it seems that speech requires little effort in comparison to other similar activities, such as playing a musical instrument. Perhaps, also, the payoff from talking is large in comparison to the effort that goes into it. In any event, it is a premise taken here that fluent speech is easy speech. Fluent speech is effortless in two distinct ways: it requires little thought, and it requires little muscular exertion. Mental effort or concentration is clearly hard to measure, but it is possible to measure amounts of time during which it may be presumed, for reasons to be discussed shortly, that thought is being devoted to speech and language production. When speech is being used in the normal, communicative way, very little time is spent thinking about the processes of speech production. Thoughts are focused on the content rather than the processes of utterance. Indeed, one of the purposes of communication is to transmit thoughts from one brain to another, and it makes sense that communicative behavior has evolved to serve that purpose most efficiently. If it were necessary to spend much time think-ing about the processes of speech production, there would be less time to think about the content of messages. So speech production is an automatic or semiautomatic behavior. Like breathing, it goes on without any con-scious effort but can be consciously controlled should the occasion demand it.

The second type of effort is muscular. Only modest amounts of muscle activity are necessary to produce speech, although of course some muscular effort is required to provide a flow of air, to open and close the glottis, and to move the tongue, lips, jaw, velum, and pharynx. There is considerably more data on muscular than on mental effort because it is so much easier to observe, although, as we shall see, the picture is not as clear as might be anticipated. Some of the difficulty arises because the actual effort involved in speech production and the effort perceived by listeners are both im-portant as far as fluency is concerned. The effort the speaker perceives himself to be putting into the speech act is as important as the effort that is actually put into it, for if the speaker perceives that too much or too little effort is being expended, for the task, the speaker may try to alter the level of effort. This occurs because the effort listeners perceive speakers to be making is a most important aspect of fluency. Listeners quickly recognize the absence of fluency when a speaker uses an unusual amount of effort in talking. Speakers who stutter, and perhaps those who do not, know this and adjust their actual effort according to what they think listeners will perceive.

One of the important clinical signs of fluency disorder is an abnormal amount of effort devoted to the production of speech. This abnormal effort may be in the form of too much thinking time or it may be in the form of too much muscular effort. Because there is a level of effort which may be judged abnormal, we need to learn what constitutes a normal amount of effort so that the clinical judgment of "abnormal" can have a point of ref-erence.

Findings

1. Alpha wave activity in locations of the brain known to be associated with speech diminishes just before a person speaks (Linebaugh, 1975).
2. Speakers take longer to abort a speech attempt and change speech direction just before utterance than at any point during utterance (Ladefoged, Silverstine, and Papcun, 1973).
3. Pauses are more frequent and longer in duration at points of high uncertainty (Goldman-Eisler, 1961; Boomer, 1970; Cook, 1971; Hawk-ins, 1971; Rochester and Gill, 1973; Cook, Smith, and Lalljee, 1974; Grosjean and Collins, 1979).

4. Pauses during oral reading occur exclusively at clause boundaries; those made during conversational speech occur intraclausally as well (Huggins, 1974).

5. Stops and fricatives require more effort than nasals and glides, as measured by intraoral air pressure (Malecot, 1955; Subtelny, Worth, and Sakuda, 1966).

6. Voiced sounds have lower intraoral air pressure than unvoiced sounds (Subtelny et al., 1966).

7. Males have lower intraoral air pressure peaks than females (Subtelny et al., 1966), no doubt because of the longer male vocal tract.

8. Children have higher pressure peaks than adults (Subtelny et al., 1966).

9. Consonants at the beginnings of words have higher intraoral air pressure values than those located at the end (Subtelny et al., 1966), probably because the closure period is longer (Oller, 1973; Klatt, 1974; Umeda, 1977).

10. Consonants introducing stressed syllables have higher intraoral air pressure values than those introducing unstressed syllables (Subtelny et al., 1966), probably because of the additional airflow that results from additional abdominal force (Netsell, 1970).

11. Intraoral air pressure decreases as the rate of speech increases (Arkebauer, 1964).

12. A speaker's perception of the effort he is using to produce speech is directly related to subglottal air pressure (Prosek and Montgomery, 1969).

13. The airway above the glottis is opened wider during more effortful productions (Tucker, 1963).

14. The contact force between opposing articulators is increased during greater speech effort (Leeper and Noll, 1969).

Theory

The two types of effort that have been mentioned—effort of thought and effort of muscle—are both important, but considerably less is known about the former because of the difficulty of observing thought. Nevertheless, we do have some information. The areas of the brain involved in speech production can be located, and Linebaugh (1975) has observed that these areas become active just before utterance, suggesting that whatever thinking time is needed to perform an utterance is expended before the utterance begins.

This interpretation of Linebaugh's data is confirmed by an interesting experiment. Ladefoged, Silverstine, and Papcun (1973) asked speakers to say "Ed had edited Id." Because the speakers knew what they were going to say, they did not have to expend any thought on the content or the structure of the sentence. The task was almost pure speech production. The speakers were asked to watch for a signal, a small light, and when this light was turned on they were to stop saying the sentence and say "psst." The experimenters measured the time that elapsed between the onset of the light signal and the onset of the "psst." They expected that the speakers would find it harder to interrupt themselves at certain points during the utterance than at others, but they were surprised to discover that this was not so. The speakers could interrupt themselves equally well at any point during the sentence, and their reaction times from the onset of the light to the onset of "psst" were the same regardless of when the light was turned on during this period.

The one exception to this was that if the light was turned on just before utterance, it took the speakers longer to stop and change direction. It seemed to the authors as if the speakers were involved in doing something at this time that was less interruptible than during the actual production of the sentence. It can only be guessed, but it seems a reasonable guess, that what they were involved in was "planning" the motoric production of the sentence. Then, the subject having made this preliminary preparation, the sentence was executed without much further thought.

The production of a sentence or clause is a complex matter, involving the careful coordination and timing of a number of different speech mechanism movements. These movements have to be made accurately with regard both to time and place. It is a little like a football team running a play. Each member of the team has to be in the right place at the right time for the play to work, and to accomplish this purpose it is useful to spend some time before the play to make sure each player is ready to perform his specific role. Then it is necessary only to make sure that everyone starts the play at the same time.

The point is that the planning of an utterance and the execution of it are two different kinds of behaviors. Planning occupies only a small proportion of the total time, but it is probably a more conscious, voluntary behavior. Execution, on the other hand, takes up more time, but is more automatic. It is also worth noting that the two types of behavior occur at different times. It seems as though we pause slightly to plan, taking a little time away from thinking about the content of the utterance to prepare for the coordinated movements, then resume thinking about content.

Consequently, the duration of pauses has been taken to be a measure of the amount of effort put into planning of the subsequent utterance. Although there is no way of being certain that this is what occurs during pauses, it is a reasonable assumption to work with. One of the difficulties with this assumption, however, is the inability to distinguish between pause time that is being used to plan for the production of speech sounds and pause time that is being used to plan the structure of sentences. That is, pause time reflects both speech fluency and language fluency.

Another way of distinguishing between speech pause time and language pause time is by the location of the pauses. It has been observed (Henderson, Goldman-Eisler, and Skarbek, 1965) that when people are asked to read aloud, their pauses occur at clause boundaries, but when they are speaking spontaneously some of their pauses occur within the clause. This suggests that speakers may interrupt themselves intraclausally to think about what they are going to say, what word they are going to use, or how to structure the rest of the sentence, but when they already know how the sentence is going to be structured and what words they are going to say, they pause only at clause boundaries. It may be that speech production planning is restricted to clause boundaries, but of course that doesn't mean that all of the time spent pausing at a clause boundary is necessarily devoted to the planning of speech production. Some of it may be used for other purposes as well. Still, it seems as though the pause that occurs at clause boundaries results from a somewhat different behavior than the pause that occurs within the clause.

Although there are still a number of uncertainties about what is occurring during pauses, it is worth restating the important fact that pauses are not distributed randomly throughout the utterances. More pauses occur and the duration of pauses is longer at points of high uncertainty (Goldman-Eisler, 1961; Boomer, 1970; Cook, 1971; Hawkins, 1971; Rochester, 1973; Cook, Smith, and Lalljee, 1974; Grosjean and Collins, 1979). Because these are locations where the information load is high, it is reasonable to conclude that the time spent during the pause is being used for an activity which is more difficult or at least takes longer when there is more information to transmit.

We are on somewhat surer ground when it comes to the muscular effort of speech production. This too is an aspect of speech fluency. We recognize quickly that the speaker who talks slowly and with evident labor, or who seems to use greater muscular force, is less fluent than the speaker whose words are produced easily.

Most people realize intuitively that it takes more effort to talk when there is loud background noise or when the person they are talking to is far away. It takes more effort to talk loudly. This type of effort, however, is probably not related to speech fluency, at least not directly, as the following facts should make clear. Prosek and Montgomery (1969) asked subjects to talk and measured the loudness of their speech. They then told the speakers how loudly they had been talking by assigning a numerical value to the loudness of the speech which was equivalent to the subglottal air pressure the speakers had been using. Then they asked the speakers to speak with greater effort and to increase their effort by multiples of the value previously assigned. When the speakers did this, their subglottal air pressure was measured again and it was found to correspond to the level of effort they had been requested to make. Consequently, speakers' perception of the effort they are using to talk is directly related to subglottal air pressure. Tucker (1963) asked speakers to talk under conditions which the subjects reported as requiring more effort. While they were talking, various measures were made, and it was found that speech perceived as more effortful involved wider mouth opening, lower jaw displacement, and a number of other differences. In combination these differences were described by Tucker as a widening of the airway.

Finally, when people are talking in a way that they perceive as more effortful, the force of contact between opposing articulators is greater (Leeper and Noll, 1969). This last observation might seem in conflict with Tucker's finding that the airway is opened more widely during speech that is perceived as effortful, but in fact it is not. It is clear that what speakers feel to be effortful speech is speech that is produced more loudly, and all three of the observations just noted—higher subglottic air pressure, a more widely opened airway, and greater force of contact between opposing articulators—increase the intensity of the sounds produced by the speaker.

The loudness of speech, or the effort used to produce it, however, does not seem to be related to speech fluency. Intuitively, we do not judge loud speech to be less fluent, even though it requires greater effort. Nor do we judge soft speech to be more fluent, even though it requires less effort. Yet there is a sense in which fluent speech can be seen and felt to be less muscularly effortful than nonfluent speech. It is consequently necessary to make a distinction between the muscular effort that is used to talk more loudly and the muscular effort that occurs when speech is not being produced fluently. To clarify this distinction, we must add to the discussion a consideration of some of the muscular activities of the airway above the glottis and the activity of the larynx itself.

Speech sounds are produced by creating a flow of air and then moving the structures of the speech mechanism in opposition to that flow. Phonation is produced by closing the glottis, or almost closing it, so that the flow of air causes the vocal folds to vibrate, but this closure also impedes the flow of air, so that there is a pressure drop across the glottis. Above the glottis, sounds are also produced by movements that result in momentary partial or complete closures and impede the flow of air. Here too there is a pressure drop across the point of closure. Because these transitory changes in air pressure reflect the movements of the speech mechanism, and because they are relatively easy to measure, it is possible to get an extremely clear picture of speech sound production by observing changes in intraoral and subglottal air pressure during speech (Netsell, 1973).

Much of the seminal work in observations of intraoral air pressure was done by Subtelny, Worth, and Sakuda (1966). They found that stops and fricatives had higher intraoral air pressure values than nasals and glides and that voiced sounds had lower intraoral air pressure than unvoiced sounds, confirming what seems intuitively obvious, that intraoral air pressure is a function of the completeness of the closure of the airway, of the duration of the closure, and of impedances introduced below the mouth during voicing, which naturally lower the subglottal air pressure.

The point here is that although considerable effort may be expended to create and sustain an adequate flow of air, and although structures are closed to impede that flow and thereby create speech sounds, in fluent speech, the speaker does not sense that there is any appreciable opposition between air flow and impedances to airflow created at the glottis and in the mouth. The nonfluent speaker, however, is aware of this opposition and of the effort that must be used to overcome it. There have not been any investigations of this phenomenon, as far as I know, but many stutterers that I have worked with clinically report a sense of effort in trying to force air through the vocal tract. It would be surprising if stutterers did not feel this sensation of pressure because their articulators, or glottises, are being held in a closed position for more than the normally brief duration and as a result air pressure builds up below the point of closure. In nonstutterers, attempts to demonstrate that sounds produced with more intraoral air pressure are perceived as more effortful have not yet been successful (Daniloff, 1973).

The differences in intraoral air pressure values for males and females and for children as compared with adults reflect the larger size of the adult male vocal tract. With a greater volume of air, the pressure builds up more slowly, and both the air and the greater tissue surface area can absorb pressure increases more easily than a small tract. This means that the male vocal tract is somewhat more elastic. It suggests also, however, that once pressure has built up to higher than normal levels, it may be more difficult, that is it may take longer, for the male tract to dissipate the extra pressure than a female tract or a child's tract. The picture is complicated even more because children talk more slowly and consequently hold their articulatory positions for a somewhat longer period of time, and this permits the buildup of pressure to occur more readily or perhaps more often. On the other hand, the child's lung volume is smaller. It is not clear what part each of these different elements plays in the intraoral air pressure values of children's speech.

Subtelny et al. (1966) also reported two other findings, which have both been confirmed by more recent investigations, findings which are important for an understanding of the role of effort in speech fluency. The first of these findings is that consonants at the beginnings of words have higher intraoral air pressure values than the same consonants located at the ends of words. This is surely just another view of the finding noted earlier that consonants at the beginnings of words are longer in duration. Because the flow of air from the lungs is essentially steady, this additional air pressure at the beginnings of words probably results from the articulators being held in an airway-impeding position for a longer than usual period of time. During the period of closure, pressure continues to build up behind the closure point, until the speech gesture moving away from the consonant is performed. The other important finding that Subtelny et al. (1966) reported is that there are greater intraoral air pressure values for consonants within stressed syllables as compared with consonants within unstressed syllables. Here too the extra intraoral air pressure agrees with the longer duration with which the closure is maintained, but in this case the flow of air from the lungs is not uniform.

Hixon (1973) has shown that there are brief "pulsatile" elevations in subglottic air pressure associated with stressed syllables. Both the additional subglottic air pressure and the additional duration of the consonants contribute to the elevated intraoral air pressure during consonants produced in stressed syllables. If intraoral air pressure can be equated or correlated with the effortfulness of speech sound production, then it is interesting to note that consonants in stressed syllables and consonants at the beginnings of words are less fluently produced in normal speakers than consonants at other locations. This is interesting because, as we shall see in the second section of this book, stutterers are more likely to stutter on sounds that occur at the beginnings of words and on sounds that introduce stressed syllables.

REFERENCES

AGNELLO, J. G., and KAGAN, H. C., *Delayed Auditory Feedback and Its Effect on the Manner of Speech Production.* Final Report, NIH Grant # 11067-01, 1966.

ALLEN, G. D., Speech rhythm: its relation to performance universals and articulatory timing, *Journal of Phonetics,* 3 (1975), 75–86.

AMERMAN, J., DANILOFF, R., and MOLL, K., Lip and jaw coarticulation for the phoneme /æ/, *Journal of Speech and Hearing Research,* 13 (1970), 147–61.

ARKEBAUER, H. J., A study of intraoral air pressure associated with the production of selected consonants. Doctoral dissertation, State University of Iowa, Ames, 1964.

BLACK, J. W., A relationship among fundamental frequency, vocal sound pressure, and rate, *Language and Speech,* 4 (1961), 196.

BOOMER, D. S., Review of F. Goldman-Eisler, Psycholinguistics: Experiments in spontaneous speech, *Lingua,* 25 (1970), 152–64.

BROWN, W., and BRANDT, J., Effects of auditory masking on vocal intensity and intraoral air pressure during sentence production, *Journal of the Acoustical Society of America,* 49 (1971), 1903–1905.

CHEN, M., Vowel length variation as a function of the voicing of the consonant environment, *Phonetica,* 22 (1970), 129–59.

CLARK, H., The importance of linguistics for the study of speech hesitations, in *The Perception of Language: Proceedings of the Symposium, University of Pittsburgh,* eds. D. Horton and J. Jenkins. Columbus, Ohio: Charles E. Merrill, 1971.

COOK, M., The incidence of filled pauses in relation to part of speech, *Language and Speech,* 14 (1971), 135–39.

COOK, M., SMITH, J., and LALLJEE, M., Filled pauses and syntactic complexity, *Language and Speech,* 17 (1974), 11–16.

DANILOFF, R., Normal articulation processes, in *Normal Aspects of Speech, Hearing and Language,* eds. T. Hixon, F. Minifie, and F. Williams. Englewood Cliffs, N.J.: Prentice-Hall, 1973.

DELATTRE, P. A comparison of syllable length conditioning among languages, *IRAL,* 4 (1966), 183–98.

FISCHER-JORGENSON, E., Sound duration and place of articulation, *Zeitschrift fur Phonetiksprachwissenschaft und Kommunikationsforschung*, 17 (1964), 757-62.

FLETCHER, S., Time-by-count measurement of diadochokinetic syllable rate, *Journal of Speech and Hearing Research*, 15 (1972), 757-62.

FOULKE, E., The perception of time compressed speech, in *Perception of Language*, eds. D. L. Horton and J. J. Jenkins. Columbus, Ohio: Charles E. Merrill, 1971.

FOWLER, C., Timing control in speech production, *Dissertation Abstracts International*, 38 (1978), 3927-28.

FROMKIN, V., The non-anomalous nature of anomalous utterances. *Language*, 7 (1971), 27-52.

GAY, T., Effect of speaking rate on vowel formant movements, *Journal of the Acoustical Society of America*, 63 (1978), 223-30.

GAY, T., and HIROSE, H., Effect of speaking rate on labial consonant production: a combined electromyographic high-speed motion picture study, *Phonetica*, 27 (1973), 203-13.

GAY, T., USHIJIMA, T., HIROSE, H., and COOPER, F. S., Effect of speaking rate on labial consonant-vowel articulation, *Journal of Phonetics*, 2 (1974), 47-63.

GOLDHOR, R. S., Sentential determinants of duration in speech. M.A. thesis, Massachusetts Institute of Technology, Cambridge, Mass., 1976.

GOLDMAN-EISLER, F., The predictability of words in context and the length of pauses in speech, *Language and Speech*, 1 (1958), 226-31.

GOLDMAN-EISLER, F., The continuity of speech utterance: its determinants and its significance, *Language and Speech*, 4 (1961), 220-31.

GOLDMAN-EISLER, F., Speech and thought, *Discovery*, April, 1962.

GOLDMAN-EISLER, F., *Psycholinguistics: Experiments in Spontaneous Speech*. New York: Academic Press, 1968.

GROSJEAN, F., and COLLINS, M., Breathing, pausing and reading, *Phonetica*, 36 (1979), 98-114.

GROSJEAN, F., and DESCHAMPS, A., Analyse des Variables Temporelles du Français Spontane, *Phonetica*, 26 (1972), 129-56.

HANLEY, T., and STEER, M., Effect of level of disturbing noise on speaking rate, duration, and intensity, *Journal of Speech and Hearing Disorders*, 14 (1949), 363-68.

HAWKINS, P., The syntactic location of hesitation pauses, *Language and Speech*, 14 (1971), 277-88.

HENDERSON, A., GOLDMAN-EISLER, F., and SKARBEK, A., The common value of pausing time in spontaneous speech, *Quarterly Journal of Experimental Psychology*, 17 (1965), 343-45.

HENDERSON, A., GOLDMAN-EISLER, F., and SKARBEK, A. Sequential temporal patterns in spontaneous speech, *Language and Speech*, 9 (1966), 207-16.

HIXON, T., Respiratory function in speech, in *Normal Aspects of Speech, Hearing, and Language*, eds. F. Minifie, T. Hixon, and F. Williams. Englewood Cliffs, N.J.: Prentice-Hall, 1973.

HOUSE, A., and FAIRBANKS, G., The influence of consonant environment upon the secondary acoustical characteristics of vowels. *Journal of the Acoustical Society of America*, 25 (1953), 105-13.

HUGGINS, A. W. F., Just-noticeable differences for segment duration in natural speech, *Journal of the Acoustical Society of America*, 51 (1972), 1270-78.

HUGGINS, A. W. F., An effect of syntax on syllable timing. Research laboratory of Electronics (QPR No. 114), Massachusetts Institute of Technology, Cambridge, Mass., 1974.

HUGGINS, A., Speech timing and intelligibility, in *Attention and Performance VII*, ed. J. Requin. Hillsdale, N.J.: Lawrence Erlbaum, 1978.

JOHNSON, W., *The Onset of Stuttering*. Minneapolis: University of Minnesota Press; 1961.

KLATT, D., The duration of /s/ in English words, *Journal of Speech and Hearing Research*, 17 (1974), 51-63.

KLATT, D., Vowel lengthening is syntactically determined in a connected discourse, *Journal of Phonetics*, 3 (1975), 129-40.

KLATT, D., Linguistic uses of segmental duration in English: acoustic and perceptual evidence, *Journal of the Acoustical Society of America*, 59 (1976), 1208-21.

KOZHEVNIKOV, V. A., and CHISTOVICH, L. A., *Speech: Articulation and Perception*. Joint Publications Research Service, 30, 543. United States Department of Commerce, 1965.

KUEHN, D. P., and TOMBLIN, J. B., The use of cineradiographic techniques for the study of articulation disorders. Paper presented at the Annual Convention of the American Speech-Language-Hearing Association, Las Vegas, Nev., 1974.

LADEFOGED, P., SILVERSTINE, R., and PAPCUN, G., Interruptibility of speech, *Journal of the Acoustical Society of America*, 54 (1973), 1105-08.

LASS, N., and SANDUSKY, J., A study of the relationship of diadochokinetic rate, speaking rate, and reading rate, *Today's Speech,* 19 (1971), 49–54.

LEEPER, H., and NOLL, J., Pressure measurements of articulatory behavior during alterations of vocal effort. Convention address, American Speech and Hearing Association, 1969.

LEHISTE, I., *Suprasegmentals.* Cambridge, Mass.: Massachusetts Institute of Technology Press, 1970.

LINDBLOM, B., Temporal organization of syllable production, *Speech Transmission Laboratory Quarterly Progress and Status Report,* Stockholm, October, 1968.

LINEBAUGH, C., Interhemispheric asymmetries in the contingent negative variation and cerebral dominance for speech production. Ph.D. dissertation, Temple University, Philadelphia, 1975.

LISKER, L., Closure duration and the intervocalic voiced-voiceless distinction in English, *Language,* 33 (1957), 42–49.

LOFQVIST, A., A study of subglottal pressure during the production of Swedish stops, *Journal of Phonetics,* 3 (1975), 175–89.

LONGHURST, T. M., and SIEGEL, G. M., Effects of communication failure on speaker-listener behavior, *Journal of Speech and Hearing Disorders,* 16 (1973), 128–40.

MACKAY, D. G., Aspects of the syntax of behavior: syllable structure and speech rate, *Quarterly Journal of Experimental Psychology,* 26 (1974), 642–57.

MALECOT, A., An experimental study of force of articulation, *Studia Linguistica,* 9 (1955), 35.

MALECOT, A., The force of articulation of American stops and fricatives as a function of position, *Phonetica,* 3 (1968), 95–102.

MALECOT, A., JOHNSTON, R., and KIZZIAR, P.-A., Syllabic rate and utterance length in French, *Phonetica,* 26 (1972), 235–51.

McCLAY, H., and OSGOOD, E. I., Hesitation phenomena in spontaneous English speech, *Word,* 15 (1959), 19–44.

McCLEAN, M., Forward coarticulation of velar movements at marked junctural boundaries, *Journal of Speech and Hearing Research,* 16 (1973), 286–96.

MILLER, G. A., Speech and language, in *Handbook of Experimental Psychology,* ed. S. S. Stevens. New York: John Wiley, 1951.

NETSELL, R., Underlying physiological mechanisms of syllable stress, *Journal of the Acoustical Society of America,* 47 (1970), 103–4.

NETSELL, R., Speech physiology, in *Normal Aspects of Speech, Hearing and Language,* eds. F. Minifie, T. Hixon, and F. Williams. Englewood Cliffs, N.J.: Prentice-Hall, 1973.

NETSELL, R., and DANIEL, B., Neural and mechanical response time for speech production, *Journal of Speech and Hearing Research,* 17 (1974), 608–18.

OHMAN, S., Coarticulation in VCV utterances: spectrographic measurements, *Journal of the Acoustical Society of America,* 39 (1965), 151–68.

OLLER, D., The duration of speech segments: the effect of position-in-utterance and word length. Unpublished Ph.D. dissertation, The University of Texas, Austin, 1971.

OLLER, D., The effect of position in utterance on speech segment duration in English, *Journal of the Acoustical Society of America,* 54 (1973), 1235–47.

OSSER, H., and PENG, F., A cross-cultural study of speech rate, *Language and Speech,* 7 (1964), 120–25.

PARNELL, M., AMERMAN, J. D., and WELLS, G. B., Closure and constriction duration for alveolar consonants during voiced and whispered speaking conditions, *Journal of the Acoustical Society of America,* 61 (1977), 612–13.

PROSEK, R., and MONTGOMERY, A., Some physical correlates of vocal effort and loudness. Convention address, American Speech and Hearing Association, 1969.

PROSEK, R., and HOUSE, A., Intraoral air pressure as a feedback cue in consonant production, *Journal of Speech and Hearing Research,* 18 (1975), 133–47.

PROSEK, R. A., MONTGOMERY, A. A., WALDEN, B. E., and SCHWARTZ, D. M., Reaction-time measures of stutterers and nonstutterers, *Journal of Fluency Disorders,* 4 (1979), 269–78.

RINGEL, R. L., and STEER, M. D., Some effects of tactile and auditory alterations on speech output, *Journal of Speech and Hearing Research,* 6 (1963), 369–78.

ROCHESTER, S., and GILL, J., Production of complex sentences in monologues and dialogues, *Journal of Verbal Learning and Verbal Behavior,* 12 (1973), 203–10.

SLIS, I., Articulatory measurements on voiced, voiceless and nasal consonants, *Phonetica,* 21 (1970), 193–210.

SLIS, I., Articulatory effort and its durational and electromyographic correlates, *Phonetica,* 23 (1971), 171–88.

SMITH, B. L., Temporal aspects of English speech production: a developmental perspective, *Journal of Phonetics,* 6 (1978), 37–67.

STARKWEATHER, C. W., Speech fluency and its development in normal children, in *Speech and Language: Advances in Basic Research and Practice,* (vol. 4), ed. N. Lass. New York: Academic Press, 1981.

STARKWEATHER, C. W., The development of speech fluency and the definition of a stuttering problem. Symposium, Northwestern University, Evanston, Ill., 1982.

SUBTELNY, W., WORTH, J., and SAKUDA, M., Intra-oral air pressure and rate of flow during speech, *Journal of Speech and Hearing Research,* 9 (1966), 498–518.

SUSSMAN, H., MACNEILAGE, P., and HANSON, R., Labial and mandibular movement dynamics during the production of bilabial stop consonants: preliminary observations, *Journal of Speech and Hearing Research,* 16 (1973), 397–420.

TIFFANY, W. R., The effects of syllable structure on diadochokinetic and reading rates, *Journal of Speech and Hearing Research,* 23 (1980), 894–908.

TUCKER, L., Articulatory variations in normal speakers with changes in vocal pitch and effort. M.A. thesis, University of Iowa, Iowa City, 1963.

UMEDA, N., Vowel duration in American English, *Journal of the Acoustical Society of America,* 58 (1975), 434–45.

UMEDA, N., Consonant duration in American English, *Journal of the Acoustical Society of America,* 61 (1977), 846–58.

VAN LANCKER, D., CANTER, G., and TERBEEK, D., Disambiguation of ditrophic sentences: acoustic and phonetic cues, *Journal of Speech and Hearing Research,* 24 (1981), 330–35.

WALKER, C., and BLACK, J., *The Intrinsic Intensity of Oral Phrases.* Joint Project Report No. 2. Pensacola, Fla.: Naval Air Station, United States Naval School of Aviation Medicine, 1950.

WEISMER, G., and INGRISANO, D., Phrase level timing patterns in English: effects of emphatic stress location and speaking rate, *Journal of Speech and Hearing Research,* 22 (1979), 516–33.

WINCHESTER, R. A., and GIBBONS, E. W., The effect of auditory masking upon oral reading rate, *Journal of Speech and Hearing Disorders,* 23 (1958), 250–52.

The Physiological
and Acoustic Bases
of Fluency

TOPICS COVERED IN THIS CHAPTER

♦ *Implications for fluency of the physical dimensions of the vocal tract*

♦ *Coordination and timing of speech movements:*
Coordinative structures
Resonant frequencies

♦ *Experimental findings related to coordination and timing*

♦ *Theory of coordination and timing:*
Reaction time
Feedback
Gestural synchrony
Dominance
Interference

♦ *Relation of coordination to rhythm*

♦ *Rhythm of speech and its relation to fluency*

♦ *Experimental findings on speech rhythm*

♦ *Theory of rhythm and fluency*

ANATOMICAL CONSIDERATIONS

This section will examine the mechanisms of speech production—the vocal tract and the central nervous system serving it—to see what, if any, contribution they may make to fluency. We all use the speech mechanism to produce speech, and some people produce speech more fluently—more easily, smoothly, and rapidly—than others. The ease with which some people speak may result from characteristics present in the mechanism they use. Of course, ease in speaking may also result from psychobehavioral effects, and in a later chapter I will examine these. But here I will look at the effect of certain properties of the vocal mechanism on speech fluency.

The Vocal Tract

Size and Mass of Moving Parts

Speech sounds are produced by continuous movements of the vocal tract. These movements produce three distinct types of acoustic result. First there is the special case of laryngeal valving. The principal function of glottal ab- and adduction is to begin and end phonation. Adjustments of the glottal opening are also important in whispered speech, glottal attack, glottal stops, and a few other sounds. Second, every movement of the vocal tract alters the shape or size of the cavities above the glottis, which changes the resonant frequencies of the tract and alters the sound. These changes result in vocalic differences, in variations of nasality, and in the clues to consonant perception in the transitional segments toward and away from consonantal positions. Third, certain movements and positions of the mechanism occlude the airway, some partially, some completely, and the occlusions result in the hissing and popping sounds we associate with most of the consonants. These movements are performed rapidly and with considerable precision, although there is some allowable variation within phonemic categories.

The structures or parts of structures that actually move—portions of the tongue, portions of the lips, the jaw, the vocal folds, sections of the pharynx, and the velum—are relatively small and light in weight by comparison with the structures involved in other body movements—head, torso, or limbs. The largest and heaviest of the moving parts of the vocal tract is the mandible; the smallest and lightest probably the vocal folds. The mass of an object is proportional to the ease with which it can be set in motion, stopped from moving, or the direction of its movement changed. We might suspect, then, that people with large or heavy mandibles might be slower talkers. This may be true for individuals of the same age and sex, but the review of the literature on normal fluency in the preceding chapters has made it evident that children, whose vocal tracts are smaller and less massive than those of adults, are usually slow talkers.

Of course, a number of factors affect the fluency of speech; the size and mass of the structures is only one. However, it should be recognized that the mass of each part of the mechanism is one influence. Specifically, the massiveness of the parts of the vocal tract will influence the speed with which movements can be initiated, and once begun, the ease with which they can be stopped or redirected. There are many compensatory forces, however. As speech is acquired, the timing and velocity of movements develops within the constraints of the mechanism as it exists at any stage of growth. Some central nervous systems are probably adept, relative to others, in making adjustments to changes in the mechanism introduced by growth.

Distances Traveled and Velocities

The distances traveled by these moving parts are small, no more than a few centimeters in any case. The most extensive movements are those of the mandible, which moves a few centimeters up and down. Because the structures are relatively small and the distances they travel relatively short, it is possible for many movements to be made in a brief period of time without requiring that the structures move at high velocities.

Muscle Lengths

The muscles of the vocal tract are short in length compared to the muscles that move other parts of the body. For the most part, this means that the vocal tract is incapable, even when muscles are fully flexed or relaxed, of moving very far. A complete flexion of any set of muscles has only a minimal spatial effect. Of course, the point of vocal tract movement is to produce sounds, and it doesn't take very much movement to generate sounds of considerable intensity.

The small size, mass, distances, and muscle lengths of the vocal tract all suggest that the production of speech sounds requires relatively little effort. The vocal tract is an energy efficient device for sound production.

Permissible Variation

The limits of acceptable variation in speech production may be seen in two ways. First, there are typically a number of different movements that will result in the same acoustic changes. Second, within phonemic and prosodic boundaries, which are established by the conventions of the linguistic community, there is a certain amount of permissible variation in the sounds. It is not clear whether this allowable variation makes it more or less easy to produce speech sounds.

THE PHYSIOLOGICAL BASIS OF FLUENCY: COORDINATION AND TIMING

Premises

First, let us try to understand what is meant by *coordination.*

Coordination of speech movements may be thought of in two different ways, according to the kinds of errors a failure of coordination can produce. The first kind of coordination has to do with the spatial precision of movements. Discoordination of this type results in movements that are imprecise with regard to placement. This kind of discoordination by itself would result in articulation errors and seems of lesser interest in a study of fluency than do other discoordinations. However, it would be wise not to put this kind of discoordination too far aside. Although spatial precision does not seem to be an aspect of fluency itself, a number of facts suggest a relation between articulation errors, at least the functional kind, and stuttering.

Furthermore, the child's developing capacity for spatially precise speech movements may affect the development of speech fluency. It may be, for example, that the rate at which a child produces words and syllables is paced by various capacities, and spatial precision of articulatory movement may easily be one of them. In other words, a child who has not yet developed the ability to produce accurately placed speech gestures will not necessarily show articulatory errors; that child may simply talk more slowly to bring the task of speaking intelligibly within the limits of a developing ability.

The other kind of discoordination has to do with precision of timing.

To be temporally coordinated, the different movements that comprise a speech gesture have to be accurate not only in placement but also in timing. It does no good to move the tongue with precision from one position to the next if the movement is too late or too early in relation to other movements. It is as if the members of a football team executed a play perfectly, except that one of the players was 3 seconds behind the rest of the team. Note that the coordination of timing is not the same thing as being able to move rapidly. *Timing coordination* refers to the ability to produce different movements and have all of them occur at the right time in relation to each other or to a starting point. Temporal precision is just as important as spatial precision.

It will be helpful, in discussing coordination, to understand the term *coordinative structure* (Fowler and Turvey, 1980). A coordinative structure is a set of body parts, muscles for moving them, and associated neural mechanisms that participate in the same act. In elevating the back of the tongue, for example, a number of muscles contract. Other muscles are more relaxed, to permit the tongueback to move easily. Each of these muscles, those contracting and those not contracting, is served by motor neurons. At the cell bodies for these neurons, information is processed, which results in the neuron signaling the muscle to contract, more or less according to the frequency with which neural impulses arrive. Muscles that will contract during a speech gesture will receive a high frequency of neural impulses at the proper moment. Muscles that will need to be relaxed during a gesture will receive, at the same moment, a low frequency of neural impulses. All the muscles involved in the gesture, those that are relaxed as well as those that are excited, and the neurons serving them, are part of the coordinative structure.

It might be noted, however, that relaxation of antagonistic muscles is somewhat more directly related to the ease with which a gesture can be made than the excitation of agonistic muscles. In other words, it seems that the capacity to relax antagonistic muscles has more to do with fluency than the capacity to contract agonistic muscles. This is corroborated by studies in which stutterers have been found to show more muscle activity in antagonistic (Freeman and Ushijima, 1978) and contralateral (Barrett and Stoeckel, 1979) muscles. It has not, however, been corroborated by studies showing that the fluency of *normal* speakers varies with their capacity to relax functionally related or antagonistic muscle sets.

Because there are many acts or movements in speech that are similar and are performed with similar groups of muscles, there is much overlapping in coordinative structures. The coordinative structure for moving the tonguetip from the position for /i/ to the position for /t/ contains many of the same muscles, neural mechanisms, and body parts as the coordinative structure for moving from /t/ to /n/. Despite this overlapping of different muscles in different coordinative structures, it is important to remember that each coordinative structure is a unique *assemblage* of muscles, neural mechanisms, and body parts. Each of these unique assemblages has properties that are different from those of other coordinative structures, and the most important of these properties are mass and stiffness.

A coordinative structure is often said to operate like a mass-spring system. Muscle tissue may be stiff or springy depending on its current tonus, and the body parts that muscles move around differ in massiveness. These variations mean that a given coordinative structure may be characterized according to its *springiness*—its tendency to return to its original length when stretched—as well as according to its *mass*—which governs its tendency to continue moving in a given direction. These two properties will have an important influence on the way a specific speech movement is performed. The more massive a coordinative structure is, the more difficult it will be for the speaker to get it moving and, once moving, to stop it or change the direction of its movement. Thus movements of the jaw are slower to start and stop than movements of the tonguetip because the jaw is more massive. However, given the time necessary to achieve movement, relatively massive coordinative structures are nonetheless able to move at high velocities. Stiffness in a coordinative structure will reduce the peak velocity of the structure, although a stiff structure may still be able to begin moving rapidly and stop moving rapidly.

In addition, every mass-spring system has a characteristic resonant frequency. That is, it moves most easily within a certain range of velocities. Furthermore, in the case of coordinative structures, springiness is adjustable by changing the background tonus of muscles, so that the resonant frequency of a speech coordinative structure is not a fixed quantity, but varies within the capacity of the individual to change background muscle tonus.

Of course, the timing of movements does not depend only on the massiveness and stiffness of the peripheral mechanisms. Certain neural mechanisms, both peripheral and central, have an important influence on the timing of movements. Different neurons transmit impulses at different speeds, according to the size of the neuron, although neural transmission is so rapid that it is unlikely to influence the speed of structural movement. A coordinative structure may contain a number of synapses, and each synapse requires additional time. A coordinative structure involving more synaptic junctures will be slower than one containing less. Also, the time taken for a signal to cross the synaptic space may be a factor in the speed of neural transmission. In addition, the neurological organization of the speech mechanism may be predisposed, through evolutionary development, to perform certain movements, such as chewing, laughing, spitting, gagging, gasping, sobbing, sighing, or yawning. These predispositions have been called "oscillators." Their presence is likely to influence the resonant frequency of the coordinative structures they use. This means, for example, that a person's jaw may be predisposed to move during speech at a frequency near that with which he or she typically chews food. This predisposition may in turn influence the rate at which the person produces syllables.

Findings

Reaction Time

1. The reaction times of normal subjects vary with the structure, the subjects' focus of attention, the hemisphere stimulated, the age and sex of the subjects, and a number of other variables (Shadden, 1979).
2. Although probably related to coordination and motor control, the relation of reaction time measures to speech in normal subjects is not known.

Feedback

3. Delayed auditory feedback disrupts speech production (Black, 1951; Lee, 1951; Brubaker, 1952; Fairbanks and Guttman, 1958; Coblenz and Agnello, 1965; Ham and Steer, 1967; Wingate, 1970).
4. Auditory masking increases loudness, raises fundamental frequency, and slows rate (Wingate, 1970).
5. Nerve blocks affect speech production minimally (Borden, 1979).

Gestural Synchrony

6. There is a strong tendency for nonspeech movements to entrain with speech movements (Kelso, Tuller, and Harris, 1983).
7. Hand gestures and other body movements such as head-nodding facilitate fluency and often coincide with stressed syllables (Condon and Ogston, 1966; Duchan et al., 1979). Furthermore, speakers use longer utterances to convey the same ideas when their hands are restrained (Hoffman, 1968).
8. Right-hand balancing tasks are disrupted by simultaneous talking more than left-hand tasks (Kinsbourne and Cook, 1971; Kinsbourne and Hiscock, 1977; Kinsbourne and Hicks, 1978; and others)
9. When one hand beats a rhythm and the other hand beats a faster counter-rhythm, performance is better when the dominant hand beats the faster rhythm (Ibbotson and Morton, 1981).
10. There is a left hemisphere advantage in pursuit-auditory tracking tasks (Sussman, 1971; Levy and Bowers, 1974; Sussman, MacNeilage, and Lumbley, 1974; Sussman, 1977; Sussman, 1979).
11. The left hemisphere reacts more quickly than the right (Hand and Haynes, 1981).

12. Alpha suppression before speech is located in the language-dominant hemisphere (Moore and Lang, 1978; Moore and Lorendo, 1980).

Interference

13. Stuttering, and the discontinuities of normal speakers, are both likely to occur at syntactic locations where language is being formulated (Starkweather and Gordon, 1983).

Theory

Reaction Time

In the "Premises" section, it was noted that the stiffness of a coordinative structure affected the peak velocity with which the corresponding speech gesture could be performed, while the mass of the coordinative structure affected the speed with which the gesture could be initiated. This means that stiffness affects the velocity of movement and the speed with which a movement can be completed but does not interfere with neural reaction time,[1] while massiveness affects mechanical reaction time (when it includes actual movement) but does not interfere with velocity.

In practice, of course, these two variables may interact. Given a limited amount of time in which to perform a movement, a structure that is massive and slow to achieve peak velocity may never reach the velocity it is capable of. Similarly, a stiffened structure may not be able to complete a movement in a given period of time, even though it initiates the movement quickly, because it cannot reach the velocity necessary to complete the movement within the time allowed. The point to be made here is that both stiffness and mass can influence the temporal coordination of a structure, although in somewhat different ways. Reaction time does not measure movement alone. Although in many reaction time studies the actual movement time is included in the measure, it should be noted that some reaction time is occupied by sensory neural transmission, some by motor neural transmission, and a substantial and important part of reaction time by central processing. This latter portion of reaction time is most highly correlated with overall reaction time (Evarts, 1966), and so would seem to be an important part of the picture.

The central nervous system plays a role in coordinating peripheral

---

[1]Neural reaction time is the time that elapses between an external stimulus and the arrival of a neural signal at the motor endplate. It is distinguished from mechanical reaction time, which is the time that elapses between an external stimulus and the initiation of a movement (Netsell and Daniel, 1974). Many studies of vocal reaction time or of manual reaction time measure from the onset of the stimulus to the onset of some external event, such as the pressing of a button or the onset of voicing. Because of this, most measures of reaction time, certainly those of vocal reaction time, involve a considerable amount of movement.

movements, and there is a long history of theory and research in this area. A full description of this area is beyond the scope of this book (see Neilson's [1980] review). However, I will attempt an overly simple summary.

Feedback

The cybernetic approach to speech motor control was believed for many years to explain speech coordination (Neilson, 1980). The theory, simply put, is that we guide our speech motor behavior from moment to moment based on information we receive about the current location of structures. This concept arose during World War II in research on weapons guidance systems, but is perhaps most easily analogized with the guidance system of a rocket, in which a trajectory is preplanned and minor adjustments are made in response to sensed deviations from this planned trajectory.

For speech, this would mean that feedback to the speaker about the status of the speech mechanism from tactile, proprioceptive, and auditory sources must be continuous, and that in response to this information, the speaker would make adjustments to achieve movements that would result in intelligible speech.

The theory is based on various findings. One is that disruptions in the feedback of speech interfere with speech production. Feedback disruption was first "discovered" by Lee (1951), who found that when normal individuals spoke with delayed auditory feedback (DAF), they showed a characteristic pattern of errors—prolonged vowels, repeated elements, emotional reactions—which Lee called "artificial stuttering." Delayed auditory feedback was also found to enhance fluency in stutterers. Others (Neeley, 1961) pointed out, however, that the kinds of errors made by normal speakers under DAF were not really very much like stuttering at all. The prolongations were in the middle of the words for the most part, and the repetitions were primarily at the ends of the words. The emotional reactions, also, bore little resemblance to the emotions of stutterers. So the term *artificial stuttering* fell into disuse. Later, Wingate (1970) suggested that the fluency-enhancing qualities of DAF resulted from the changes the condition produced in the stutterers' speech, which were not much different from those the condition produced in nonstutterers—prolonged elements being a salient type.

For speech to be controlled by feedback, there must be a substantial amount of sensory-motor integration: the information received from the sensorium would need to be received, recognized, sorted, filtered, processed, and assigned to output devices, all in extremely short periods of time. It was known that disruptions of auditory feedback such as those provided by background noise and DAF produced changes in speech. Investigators subsequently found evidence for the existence of sensory-motor control systems, lateralized on the language side of the brain (Sussman, 1971, 1977, 1979; Sussman, MacNeilage, and Lumbley, 1974).

Then there was a refutation of servomechanism control for several reasons. The fact that disruptions in feedback caused changes was not sufficient evidence for the theory that normal speech depended on feedback, and the speed required for the information to be received, processed, and acted upon seemed too demanding of the system (Borden, 1979). Hybrid theories were later suggested, involving combinations of external and internal feedback for different types or levels of movements (Borden, 1979; Neilson, 1980).

Current thinking emphasizes the role of peripheral mechanisms (coordinative structures, oscillators) in setting up a kind of equilibrium that enables the mechanism to achieve a sensory goal without the necessity of checking continuously with central control centers (Fowler and Turvey, 1980).

Dominance

Lateralization of sensory-motor integration tasks has been shown (Sussman and associates; Neilson, 1980). Lateralization of reaction time has been shown (Hand and Haynes, 1981). Lateralization of alpha suppression in the motor areas before speech has been shown (see Moore's work).

Interference

So far, I have been describing the coordination of motor control as if it were independent of language function, but it is important not to adopt as a premise the idea that these functions are independent. Broadbent (1974) has described the concept of interaction and interference in the central nervous systems. When different functions are simultaneously performed they may interfere with each other. Kinsbourne and Hicks (1978) have elaborated on this idea, going so far as to suggest that close interconnections between two functionally distinct areas may demand more energy to dissociate them during simultaneous performance of the two functions. Kinsbourne and Cook (1971) asked subjects to balance a dowel on an index finger while they were repeating sentences and during silence. The subjects performed less well using their right index fingers when they were talking at the same time. But their performance using the left index finger was not disturbed by the same condition. A number of replications have been successful (Hicks, 1975). Interference effects have also been observed in children (Kinsbourne and McMurray, 1975; Kinsbourne and Hiscock, 1977).

The implications of these studies for coordination of speaking are interesting. The fact that language must be formulated and speech sounds produced simultaneously suggests that there is a potential for a kind of interference with speech production by the language formulation that accompanies it. The possibility for such interference seems enhanced when one considers that the language is being formulated considerably in advance of the speech sound production for the same sentence. The analysis of spoonerisms and similar errors (Fromkin, 1971) shows that there is such a time discrepancy.

Coordination of speaking, then, involves more than motoric coordination. It also involves coordination of the motoric task with other aspects of expressive communication, of which language formulation is one. This coordination may be of a different kind; it may involve the prevention of or surmounting of inherent internal central nervous system interference.

If individuals differ in their ability to overcome the potentially disruptive effects on speaking of the interference of language formulation, then it follows that some, who are low on the continuum, may find their speech sound production disrupted by language formulation, or vice versa. This kind of central nervous system interference may help to explain the fact that discontinuities of speech, in stutterers and in nonstutterers, are likely to be located at places where language formulation is occurring (Starkweather and Gordon, 1983). It should also be mentioned that tasks involving lesser amounts of language formulation have been shown to evoke less disfluency in stutterers (Andrews et al., 1982).

The Relation of Coordination to Rhythm

An important element in the central control of speech, or any other, movement is the ability to anticipate the future status of the system. This element was investigated in studies of tracking tasks by Sussman and his colleagues cited earlier, and has been investigated by many others. The ability to anticipate the future status of the speech mechanism during speech production may depend not just on the memory of past speech experiences but also on the rhythm of speech. (The rhythm of fluent speech is discussed on pp. 62–72.)

This rhythm depends on the speaker's central capacity to generate a temporal structure and allocate peripheral speech movements to it. If the rhythm were regular and constant, as in a song, or when talking to the beat of a metronome, this might not be difficult, but speech rhythm is not so regular—the number of unstressed syllables per "beat" of speech can vary—nor is it so constant—the rate of speech varies according to sentence length, possibly according to the speaker's emotional state and possibly according to the social situation. And the rate of articulatory movements, which may be timed by a central regulating rhythm, varies according to location within the clause and is affected by word boundaries, syllabic stress, and some other factors (see pp. 62–72). This means that the speaker's ability to use his or her sense of rhythm, to adapt it to the rhythmic needs of speech, which change from moment to moment, is probably a more important capacity for fluency than the simple presence of a central rhythmic "clock."

Conclusions about Coordination and Rhythm

What happens when coordination is insufficient? What kind of errors occur? A speaker, lacking the coordination to perform accurately *timed* movements might compensate for this difficulty in two ways. The first way is to slow down the rate at which gestures are produced. (So, although speed of movement and temporal coordination are not the same thing, it is possible that a slow rate of movement is a consequence of poor coordination.) But the second way a speaker could compensate for poor timing coordination is by repeatedly stopping and starting over again. This strategy might be adopted because it enables a speaker to return to a status in which all gestures are coordinated temporally, that is, before any movements have been made.

Why should poorly coordinated timing result in slower or repeated movements? Why wouldn't there simply be errors? The answer to this question is that the purpose of communicating is to share thoughts, and this requires as a sine qua non that speech be intelligible. Many studies have demonstrated that speakers who lack the equipment to perform the typical movements of speech make adjustments so that the movements they make result in an acoustic product that performs the communicative function, a product that is as close as possible to the conventionally shared sound system we use to communicate with. The same principle might apply to timing. Given that a speaker lacks the ability to coordinate the timing of utterance, that speaker would first of all strive to communicate, to convey information. The two strategies noted earlier, slowing down, and stopping and restarting, seem reasonable ways to go about achieving communication when using a speech mechanism that lacks normal coordination.

It may be then that a physiological weakness of coordination in speaking may manifest itself as a lack of fluency—slowed rate, repeated elements, hesitation, even perhaps evidence of unusual amounts of effort in speaking. This is really just another way of saying that disfluency is a sign of temporal incoordination, or that the physiological basis of fluency is temporal coordination.

Although this chapter deals with normal processes, it is worth noting that stutterers show evidence of being incoordinated in subtle ways: they show slower and less regular diadochokinetic movements (Blackburn, 1931), and they show slower reaction time (RT) than nonstutterers (Adams and Hayden, 1976; Starkweather, Hirshman, and Tannenbaum, 1976), but these effects could also be the result of the disorder. The kind of evidence that would support this position is positive correlations between measures of coordination, such as DDK or RT, and speech rate, pause time, coarticulation, segment duration, continuity, or effort *in normal speakers*. This evidence is lacking. Consequently, the idea that coordination serves fluency remains theoretical.

There are some connections, however, between fluency and coordination. Stutterers seem to be lacking full dominance for speech (Neilson, 1980), and dominance seems related to coordination. But again, the relationship between *normal* fluency and coordination is not established. Evidence is lacking that nonstuttering speakers who lack dominance are also slower of speech, more discontinuous, or use more effort in talking. Similarly, synchrony between speech and gesture occurs (Condon and Ogston, 1966; Duchan et al., 1979), and may even be difficult to inhibit (Kelso, Tuller, and Harris, 1983), but the only evidence that it enhances fluency in normal speakers is Hoffman's (1968) study, which shows that speakers take more time when their hands are restrained. This is an interesting piece of information, but it is not sufficient to make the case that hand or body gestures enhance fluency in normal speakers.

THE ACOUSTIC BASIS OF FLUENCY: SPEECH RHYTHM

Premises

There is a certain rhythm to speech. It is not like the rhythm in a song, which is a regular rhythm divided into regular subdivisions. It is not even like the rhythm in a poem. In poetry, at least in the rhythmic kind such as: "This is the forest primeval/ The murmuring pines and the hemlocks," the accented and unaccented syllables are arranged in a regular pattern. In the preceding example, they form the pattern |ʋʋ|ʋʋ|ʋʋ|ʋʋ|ʋʋ|ʋ.

The kind of rhythm found in ordinary spoken speech is much less regular, although it has some regularities, which provide structure. Speech rhythm can be heard by itself without the distraction of meaning by tuning in a radio station so badly that the signal is seriously distorted. When just the right amount of distortion is reached, the speech is incomprehensible but variations of intensity can still be recognized. At this point, each syllable will be heard and stressed syllables can be distinguished from unstressed ones. Speech heard at a great distance or across acoustic barriers may preserve the rhythm even though it is unintelligible. In these circumstances, the sound is recognized to be speech partly because of the characteristic rhythm. In the sentence "May I take you out to dinner tonight?" the pattern of stressed and unstressed syllables is: ʋʋ|ʋ|ʋ|ʋʋ|. The sentence "No thanks. I've made plans for the evening." shows the pattern ||. |ʋ|ʋʋ|ʋ. A longer example from a superior speaker is provided below.*

Today has more of a central theme.

ʋ | ʋ   ʋ   ʋ ʋ | ʋ |

*By permission of George Jellinek.

We ended with this last movement of

ᴜ| ᴜ   ᴜ   ᴜ | | ᴜ   ᴜ

the Brahms, which has a certain

ᴜ | ᴜ   ᴜ ᴜ | ᴜ

Hungarian flavor. But it would be

ᴜ | ᴜᴜ | ᴜ | ᴜ   ᴜ   ᴜ

nice after intermission to continue

| | ᴜ ᴜ ᴜ | ᴜ   ᴜ ᴜ | ᴜ

that Hungarian flavor, and so I opted

| ᴜ | ᴜᴜ | ᴜ   ᴜ   ᴜ | | ᴜ

for the suite extracted from the opera

ᴜ   ᴜ | ᴜ | ᴜ   ᴜ   ᴜ | ᴜ ᴜ

by the present day or I should say the

ᴜ   ᴜ | ᴜ   ᴜ ᴜ | ᴜ | ᴜ

twentieth century Hungarian master,

| ᴜᴜ | ᴜ ᴜ   ᴜ | ᴜᴜ | ᴜ

Zoltan Koldaly, namely Háry János.

| | ᴜ | ᴜ | ᴜ | ᴜ | ᴜ

It should be really called, uh, Jaños

ᴜ | ᴜ | ᴜ | | | ᴜ

Háry in this country but somehow it

| ᴜ ᴜ | | ᴜ ᴜ | ᴜ   ᴜ

never is. He was as you know the baron

| ᴜ ᴜ   ᴜ | ᴜ ᴜ | ᴜ | ᴜ

Munchausen of Hungarian folk lore.

| | ᴜ ᴜ   ᴜ | ᴜᴜ | |

It's colorful. It is Hungarian, and

ᴜ | ᴜ ᴜ ᴜ | ᴜ | ᴜᴜ ᴜ

therefore, there is coherence. One

| ᴜ | | ᴜ | ᴜ |

of the three C's that I mentioned

U   U | | U | | U

earlier. Namely caliber, contrasts, but

| UU | U | UU | U   U

coherence, there is coherence with what

U | U   U | U | U   U   U

we just heard. It begins like this and

U | | U   U| U | U

incidentally this takes a little expla-

U U| U U   U | U | U| U

nation that the audience should know,

| U   U   U | UU   U |

and there should be some word, if not

U   U | U | | U   U

in the program notes maybe announced by

U   U | U | | U | U |

the conductor. It's time he turned

U U | U   U | U |

around and showed that he's human.

U | U | U   U | U

Namely, the Hungarian superstition to

| U U   U | UU | U |U   U

the effect that if anyone sneezes while

U U| U U | U U | U   U

telling a tale, the veracity is thereby

| U   U | U   U| UU U | U

established. And so it begins with a

U |U   U | U U| U   U

gigantic orchestral sneeze, like this.

U| U U | U | | |

An analysis of this passage revealed the following: There were 116 stressed and 188 unstressed syllables, for a total of 304. They were produced in 81 seconds, for an average rate of 3.75 syllables per second. Of the stressed syllables, 88 were preceded and followed by unstressed syllables. Only 14 times did 2 stressed syllables occur together. Of the unstressed syllables, 44 were preceded and followed by stressed syllables. There were 29 pairs of double unstressed syllables together, 22 runs of 3 unstressed syllables together, and 5 runs of 4 unstressed syllables together. So 61.8 percent of the syllables were unstressed, and if there were no structure but instead a random distribution of the syllables, the probability of an unstressed syllable's occurring next would always be .618, that of a stressed syllable always .382.

However, the structure of speech rhythm reduces these probabilities considerably. Given that a stressed syllable has occurred, the probability that the next syllable will be stressed is only 14/304, or .046. Given that an unstressed syllable has already occurred, the probability that the next one will also be unstressed is 29/304, or .09. Given that there have already been two unstressed syllables in a row, the probability that the next one will also be unstressed is 22/304, or .07. And given that three in a row have already occurred, the probability that the fourth one will be unstressed is 5/304, or .016. These probabilities are just a way of expressing the structure of rhythm; they should not be construed as descriptive of the way listeners anticipate future events. And of course, the probabilities just mentioned are taken from one sample, which may not be perfectly representative of the trends, although it is unlikely to be too far off.

Just from looking at these three examples the tendency of English speech rhythm to alternate single or small groups of stressed and unstressed syllables can be appreciated. This tendency is the structure of English rhythm—a stressed syllable, occasionally two, followed typically by a small cluster of one, two, or three, rarely more, unstressed syllables. It is a valuable exercise to transcribe a passage of natural speech, spontaneously produced, and assign values of stress to the transcribed syllables as you listen to the tape. If this is done, it will be apparent that some syllables are not so easy to decide on. It may seem as though some syllables are between stressed and unstressed, and one is tempted to suggest that there may be three levels, perhaps even more than three levels of stress. In actuality, the duration, intensity, and fundamental frequency of syllables varies along a continuum, and listeners perceive as stressed those syllables that are salient relative to their neighbors. That is, a syllable is heard as stressed if it is louder, longer, and higher pitched than neighboring syllables, and although there is an occasional syllable that is ambiguous, not much is really lost by describing stress as consisting of two levels. For our purposes two levels will suffice, because this simplification makes it easier to understand the structure of English speech rhythm.

Languages differ in their rhythm. English is called a "stress-timed" language, that is, the stressed syllables are perceived as the "beats." Some other languages, Japanese is an example, are "syllable-timed," that is, the syllables are the "beats." But many languages are hard to classify as either stress-timed or syllable-timed. For English speakers, it can be difficult to appreciate the nature of syllable-timed speech. In stress-timed speech, the "beats" seem to fall on the stressed syllables. In syllable-timed speech, the beats fall on each syllable. Rhythmic poetry, read as sing-song doggerel, is syllable-timed: "Roses are red, vi'lets are blue." It is because the lines are recited in syllable-timed speech that the second syllable in *violets* has to be dropped completely in order to preserve the strict (syllable-timed) meter. But English, as it is spoken, is not like this. We do not expect every syllable to be given full weight. To the contrary, we expect many syllables to be unstressed, truncated and deemphasized, often to the point that they are completely lost—consider the typical pronunciations of words such as "Frederick," "elementary," and /dʒitʃet/ for "Did you eat yet." We do seem to expect, or at least to "hear," equal intervals of time between stressed syllables, on which the "beats" of English occur. However, an examination of the findings will make it clear that even this perception is not quite true, although it is not quite false either.

Findings

1. Although it may seem that there are equal amounts of time between adjacent stressed syllables in English, there is in fact more time between stressed syllables that are separated by a greater number of unstressed ones (Allen, 1968). This really shouldn't be surprising, in spite of our perceptions, because there is a limit to how much an unstressed syllable can be shortened. However, it appears that we try to equalize the time between adjacent stressed syllables, because the time between two stresses is not proportional to the number of unstressed syllables. Two stressed syllables take up a little less than twice the amount of time of one, and three consecutive unstressed syllables are squeezed a little further, taking up less than a third more of the time consumed by two consecutive unstressed syllables. So there is a tendency to speed up when there is a long run of unstressed syllables. Speakers seem to try to create equal temporal intervals between stresses, and listeners seem to hear speech this way, even though the ideal is not reached in actual production.

2. The perception of whether a syllable is stressed or unstressed depends not only on the acoustic characteristics of the syllable itself but also on the temporal, rhythmic context (Huggins, 1972). Huggins discovered this by altering the duration of speech segments and then varying the relative stress of the syllables in which the altered segments were located and that of neighboring syllables. The altered segment durations were less likely to be noticed by the listeners when the relative stress of the syllables was normally placed.

3. Ladefoged (1967) has shown that the production of stress requires additional psychological effort. This fact is clearly of some interest to an understanding of fluency because of the important role speech effort plays in fluency.
4. Fonagy (1968) found that when people whisper they compensate for the loss of frequency and amplitude variation by exaggerating stress.
5. Blesser (1969) distorted speech so that spectral characteristics were removed but temporal patterning and fundamental pitch contour were preserved. Subjects were able to converse with each other despite the distortion. The mistakes they made preserved the rhythm of the original, e.g., "Hoist the load to your left shoulder" was heard as "Turn the page to the next lesson." Blesser concluded that syntax was encoded into prosodic features.
6. Segmental rhythm (the preceding findings have dealt with suprasegmental rhythm) reflects word boundaries—compare "great rain" and "gray train," or "six tars" with "sick stars." Allen (1968) uses the word *rhythm* to refer to segmental timing variations.
7. In speeded speech, syllables are further unstressed (Gay, 1978).
8. Speech produced in time to a regular rhythm, like a metronome, contains fewer disfluencies (Silverman, 1971) and is subjectively easier to produce.

Theory

My purpose in this section is to come to an understanding of the role played by rhythm in fluency. This role is a little different from that of rate, continuity, and ease, which have been described earlier. Rate, continuity, and ease were elements, aspects, or dimensions of fluency. Rhythm plays a different role. Rather than being a *dimension* of fluency, rhythm seems to *promote* or *enhance* fluency. Specifically, it seems that speech rhythm serves fluency by making it easier for us to talk faster. It does this in several ways— unstressed syllables are shorter and thus require less time. In addition, rhythm assists in rapid speech production by providing a means for us to anticipate upcoming movements.

To document this idea, several facts have to be considered. First, for the most part, researchers have been interested in the stressed syllable. This is natural because the stressed syllable is more salient, both acoustically and physiologically. But it may be more instructive, for an understanding of fluency, to look at the unstressed syllables. Unstressed syllables take up less time and thus make a faster rate of speech possible. In this sense, the unstressed syllables are more fluent. Furthermore, Gay (1978) has shown that when speakers are asked to produce speech at faster than normal speeds, one of the ways they accomplish the goal is to shorten the duration of syllables, reduce their intensity, and produce vowels that are a little farther away from their target formant structure. These are all changes that can be described as unstressing. They are the same changes that are made to unstress a syllable. Unstressed syllables of course take up less time and thus facilitate a rapid rate of information exchange. Furthermore, there is a heavier load of information on the stressed syllables (Lieberman, 1963). It is specifically those syllables that do not carry a very heavy load of information, the ones that can most easily be sacrificed to speed, that are unstressed. The tendency we have to speed up during a long run of unstressed syllables (Allen, 1968) might be seen as part of the same phenomenon.

There are, however, some other ways speech rhythm makes it possible for us to talk faster. Allen (1968) theorizes that rhythm is imposed on speech for the same reasons that any movement might be organized temporally, to facilitate execution. Like counting the beats of a measure while learning a new dance step, the rhythm of speech makes it easier for speakers to perform speech movements at the appropriate time and to coordinate them with other movements involved in the same production. Allen offers very little evidence for this idea, although it has strong intuitive appeal. It might be noted, however, that when speech rhythm is made more regular, as it is when speaking in time to a metronome or singing, there is a tendency to speak with fewer discontinuities. This is true for stutterers (Johnson and Rosen, 1937; Barber, 1939, 1940; Van Dantzig, 1940; Bloodstein, 1950; Greenberg, 1970) as well as for nonstutterers (Silverman, 1971). However, this way of talking, which is essentially syllable-timed speech, typically slows speech and in that sense makes it less fluent. However, the effect, at least with stutterers, seems not to depend on the slowing down of speech (Fransella and Beech, 1965).

Allen (1968) premises this idea on the assumption that rhythm conveys no information. He refers to "the fact that rhythm conveys very little information during speech" (p. 229). Martin (1972), however, says that "rhythmic patterning carries a heavy information load in ordinary connected speech" (p. 500), and he presents a number of facts in support of the idea, for example, the studies by Blesser (1969) and Fonagy (1968) referred to above. Although Martin's and Allen's views are contradictory, it is not clear whether the truth of the matter is relevant to understanding rhythm's role in speech fluency. That is, speech rhythm seems to serve fluency in several ways. One of these ways is the coordination of movement, as Allen has suggested, and this idea does not seem to depend on the premise that speech rhythm contains no information.

Martin's idea (1972) is that the rhythm of language is a kind of temporal structure, a convention held jointly by speakers of the language. Because the rhythm is conventionally held, the listener is able to anticipate the rhythm of words that the speaker has not yet uttered. This prepares the listener in a number of ways. It reduces the uncertainty of *when* specific speech events, for example, stressed syllables, are going to occur. This might facilitate the focus of attention on information-bearing elements, such as content words (Lieberman, 1963). As Martin (1972, p. 488) puts it, "since rhythmically patterned sounds have a time trajectory that can be tracked without continuous monitoring, perception of initial elements in a pattern allows later elements to be anticipated in real time." One of the "elements" that rhythm enables the listener to anticipate may be the syntactic structure, as the analysis of errors in Blesser's study, described above, suggests.

Martin's (1972) theoretical position is summarized in the following quotation (p. 503):

> ... the perception of early events in a sequence generates expectancies concerning later events, in real time. When the events are sounds produced by continuous movements, the perception of these includes cues as to the movement dynamics involved in their production. Hence it is not simply, or not only, that discrete arrival times of accented syllables are induced from earlier timing relationships but also that the total array of time-varying cues in the continuous flow of speech will project ahead the general outline of the remaining prosodic contour. These cues telegraph not only tempo changes but more generally the whole thrust of the pattern of sounds yet to come. It is on this basis that one might say not that the listener "follows" the speaker but rather that the listener, given initial cues, actively enters into the speaker's tempo.

It is interesting that Allen's theory of speech rhythm explains how rhythm helps the speaker produce speech more quickly, while Martin's explains how rhythm enables the listener to decode speech more quickly. These two theories are consequently not only compatible, they are complementary. Speech is of course an interactive process in which both speaker and listener participate simultaneously, their roles shifting as turns are taken, so it is not surprising that an element of speech increases the speed of both producing and receiving speech.

The findings relating gestural synchrony to stressed syllables would seem to confirm Martin's theory, although he doesn't cite this material. A speaker's hand or body gestures tend to coincide with the rhythm of the syllables that are being produced (see the following section). This gestural synchrony (we may call it self-synchrony) doesn't seem surprising. It is most natural to move synchronously, in fact it is difficult not to. A pianist nods and bows at the beginnings of musical phrases, and athletes often accompany their efforts with words or shouts produced at critical moments. Children, concentrating on performing a difficult manual task, often protrude and move their tongues. Adults may inhibit this tendency only partially and clench their jaws.

It is surprising, however, for many people to learn that the movements of listeners tend to be in synchrony with the syllabic rhythm of speech produced by someone who is talking to them. The listener's body seems to respond to the rhythm of the speaker's words, almost as if in a dance. Condon and Sander (1974) demonstrated that this rhythmic response of listeners to speech rhythm was, astonishingly, present in babies less than a week old and that the tendency to move in synchrony was restricted to speech rhythms. The babies did not move in time to rhythmic sounds that were not human speech.

The role of rhythm in promoting fluency may be summed up by noting three factors cited by Bruner (1973) as criteria of motor skill learning— speed, efficiency, and anticipation. For speech motor skill, which is what fluency is, this translates into rate, ease, and rhythm. However, the rhythm of speech is special in two ways—first, it is not a strictly regular beat and second, the tempo of the rhythm changes during utterance in relation to word and clause boundaries. This means that, if rhythm is used to assist the motor execution of speech by helping speakers anticipate movements, they must be able to adjust the tempo of the rhythm continuously as they talk. Consequently, the ability to adjust one's motoric output while the tempo of the rhythm changes is a prerequisite to fluent speech production. (This is one of those "prerequisites" derived from logical analysis. Sometimes they turn out not to be prerequisite in reality.) Several preliminary studies (Starkweather, 1983) indicate that speakers are able to follow rhythms, using them to anticipate and produce temporally accurate speech movements, as the tempos of the rhythms increase and decrease.

REFERENCES

ADAMS, M. R., and HAYDEN, P., The ability of stutterers and nonstutterers to initiate and terminate phonation during production of an isolated vowel, *Journal of Speech and Hearing Research*, 19 (1976), 290–96.

ALLEN, G. D., The place of rhythm in a theory of language, *Working Papers in Phonetics*, No. 11. Los Angeles: University of California, 1968.

ANDREWS, G., HOWIE, P., DOZSA, M. and GUITAR, B., Stuttering: speech pattern characteristics under fluency-inducing conditions, *Journal of Speech and Hearing Research*, 25 (1982) 208–16.

BARBER, V. A., Studies in the psychology of stuttering: chorus reading as a distraction in stuttering, *Journal of Speech Disorders*, 4 (1939), 371–83.

BARBER, V. A., Rhythm as a distraction in stuttering, *Journal of Speech Disorders*, 5 (1940), 29–42.

BARRETT, R. S., and STOECKEL, C. M., Unilateral eyelid movement control in stutterers and nonstutterers. Convention address, American Speech and Hearing Association, 1979.

BLACK, J. W., The effect of delayed sidetone upon vocal rate and intensity, *Journal of Speech and Hearing Disorders*, 16 (1951), 56–60.

BLACKBURN, B., A study of the diaphragm, tongue, lips, and jaw in stutterers and normal speakers, *Psychological Monographs*, 41 (1931), 1–13.

BLESSER, B., Perception of spectrally rotated speech. Ph.D. dissertation, Massachusetts Institute of Technology, Cambridge, Mass., 1969.

BLOODSTEIN, O., Hypothetic conditions under which stuttering is reduced or absent, *Journal of Speech and Hearing Disorders*, 15 (1950), 142–53.

BORDEN, G., An interpretation of research on feedback interruption in speech, *Brain and Language*, 7 (1979), 307–19.

BROADBENT, D., Division of function and integration of behavior, in *The Neurosciences: Third Study Program*, eds. F. O. Schmitt and F. G. Worden. Cambridge, Mass.: Massachusetts Institute of Technology Press, 1974

BRUBAKER, R., An experimental investigation of speech disturbance as a function of the intensity of delayed auditory feedback. Ph.D. dissertation, University of Illinois, Urbana, 1952.

BRUNER, J. S., Organization of early skilled action, *Child Development*, 44 (1973), 1–11.

COBLENZ, H., and AGNELLO, J. G., The effects of delayed auditory feedback on the manner of consonant production. Convention address, American Speech and Hearing Association, 1965.

CONDON, W. S., and OGSTON, W. D., "Soundfilm analysis of normal and pathological behavioral patterns, *Journal of Nervous and Mental Disease*, 143 (1966), 338–47.

CONDON, W., and SANDER, L., Neonate movement is synchronized with adult speech: interactional participation and language acquisition, *Science*, 183 (1974), 99–101.

DUCHAN, J., OLIVA, J., and LINDNER, R., Performative acts defined by synchrony among intonational verbal and nonverbal systems in a one-and-a-half-year-old child, *Sign Language Studies*, 22 (1979), 75–88.

EVARTS, E., Pyramidal tract activity associated with a conditioned hand movement in the monkey, *Journal of Neurophysiology*, 29 (1966), 1101–27.

FAIRBANKS, G., and GUTTMAN, N., Effects of delayed auditory feedback upon articulation, *Journal of Speech and Hearing Research*, 1 (1958), 12–22.

FONAGY, I., Accent and intonation in whispered speech, *Phonetics*, 20 (1968), 177–92.

FOWLER, C., and TURVEY, M., Skill acquisition: an event approach with special reference to searching for the optimum of a function of several variables, in *Information Processing in Motor Control and Learning*, ed. G. Stelmach. New York: Academic Press, 1980.

FREEMAN, F., and USHIJIMA, T., Laryngeal muscle activity during stuttering, *Journal of Speech and Hearing Research*, 21 (1978), 538–62.

FROMKIN, V., The non-anomalous nature of anomalous utterances, *Language*, 47 (1971), 27–52.

GAY, T., Effect of speaking rate on vowel formant movements, *Journal of the Acoustical Society of America*, 63 (1978), 223–30.

GREENBERG, J. B., The effect of a metronome on the speech of young stutterers, *Behavior Therapy*, 1 (1970), 240–44.

HAM, R., and STEER, M. D., Certain effects of alterations in auditory feedback, *Folia Phoniatrica*, 19 (1967), 53–62.

HAND, R., and HAYNES, W. O., Linguistic processing and reaction time differences in stutterers and nonstutterers, *Journal of Speech and Hearing Research*, 26 (1983), 181–85.

HICKS, R. E., Intrahemispheric response competition between vocal and unimanual performance in normal adult human males, *Journal of Comparative Physiology and Psychology*, 89 (1975), 50–60.

HICKS, R. E., BRADSHAW, G. J., KINSBOURNE, M., and FEIGIN, D. S., Vocal-manual trade-offs in hemispheric sharing of performance control in normal adult humans, *Journal of Motor Behavior*, 10 (1978), 1–6.

HOFFMAN, S. P., An empirical study of representational hand movements. Ph.D. dissertation, New York University, New York, 1968.

HUGGINS, A., On the perception of temporal phenomena in speech, *Journal of the Acoustical Society of America*, 51 (1972), 1279–90.

IBBOTSON, N., and MORTON, J., Rhythm and dominance, *Cognition*, 9 (1981), 125–38.

IZDEBSKI, K., and SHIPP, I., Voluntary reaction times for phonation initiation. Convention address, Acoustical Society of America, 1976.

JOHNSON, W., and ROSEN, L., Effects of certain changes in speech patterns upon the frequency of stuttering, *Journal of Speech Disorders*, 2 (1937), 101–4.

KELSO, J. A. S., TULLER, B., and HARRIS, K. S., Control and coordination of movement, in *The Production of Speech*, ed. P. MacNeilage, New York: Springer-Verlag, 1983.

KENT, R. D., and FORNER, L. L., Speech segment durations in sentence recitations by children and adults, *Journal of Phonetics*, 8 (1980), 157–68.

KINSBOURNE, M., and COOK, J., Generalized and lateralized effects of concurrent verbalization on a unimanual skill, *Quarterly Journal of Experimental Psychology*, 23 (1971), 341–45.

KINSBOURNE, M., and McMURRAY, J., The effect of cerebral dominance on time-sharing between speaking and tapping in preschool children, *Child Development*, 46 (1975), 240–42.

KINSBOURNE, M., and HISCOCK, M., Does cerebral dominance develop? in *Language Development and Neurological Theory*, eds. S. J. Sealowitz and F. A. Gruber. New York: Academic Press, 1977.

KINSBOURNE, M., and HICKS, R. E., Mapping cerebral functional space: Competition and collaboration in human performance, in *Asymmetrical Function of the Brain*, ed. M. Kinsbourne. Cambridge, Mass.: Cambridge University Press, 1978.

LADEFOGED, P., Linguistic Phonetics, *Working Papers in Phonetics*, No. 6. Los Angeles, University of California at Los Angeles, 1967.

LEE, B. S., Artifical stuttering, *Journal of Speech and Hearing Disorders*, 16 (1951), 53–55.

LEVY, C., and BOWERS, D., Hemispheric asymmetry of reaction time in a dichotic discrimination task, *Cortex*, 10 (1974), 18–25.

LIEBERMAN, P., Some effects of semantic and grammatical context on the production and perception of speech, *Language and Speech*, 6 (1963), 172–79.

MARTIN, J., Rhythmic (hierarchical) versus serial structure in speech and other behavior, *Psychological Review*, 79 (1972), 487–509.

MOORE, W. H., JR., and LANG, M. K., Alpha asymmetry over the right and left hemispheres of stutterers and control subjects preceding massed oral readings: a preliminary investigation, *Perceptual and Motor Skills*, 44 (1977), 223–30.

MOORE, W. H., JR., and LORENDO, L. C., Hemispheric alpha asymmetries of stuttering males and nonstuttering males and females for words of high and low imagery, *Journal of Fluency Disorders*, 5 (1980), 11–26.

NEELEY, J. N., A study of the speech behavior of stutterers and nonstutterers under normal and delayed auditory feedback, *Journal of Speech and Hearing Disorders*, Monograph Supplement #7 (1961).

NEILSON, M., Stuttering and the control of speech: a systems analysis approach. Ph.D. dissertation, University of New South Wales, 1980.

NETSELL, R., and DANIEL, B., Neural and mechanical response time for speech production, *Journal of Speech and Hearing Research*, 17 (1974), 608–18.

PORTER, R., and LUBKER, J., Rapid reproduction of vowel-vowel sequences; evidence for a fast and direct acoustic-motoric linkage in speech, *Journal of Speech and Hearing Research*, 23 (1980), 593–602.

SHADDEN, B. Ph.D. dissertation, University of Tennessee, Knoxville, 1979.

SILVERMAN, F. H., The effect of rhythmic auditory stimulation on the disfluency of nonstutterers, *Journal of Speech and Hearing Research*, 14 (1971), 350–55.

STARKWEATHER, C. W., Tracking a changing tempo. Convention Address, American Speech and Hearing Association, 1983.

STARKWEATHER, C. W., HIRSHMAN, P., and TANNENBAUM, R., Latency of vocalization: stutterers v. nonstutterers, *Journal of Speech and Hearing Research*, 19 (1976), 481–92.

STARKWEATHER, C., and GORDON, P., Stuttering: The Language Connection. Short course, American Speech and Hearing Association, 1983.

SUSSMAN, H., The laterality effect in lingual-auditory tracking. *Journal of the Acoustical Society of America*, 49 (1971), 1874–80.

SUSSMAN, H., Respiratory tracking of dichotically presented tonal amplitudes, *Journal of Speech and Hearing Research*, 20 (1977), 555–64.

SUSSMAN, H., Evidence for left hemisphere superiority in processing movement-related tonal signals, *Journal of Speech and Hearing Research*, 22 (1979), 224–35.

SUSSMAN, H., MACNEILAGE, P., and LUMBLEY, J., Sensorimotor dominance and the right ear advantage in mandibular-auditory tracking, *Journal of the Acoustical Society of America*, 56 (1974), 214–26.

TIFFANY, W. R., The effects of syllable structure on diadochokinetic and reading rates, *Journal of Speech and Hearing Research*, 23 (1980), 894–908.

VAN DANTZIG, M., Syllable-tapping: a new method for the help of stammerers, *Journal of Speech Disorders*, 5 (1940), 127–32.

WINGATE, M. E., Effect on stuttering of changes in audition, *Journal of Speech and Hearing Research*, 13 (1970), 861–73.

The Development
of Fluency in Children

INTRODUCTION

Premises

The findings related to fluency development, which will be listed shortly, make it clear that children's speech becomes increasingly fluent as they mature. When children first begin to use speech to convey ideas, their speech lacks fluency. It is produced slowly, and many of the features of normal rhythm are missing. As their fluency increases, children also learn to deal with lapses of fluency, such as discontinuities, in more sophisticated ways. This growing ability to talk more easily stems from several capacities upon which fluent speech hypothetically depends. These hypothetical capacities will be described shortly. However, it is a premise of this chapter that this growing capacity to talk more easily is paralleled by increasing demands for fluent speech, demands placed on children by the people they communicate with and by themselves. A second premise is that when the child's capacity for fluency exceeds the demands, the child will talk fluently, but when the child lacks the capacity to meet demands for fluency, stuttering, or something like it, will occur.

Fortunately, in most children the capacities for fluency develop as rapidly as the demands, and increasingly fluent speech—a faster rate, more adult rhythm, and more sophisticated and conventional techniques for dealing with breaks in continuity—is the result. They also show increased coarticulatory undershoot, longer utterances, and possibly use less effort in talking. In short, all elements of fluency seem to grow.

Some children, of course, do not develop the capacity for fluent speech as rapidly as others, and at times the demands for fluency made by their environments are too much for them to handle. When this is the case, fluent speech breaks down. Environmental demands may exceed capacity only now

75

and then. Indeed, it seems to be a common feature of adult speech that, once in a while, the demand we place on ourselves to produce information at a rapid rate exceeds our capacity to produce it. But when demands for fluency in children's environments *chronically* exceed their capacity for fluent speech production, they will lack full fluency more often.

These frequent episodes are likely to cause children to try harder to get words out faster, particularly words that have been produced discontinuously, to struggle with them, forcing and pushing with increased air pressure, and to tense the speech musculature so that it is stiff, slow-moving, uncoordinated, and tremulous. Forcing and struggle do not produce the desired result, and in fact are likely to slow even further the rate at which such children produce information. At this point, parents may react with alarm or distaste, showing their disapproval verbally or nonverbally. The children react further, struggling to talk as they feel they should. During this period of development, speech behavior is being learned. The child is learning how to talk semiautomatically. When the patterns of struggle, tension, and emotional reaction have become habitual and semiautomatic, stuttering has developed.

In this chapter both the demands and the capacities for speech fluency will be considered. Growth in the capacity for fluent speech comes from several areas. There is increasing control over the movements of the vocal tract. This control develops in several ways. First there is growth in the child's ability to move rapidly and to react rapidly to stimuli. Second, there is an increase in the child's ability to coordinate the simultaneous movements of different parts of the vocal tract. Third, the ability to plan and then execute a sequence of movements may also develop.

Another capacity for fluency comes from rhythm. Although we know little about it, the sense of speech rhythm may develop and make it easier for a child to anticipate the movements of speech production. An ability to anticipate the movements of speech will give a sense of motoric confidence similar to the confidence a well-practiced athlete or musician feels when performing a task with superior skill.

The increased demands for fluency also come from many sources, both internal and external. One of the growing demands for fluency comes from the child's development of language skill. Increased syntactic, semantic, phonologic, and pragmatic knowledge all contribute to this demand for fluency. As children's syntax develops, their sentences become longer and structurally more complex. This requires that their ability to plan and execute a longer sequence of speech movements also develops. Because the length of utterance is correlated with the rate of speech, the child must also deal with a demand to increase the speed with which the vocal tract parts move. Thus increased syntactic knowledge is a demand on motor speech production.

Semantics also develops, as reflected in a greater number of lexical items to choose from when encoding a sentence. Any given word has a probability of occurrence that may be expressed as a fraction with a denominator determined by the total vocabulary. Thus, when a child only knows three words, the probability of using each word is high (.33). With a vocabulary of 100 words, any individual word is less certain to be used (.01). This increased uncertainty of each lexical item the child uses makes it more difficult and time-consuming to plan an utterance. It is a demand on fluency. The result of this increasing demand would be a gradual increase in the duration and frequency of pauses in speech were it not for the child's simultaneously increasing ability to select quickly those lexical items appropriate to intended meaning. Thus, word-finding skill is a *capacity* for fluency, but vocabulary is a *demand*.

As children's knowledge of the rules of phonology increases, they become interested in using longer words and phrases and more difficult combinations of sounds to express intentions. The additional length and complexity of these strings of words and sounds places a demand on children's motoric skill to produce the strings they have the knowledge to use. They may be able to plan a motoric pattern, but lack the fluency to execute it at normal speed.

Children's pragmatic knowledge also grows, and this too places a demand on the fluency of speech. The speech of young children is characterized by spontaneity. At two or three years of age, their speech is a verbalization of their current thought or activity. With increased maturity, speech becomes more controlled and directed to more specific purposes. Growth in the area of pragmatics seems to diminish the spontaneity of children's speech. One of the earlier pragmatic skills to develop is turn-taking. Young children do not wait their conversational turn before talking until they have learned this fundamental consideration. At this level, their speech is nonspontaneous only to the extent that they must inhibit themselves from talking until it is their turn.

At more advanced levels, spontaneity is further decreased by the use of speech for different pragmatic purposes. For example, older children are expected to talk on demand, reciting stories and giving narrative accounts of past events. These little speeches are a more formal, controlled way of talking. They differ from the more spontaneous utterance of thoughts in a conversation. Older children have no difficulty with "demand" speech, but a certain level of maturity is necessary before a child feels comfortable talking on demand. As children mature, they are expected to adopt a more mature role, and take more responsibility for themselves. Maturing children are also expected to carry more of the burden of a conversation, asking more of the questions and assuming the conversational lead to an extent commensurate with their age. Finally, as the last stage of pragmatic development occurs, children become more aware of the knowledge and intentions of others and are able to consider what others know in planning their utterances. They even learn what kinds of information will be interesting to listeners and inhibit themselves from talking about topics that other people will not be interested in. So increased pragmatic knowledge places a demand on fluency by diminishing spontaneity and increasing the need to control the content and form of language.

It is not just the growth in language skill that places demands on children for fluency. The people with whom children communicate—their parents, siblings, relatives, peers, and teachers—also place demands on them. Children have a natural tendency to use speech and language that is similar to that used by those they are talking to. Consequently, parents and siblings who talk rapidly inadvertently place a demand on a child to talk rapidly. Rapid turn-taking and a fast rate both suggest to a child that there is little time in which to say what they want to say. In a more general sense, a child comes to understand how much time is available for any activity according to the urgency with which parents and other important people undertake daily activities. Thus, a rushed household places a demand on a child to do everything rapidly, including talking. Children's desire to match parental behavior may also be seen in the level of language they use. When parents talk to their children using sophisticated language—syntactically complex and with an advanced vocabulary—the children try to use the same forms. Often, the children are quite capable linguistically, and readily use sentences that show mature syntactic forms and adult vocabulary. However, the longer utterances and the larger pool of words to be used place demands on children's motor speech production which may be beyond their capacity.

It is evident that for most children capacities grow faster than demands because the rate and continuity of their speech increases. In the material that follows I will be considering both sides of fluency development—the increased demands made by a developing language system and the changing expectations of listeners together with the increased capacities children develop to deal with those demands. Most importantly, I will look at the behavioral result of these parallel changes; that result is the increasing fluency of growing children.

THE DEVELOPMENT OF SPEECH CONTINUITY

Findings

1. From twenty-nine months, to thirty-three months, to thirty-seven months, discontinuities decline from 6.5 percent, to 5.10 percent, to 4.10 percent (Yairi, 1981).

2. Discontinuities decline from 14.6 percent to 9.1 percent from ages two to four but then remain the same from four to six years (Wexler and Mysak, 1982).

3. From three and a half to five years, discontinuities decline from 11.9 percent to 9.5 percent (DeJoy and Gregory, 1975).

4. Kindergarten and first-grade children's speech is approximately 2 percent more discontinuous than that of high-school children (Kowal, O'Connell, and Sabin, 1975).

5. Certain types of discontinuities do not decrease with age. Revisions do not decline or decline only slightly from two to six years (Wexler and Mysak, 1982), from two to three years (Yairi, 1982) or from three and a half to five years (DeJoy and Gregory, 1975). Parenthetical remarks increase from kindergarten to senior year of high school (Kowal, O'Connell, and Sabin, 1975). Phrase repetitions do not decline from two to three years (Yairi, 1982).

6. Two-year-olds showed a frequency of disfluency ranging from 0 to 25 per 100 words, with a mean of 6.49 (boys 7.95, girls 5.24) and a standard deviation of 5.04 (boys 6.39, girls 3.35), when whole and partword repetitions, phrase repetitions, interjections, revisions, disrhythmic phonations, and tense pauses are counted. The sex differences are not significant, although the boys are systematically more disfluent and there are more boys than girls among the more disfluent children (Yairi, 1981).

7. Two types dominate the discontinuities of two-year-olds; (1) repetitions of small units (parts of words and whole words of one syllable) and (2) interjections and revision (Yairi, 1981).

Theory

Kowal, O'Connell, and Sabin (1975) conducted a stratified study of speech continuity (and other aspects of speech fluency) in 168 normal children. They asked twelve boys and twelve girls at each of seven age groups from kindergarten through senior year of high school to describe a series of "Snoopy" cartoons while their speech was recorded. Afterward, the recordings were analyzed for the number of syllables, the number and type of discontinuities, the rate of speech in syllables per second, the number of syllables per unfilled pause, and the duration of unfilled pauses per syllable. Figure 4–1 shows the mean percentage of discontinuities per syllable for each of the seven age groups. Discontinuities consisted in this study of filled pauses ("um," "uh," "hm"), false starts, repeated words or parts of words, and parenthetical remarks. It is clear that there is only a modest change in the frequency of discontinuities from kindergarten through high school. There is a downward trend, but it is small—about 2 percent. The

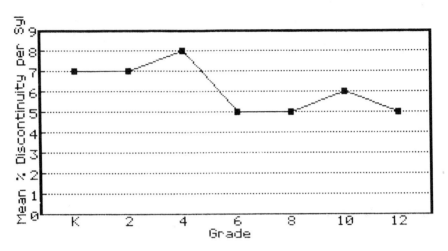

FIGURE 4-1 The development of speech fluency: the frequency of all types of discontinuities.

number of discontinuities per syllable does not seem to be an aspect of *
normal speech fluency that shows very much development. This seems odd
because other measures, which we will come to shortly, do show developmental changes. It seems, from these data, that the frequency with which
discontinuities occur is not a good index of fluency development during
the school years.

One reason why children's speech seems not to become more continuous during the school years is that there are several different types of
discontinuities, and developmental effects are masked over when all discontinuities are lumped together as a single category. Figures 4–2 through
4–5 show the number of discontinuities per thousand syllables for individual types of discontinuities. Filled pauses per 1,000 syllables are shown in
Figure 4–2. A modest decline can be seen. In absolute terms, the frequency
of filled pauses only declines 7 per 1,000 (0.7 percent) during 12 years of
development. Figures 4–3 and 4–4 show the frequency of false starts and
repetitions. Both show a noticeable decline, false starts from 31 per 1,000
in kindergarten to 10 per 1,000 in senior year, or a net change of 2.1 percent. Repetitions decrease abruptly from 25 per 1,000 in kindergarten to
15 per 1,000 in second grade (a change of 1 percent), and then further to
about 4 per 1,000 in senior year, an additional 1.1 percent change. By senior year, repetitions are about one-sixth of the kindergarten level and very
low in absolute terms. In fact, the frequency of repetitions is negligible after
second grade.

Note that the category of repetitions in these data includes whole word
as well as part-word repetitions. Kowal, O'Connell, and Sabin commented
in their paper that the part-word repetition made up a sizable proportion
of the total number of repetitions in the kindergarteners and second-grad-

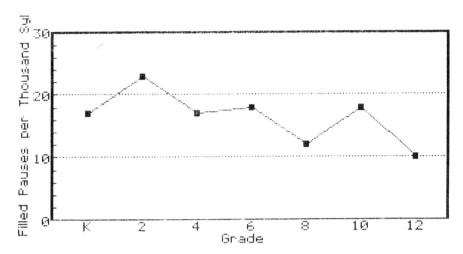

FIGURE 4-2   The development of speech fluency: the frequency of filled pauses by grade level in schoolchildren.

ers but that this type of discontinuity had all but dropped out of the picture by fourth grade.

The increase in false starts that occurs at fourth grade is an interesting reversal of the developmenal trend. It may be at this time in development that children begin trying to talk more correctly, under the influence of the formal teaching of grammar for purposes of written composition. It may be that as they try to edit their speech, they become more hesitant and correct themselves more often.

FIGURE 4-3   The development of speech fluency: the frequency of false starts by grade level in schoolchildren.

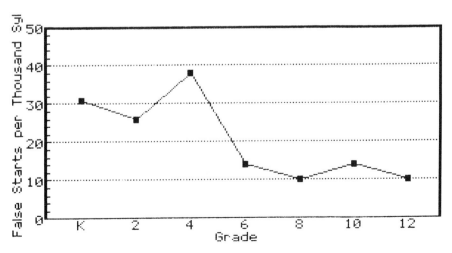

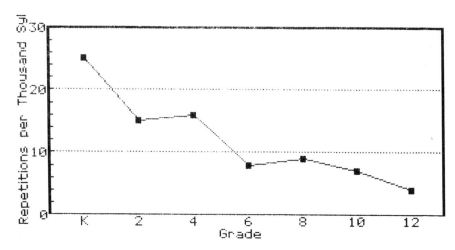

FIGURE 4-4 The development of speech fluency: the frequency of repetitions by grade level in schoolchildren.

Figure 4–5 shows the frequency of parenthetical remarks throughout the school years, and it is apparent why the frequency of all discontinuities does not show a developmental trend. While filled pauses are staying about the same, and while false starts and repetitions are declining, the frequency of parenthetical remarks is increasing from only 2 per 1,000 syllables in kindergarten to 25 per 1,000 syllables in senior year.

DeJoy and Gregory's findings confirm those of Kowal, O'Connell, and Sabin. They compared 3½- with 5-year-old males. The 3½-year-olds showed significantly more part-word repetitions, word repetitions, phrase repeti-

FIGURE 4-5 The development of speech fluency: the frequency of parenthetical remarks by grade level in schoolchildren.

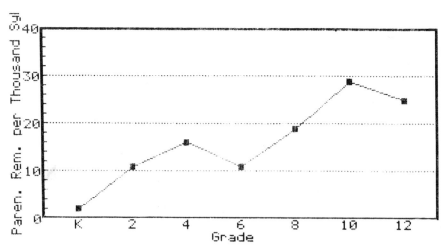

tion, incomplete phrases, and disrhythmic phonations than the 5-year-olds. But they showed significantly less grammatical pauses, and there were no significant differences between the two groups in the number of ungrammatical pauses, revisions, and interjections. The results are shown in Figure 4–6.

One can conclude that the frequency of discontinuities, when all types are taken together, does not show much of a developmental trend. The kindergartener is not much less fluent than the high school senior in this respect. But there is development in the type of discontinuities that schoolchildren show. Certain types, such as false starts and repetitions, are more common in younger than in older children. These types might be considered immature, particularly the repetitions, and most particularly the part-word repetitions. Part-word repetitions are also special because, unlike other types of discontinuity, their development corresponds with other important measures of fluency, as we shall see. With development, these immature types of discontinuity are replaced with more sophisticated types, of which the parenthetical remark—"well," "you know," "I mean,"—is typical. After the school years, it is possible that discontinuities may get even more sophisticated, but we don't know that from these data. Table 4–1 shows the distributions of these different types of filled pauses for school-aged children. The data were taken from Kowal, O'Connell, and Sabin's (1975) study, smoothed so as to diminish sampling error, and the missing grades interpolated.

Davis (1939), looking at the frequency of repetitions in preschool children two to five years old, found that this type of discontinuity occurred at a mean frequency of 49 per 1,000 for the group as a whole, which would

FIGURE 4-6   The development of speech fluency: the distribution of types of discontinuities in three-and-a-half- and five-year-old children.

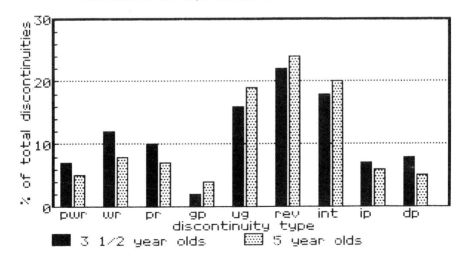

TABLE 4-1   Discontinuity Profiles for Schoolchildren

GRADE	MEAN FREQUENCY PER 1,000 SYLLABLES				
	FP	FS	R	PR	TOTALS
K	18	29	23	4	73
1	19	28	20	7	74
2	20	27	18	10	74
3	19	26	16	12	73
4	19	26	14	14	72
5	18	22	12	14	65
6	17	18	10	14	59
7	17	15	9	17	57
8	17	12	8	20	55
9	16	12	8	23	57
10	16	12	7	26	59
11	14	11	6	26	56
12	13	11	5	26	54

FP = filled pauses, FS = false starts, R = repetitions, PR = parenthetical remarks.

fall very nearly on a curve projecting backward from the graph in Figure 4-4 that shows Kowal, O'Connell, and Sabin's data for older children. In other words, Davis' data for younger children seem to agree with what Kowal, O'Connell, and Sabin (1975) would have found had they sampled younger children.

Yairi (1981) recorded the spontaneous speech of thirty-three normal children ranging in age from twenty-four to thirty-three months. Speech samples were elicited by an adult whom the child did not know, using toys, pictures, and questions. An attempt was made to obtain samples of 500 words, and for most (twenty-six) of the subjects samples of this length were obtained. The other samples did not fall far short. Eight categories of discontinuity were counted: part-word repetitions, single-syllable word repetitions, polysyllabic word repetitions, phrase repetitions, interjections, revisions and incomplete phrases, disrhythmic phonations (mostly sound prolongations and broken words), and tense pauses ("audible tense vocalization between words").

The clearest finding of this study was the variability among subjects in the number of discontinuities produced. A third of these two-year-olds produced 0, 1, or 2 discontinuities per 100 words. We would have to conclude from this fact alone, that a third of two-year-olds speak as continuously as most adults. Another third produced between 3 and 7 discontinuities per 100 words, and of the remaining group, eleven produced between 8 and 13 discontinuities per 100 words. One subject produced 25 discontinuities per 100 words. Figure 4-7 displays the frequency distribution of discontinuities per 100 words in the children observed by Yairi

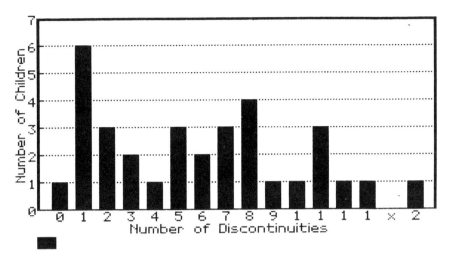

FIGURE 4-7   The development of speech fluency: the frequency distribution of discontinuities in two-year-olds.

(1981). To see if Yairi's observations are consistent with those of Kowal, O'Connell, and Sabin, it is necessary to make some adjustments. Yairi did not count parenthetical remarks, and when this category is subtracted from Kowal, O'Connell, and Sabin's data, the remaining totals show evidently that in the kindergarteners, 6.8 percent of syllables contained discontinuities of approximately the same type as in Kowal, O'Connell, and Sabin's study. When Yairi looked at children who were three years younger, he found 6.9 percent of disfluent *words*. So Yairi's children were considerably more fluent, perhaps twice as fluent as children three years older in Kowal, O'Connell, and Sabin's study. The discrepancy is substantial. The methods of obtaining the speech samples were comparable. The only conclusion is that the two studies sampled different populations. Considering the extreme variability Yairi reported for his group, it seems probable that differences in the populations sampled may have been responsible for the discrepancy.

There is one respect, however, in which Yairi's observations do confirm those of Kowal, O'Connell, and Sabin. The frequency of repetitions of small units—small words and part of words—occupies a large proportion of the discontinuities in younger children. No direct comparison is possible because Kowal, O'Connell, and Sabin did not report separate figures for part-word and other types of repetitions, but the thrust of their observations was clearly the same as Yairi's.

Wexler and Mysak (1982) counted the frequency of various types of discontinuities in thirty-six two-, four-, and six-year-old children. They found a tendency for children's speech to become more continuous from age two to age four but not from age four to age six. Revisions and incomplete phrase showed no developmental trend, while word repetitions, disrhythmic phonations, and tense pauses tended to decline from age two to age four but not from age four to age six. Interjections, part-word repetitions, and phrase repetitions declined steadily. Variability of continuity declined from 5.7 to 3.2 standard deviations between age two and age four but increased from 3.2 to 4.1 at age six.

What kind of behavior are these discontinuities? Are they stumbles in the forward flow of speech, errors of speech production, or do they result from a more purposeful intention? The parenthetical remark—"well," "you know," "what I mean to say"—and the filled pause or interjection—"uh"—are surely more than stumbles. As behaviors, they result in our being able to stall for time so as to keep talking while we think or plan or edit. They may not have very much meaning—indeed, their purpose is to fill up time at a point when the speaker has nothing meaningful ready to produce—but the parenthetical remark is a coordinated and studied use of language. It appears to be a more elaborate version of the filled pause, a speaker's way of keeping the floor while gaining a little more time to produce the next utterance. So the filled pause and the parenthetical remark do not seem to be errors. In fact they are rather more like corrections, or at least they provide the time for corrections of thought or of language to occur before utterance. The language that parenthetical remarks are composed of suggests this purpose, even though they are used without much regard for their meaning: "Do you know what I mean?" "Understand?" "I mean, I mean."

The actual consequence of these discontinuities is additional preparation time. If we can accept the idea that the parenthetical remarks serve a correcting function by providing speakers with time to revise or better plan utterance, it should not be difficult to see the false start, revision, and incomplete phrase also as corrections, essentially the same kind of correction as the parenthetical remark, except that the error isn't quite detected until after utterance has begun. A speaker begins to say something in a certain way, gets part way into the utterance and realizes that the beginning of the sentence would lead to an ungrammatical ending, express an incongruous thought or an illogical conclusion, or state a position that could not be defended, would be socially inappropriate, might lead to a word of uncertain meaning, or make any of a number of other "mistakes." Before going any farther, the speaker stops and starts over again on a better course. Surely that can be seen as a correction, not an error.

The tense pause and disrhythmic phonations are briefer and harder to ascertain. They may be very small stalls or they may be stumbles. In any event, they are a less frequent category. Repetitions, the form of discontinuity found in the youngest children, may be errors. But even in the case of repetitions, it is not clear that they are errors. When young children repeat whole words or phrases they may be stalling for time in just the same way older children stall for time by saying "uh" or "Ya knowwaddimean." I suspect that when I told my son at the age of six that he couldn't have an ice cream bar just before dinner, and he came back with the fast argument "But, but, but, but, but I'll eat my dinner anyway," he repeated "but" because he had learned that the fast argument is compelling. So he started up right away, but unfortunately he couldn't think of a good argument very quickly. So he got going, then stalled for time, until the argument arrived. The urgency of the argument preceded its formulation. It seems then that all of the discontinuities that are vocalized, with the possible and important, exception of the part-word repetition, represent corrections, or a correcting function, rather than stumbles, slips, or errors in the production of speech.

It should be noted that these discontinuities also help the listener in a number of different ways. They are conversational devices. Without putting too fine a point on it, discontinuities signal to the listener that the speaker continues to be interested in maintaining his or her conversational turn but needs a moment more time. Considering this function, perhaps such discontinuities should be considered as a legitimate aspect of language pragmatics.

The odd thing about these discontinuities is the persistent belief that they are errors of speech. Of course, there are superior speakers who show very few of these discontinuities—superbly fluent, they never need to stall for time or correct themselves because they get it right the first time. And typically these individuals serve as models; they are the broadcasters, newsmen, and disc jockeys. But the individual fluency varies greatly, and it is just as inappropriate to consider these discontinuities as errors as it would be to conclude that I can't carry a tune because I lack the musicianship of Pavarotti.

Furthermore, we should not reject the idea that it may be bad for children to be told to correct these corrections. Not that such admonitions will necessarily cause the children to become stutterers. But it will probably make their young lives more difficult than necessary. They may try to talk faster to rush by discontinuities, or push hard to get the words out, or just get very tense muscularly as they try to make their speech mechanisms do something they are not yet equipped to do. In some children, these misguided attempts at correction may lead to other behaviors which are even less desirable, and which may require further correction, and so on, down a rapid spiral to a dark and tightly centered place with little chance of extrication except giving up the attempt at speech.

LANGUAGE ACQUISITION AND THE DEVELOPMENT OF CONTINUOUS SPEECH

Muma (1967) investigated the language used by normal children who were disfluent speakers. He looked at samples of speech taken in free-play situations from four-year-old children who were later categorized as highly fluent or highly disfluent (discontinuous). In most respects the two groups used similar language, but the highly disfluent group used language that was slightly less complex. It was not clear from the results whether the children were disfluent because they were unable to use complex sentences or whether they used simple sentences to avoid being disfluent. Looking at the relation between language and normal fluency from another perspective, Caldwell (1971) administered two tests of comprehension to four-year-olds. Those children who showed good understanding of the syntax and morphology of spoken language were likely to have fewer discontinuities in their speech than those whose comprehension was less well developed. There seems, then, to be some connection between a normal child's fluency and the complexity of the language that he or she can use and understand.

The linguistic location of discontinuities in the speech of children reveals important information about what causes children to produce them. Helmreich and Bloodstein (1973) examined the free speech of four-year-olds and found that their discontinuities were likely to be located on pronouns and conjunctions and likely not to be located on nouns and verbs, suggesting that discontinuities are most common at the beginnings of syntactic units. Similarly, E-M. Silverman (1974; 1975) found that the discontinuities of preschool-aged boys were likely to be located on monosyllabic rather than polysyllabic words. Bernstein (1981) also found a tendency for discontinuities in the speech of normal preschool to second-grade children to occur at constituent boundaries of sentences rather than within the structure of the sentence.

Certain sentences are more evocative of discontinuity than others. DeJoy and Gregory (1973) found that discontinuities were likely to occur on longer than on shorter sentences. But it may not be just the length of the sentence that causes children to speak discontinuously. Interesting evidence for a grammatical effect comes from a study by Haynes and Hood (1978). They asked five year olds to produce sentences that had been modelled by an adult. The children didn't imitate the modeled sentences. They produced a new sentence of the same structure. The experimenters were able to use this method to control the complexity of the sentences the children produced without having them simply imitate. As the children produced sentences that were more and more complex, they became more disfluent. Another study confirmed the importance of sentence complexity on the continuity of speech. Pearl and Bernthal found that in the speech of three- and four-year-olds, the number of discontinuities increased as the

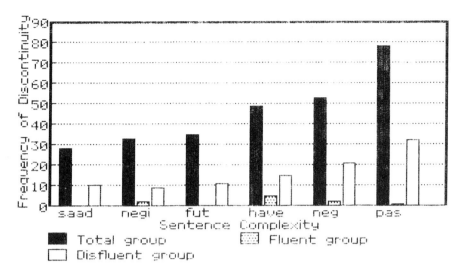

FIGURE 4-8   The development of speech fluency: the relation between discontinuity and sentence complexity.

complexity of the sentence increased. The results, shown in Figure 4–8, are striking. They make it evident that there is a linear relationship between the probability of discontinuous speech and the complexity of the sentence. However, it is difficult to separate the effect of formulating syntactically complex sentences from the effect of organizing and executing motorically long sentences. Complex sentences are invariably longer. Gordon (1982) solved the problem in an ingenious way. She compared the frequency of discontinuities in a modeling task with the frequency of discontinuities in an imitation task, while varying the complexity of the sentences. The results, illustrated in Figure 4–9, showed that complexity had the effect of evoking more discontinuities when the sentences were modeled but not when they were imitated. Because formulation was involved only in the modeling task, and length was the same in the two conditions, this suggested that the reason sentence complexity causes children to be disfluent is the additional demands that language formulation places on their young systems.

    An important detail in this picture was provided by an experiment that Colburn (1979) reported. She followed four children as they developed from one-word through multiword utterances. One of her observations was that "developmental disfluencies reflected a type of practice effect for children beginning to learn syntax, and disfluencies fell proportionally on those structures that children were beginning to use productively in their speech rather than those that were novel, or new." In other words, when a child first began to use a new form, it was not likely to be spoken discontinuously, but as soon as the child began to use it more often, for productive, com-

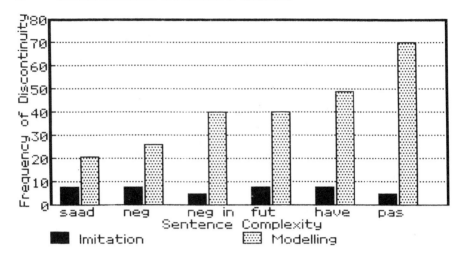

FIGURE 4-9   The development of speech fluency: the role of language formulation in determining the relation between discontinuity and sentence complexity.

municative purposes, it was likely to be spoken discontinuously. Colburn called this a "practice effect," but this is an interpretation of the evidence. It isn't certain that it is the practicing of forms that causes them to be spoken discontinuously. It could be the reliance on semiautomatic execution that accompanies the use of a form in communicative utterance. It could even be the rate at which forms are produced, because this increases as forms are used with more practice. Nevertheless, it is an important part of the puzzle to know that the earliest use of a form is likely to be produced without discontinuity, perhaps slowly, perhaps with effort, but not with discontinuity. Discontinuous performance characterizes the more practiced use of a form.

As children mature, they learn to produce speech that is more continuous, but in the process of developing the skill of producing continuous speech, they encounter some barriers interposed by the simultaneous development of language skills. Specifically, the need to formulate language quickly and semiautomatically, to use it productively in ordinary conversation, seems to place a demand on the motor speech production system. Perhaps this demand arises because of interference between the two CNS functions. The work of Kinsbourne and his colleagues, reviewed earlier, at least suggests this possibility.

THE DEVELOPMENT OF RATE

The rate at which speech is produced is an important aspect of fluency, and as with other fluency measures, rate shows clear developmental trends.

These trends are evident in several different measures—pause duration, length of utterance, syllables per second, and segment duration.

Pause Duration

Findings

1. The duration of unfilled pauses diminishes rapidly from kindergarten to second grade and then continues to diminish more gradually during the rest of the school years (Kowal, O'Connell, and Sabin, 1975).
2. During most of the school years, the duration of unfilled pauses in males is longer than the duration of unfilled pauses in females (Kowal, O'Connell, and Sabin, 1975).

Theory

Kowal, O'Connell, and Sabin (1975) observed the duration of unfilled pauses in schoolchildren's speech. They defined unfilled pauses as any silence longer than 270 msec. As a result, some of the longer juncture pauses were probably included in their data. It is clear from Figure 4–10 that the length of unfilled pauses shows a dramatic course of development. Developmental changes are precipitous between kindergarten and second grade, but from then on they are quite leisurely. This is similar to the course of development shown by the frequency of part-word repetitions. Also, there are significant differences between the sexes in the duration of unfilled pauses at all age levels except 8th grade, the boys producing longer unfilled pauses than the girls. Figure 4–10 also shows that the standard deviations parallel the central tendencies closely, indicating that the shorter pauses

FIGURE 4-10   The development of speech fluency: the duration of unfilled pauses by grade level in schoolchildren.

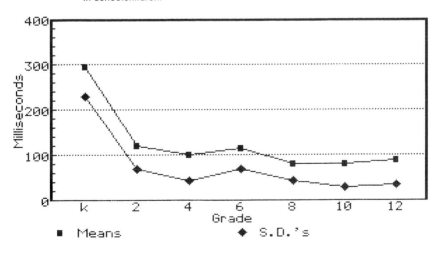

have little room for variation, probably because of the tendency, even in children, to produce speech as rapidly as possible.

Several of Kowal, O'Connell, and Sabin's observations suggest that the duration of unfilled pauses is an excellent measure of fluency development: (1) it directly influences the rate of speech; (see Chapter 2), (2) it shows strong developmental trends that parallel another fluency measure of known clinical importance (part-word repetitions); and (3) it shows a clinically important difference between the sexes. Unfilled pause duration presents one difficulty as a measure of speech fluency—it is not independent of language fluency. Children with abnormally long unfilled pauses may be using the extra time to plan language, not speech. In fact, the duration of unfilled pauses probably reflects both speech and language fluency, which would account for the fact that it shows a more rapid developmental pattern than other fluency measures and distinguishes between the sexes. Perhaps when neither speech fluency nor language fluency alone has a strong developmental trend or distinguishes between the sexes, the two together may still do so.

Because pause durations are related to fluency in several important ways, it is useful to know how they develop in normally speaking children as a basis for making clinical judgments about the fluency of chidren. Despite the small size of Kowal, O'Connell, and Sabin's sample, which is insufficient for true normative comparisons (the authors did not intend the data to be used this way), it still offers the best information available on the development of this important aspect of fluency. Consequently, Table 4–2 is presented, showing data which have been smoothed to reduce sampling error and interpolated for the missing grades for the development of pause durations in normal children.

Table 4–2 should be used to compare the pause durations of an individual child only with great care, particularly in the early grades, when

TABLE 4–2   Duration of Unfilled Pauses per Syllable, by Grade

GRADE	MEAN	STANDARD DEVIATION
K	250	197
1	204	152
2	159	107
3	134	82
4	109	58
5	105	57
6	102	56
7	94	51
8	86	46
9	82	40
10	79	33
11	82	34
12	85	34

the variability is quite large. With these cautions in mind, clinicians might want to conclude that children who pause on the average for more than one standard deviation of the value shown in this table for their age appear to be less fluent than their peers.

Syllable Production

Findings

1. The length of utterance, as measured by the number of syllables per unfilled pause,[1] increases sharply from kindergarten to second grade, then levels off for four years, following which there is another sharp increase between sixth and eighth grade and then only modest changes thereafter (Kowal, O'Connell, and Sabin, 1975).

2. Phrase-final lengthening of syllables may be present with essentially adult values (Oller, 1973) in the speech of two-year-old children (Oller and Smith, 1977; Smith, 1978), although some authors have suggested a later development of this trait (Keating and Kubaska, 1978).

3. The rate of speech in syllables per second is faster for longer than for shorter utterances, both in adults (Malecot, Johnston, and Kizziar, 1972) and in preschool children (Amster, 1984).

4. The rate of speech in preschool children is slow and lacks the features of adult speech rhythm (Allen and Hawkins, 1980).

5. The rate of speech in preschool children shows clear developmental trends, even when the effect of increasing utterance length is factored out (Amster, 1984).

6. The rate of speech in syllables per second increases steadily during the school years (Kowal, O'Connell, and Sabin, 1975).

7. Mothers talk more rapidly to preschool boys than to preschool girls (Hutt, 1985).

Theory

Speech has many levels of organization—words are nested within utterances, syllables within words, sounds within syllables, and individual gestures within sounds. The rate of speech is seen a little differently at each of these levels of organization.

The most complex level is the utterance, and the length of an utterance is related to the rate at which it is produced. This relation seems to be determined by the amount of information the utterance contains. Although a longer utterance typically contains more information than a shorter one, the amount of information in each word of a longer utterance is less than that in a shorter utterance because of the additional redundancy of the context. This can be demonstrated easily by deleting every nth word

---

[1]This is a measure of utterance length for syllable production, not to be confused with mean length of utterance for morphemes, which is a language production measure.

in utterances of varying lengths. The longer utterances are not so injured by the deletions as the shorter ones. One can supply the missing item more readily in a longer utterance because of the additional context. Context is redundancy. So there is less information in each word of a longer utterance than there is in a shorter one. It may be for this reason that the rate of speech in syllables per second is faster in longer than in shorter utterances (Malecot, Johnston, and Kizziar, 1972; Amster, 1984).

If the relation between utterance length and articulatory rate is indeed a result of the speaker's expectation that information should flow at an acceptable rate, the presence of the correlation between utterance length and rate in preschool children (Amster, 1984) is particularly interesting. It suggests that cultural norms for information flow are already present in the preschool population. The implications of this idea for stuttering development are substantial. If preschool children expect to produce information at a certain rate, it is not surprising that they would struggle and force their way through disfluencies to meet the cultural standard of information flow.

There is plenty of information about the length of children's utterances. For the most part, this information has been concerned with language development, and the unit of utterance length in these studies has been the morpheme, but some work has been on the length of children's utterances in syllables. Kowal, O'Connell, and Sabin (1975) measured the length of utterance by counting the number of syllables between each unfilled pause (> 250 msec). The results are shown in Figure 4-11. Developmental changes are evident, the length of utterance increasing with age, as might be expected. There were no sex differences in this measure, which

FIGURE 4-11 The development of speech fluency: the length of utterance by grade level in school-children.

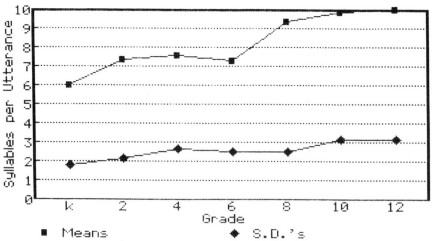

is surprising in light of the language development literature and the presence of a sex difference for utterance length in adults (Malecot, Johnston, and Kizziar, 1972). However, it may be that in children the length of utterance in syllables is more closely related to respiratory needs than it is in adults. That is, the child's ability to coordinate respirations with syntax may still be in the process of development as late as the school years.

The standard deviations for utterance length in syllables show very modest increases throughout the school years, reflecting the fact that, as the child becomes capable of constructing longer and more complex sentences, a few very long sentences are produced. Although utterance length undoubtedly reflects speech fluency in the growing child, it is clearly not independent of language fluency, a fact which must be borne in mind when assessing a child's utterance length in this way.

Utterance length is something we need to be concerned with because it reflects speech fluency, even though it is not independent of language fluency. But we also need to be concerned with utterance length because it is correlated with rate (Malecot, Johnston, and Kizziar, 1972). It is a matter for speculation why speakers tend to produce longer utterances more quickly. It may be that there are social expectations determining how much time people believe they can take when it is their turn to talk. When they have a longer utterance to make, they go faster so as to get it all in within the time they believe they should take.

The correlation of utterance length with rate, as reflected in segment duration, also shows development. DiSimoni (1974) did an experiment in which he showed that the duration of bilabial consonant closure is more likely to be affected by utterance length in older than in younger children. Regrettably, he did not report the actual correlations, so definitive information about the growth in this relationship is lacking. In addition, the study was done with only one speech sound. It is interesting, however, that even one sound's duration is more affected by utterance length in older than in younger children. It seems unlikely that such a relation could reflect physiological maturation, which suggests that the continuing experience the children have in speaking is responsible for this aspect of development.

The relation between utterance length and rate is important because it seems to be a speech production, not a language formulation, effect. The rate at which a person speaks depends on capacities for language as well as speech, and the additional complexity of longer utterances requires more planning, which is reflected in longer pauses preceding longer utterances. However, the speed with which utterances are executed seems to reflect speech production capacity, and the speed of execution is more rapid for longer than for shorter utterances. This suggests that the planning of an utterance and the execution of it are different kinds of behavior.

The relation between utterance length and rate is also interesting because longer utterances are more likely to be stuttered (Soderberg, 1967).

That is, the longer utterances demand more rapid production, and children stutter because they are trying to produce speech more rapidly than their mechanism can.

The next level at which rate can be assessed is the word level. Smith (1978) compared the duration of nine words in the speech of two- and four-year-old children with that of adults. The duration of words was a direct function of the subjects' age. When the results from all nine words are averaged together, the following emerges:

Adult		Four-Year-Olds		Two-Year-Olds	
M	**SD**	**M**	**SD**	**M**	**SD**
532	53.6	612	53.4	697	106.7

This is interesting because the means are clearly not parallel to the standard deviations. This means that the difference between the four-year-olds and the adults cannot be attributed to the adults' superior control. And probably only a portion of the difference between the younger and older children can be attributed to developing control. Instead, it is evident here as elsewhere that the speech of children simply gets faster and faster with increasing age, and it seems likely from the data in this study that the speech rate of children approaches closer and closer to the fastest rate they can manage.

The sexes were compared in Eilers' study (1975), and although there were few significant differences, the trends were interesting. In the adults, female word durations were longer than males for each of the nine words but not to a significant degree (the average difference was 51 msec). But in the children, the males tended to have longer durations (eight of the nine words for the two year olds, six of the nine words for the four-year-olds). This could be interpreted as meaning either that the demand for change is greater in males, because they have to end up talking a little faster, or that the capacity for rapid speech is less in male children, or both.

The word is more of an informational unit than a speech production unit. Consequently, words per minute is a measure of the amount of information a speaker is producing. It is related to but not the same as the rate at which syllables are produced. The more syllables a word contains, the more rapidly each syllable in the word is produced (Klatt, 1973; Darley and Spriestersbach, 1978). As with utterance length, the additional speed with which speech gestures are made in longer words may be responsible for the fact that stutterers are more likely to stutter on longer than on shorter words (Soderberg, 1966).

The next level is the syllable. Utterance duration and word duration seem to depend heavily on the amount of information contained in the utterance, but syllables per second seems independent of content, as long as the sample is large enough to contain a large variety of syllables. For this reason, the number of syllables per second is the most common measure of speech production rate.

The rate of speech in adults is 5 to 6 syllables per second (Walker and Black, 1950). Kowal, O'Connell, and Sabin (1975) measured the rate of speech in syllables per second in schoolchildren telling stories about "Snoopy" cartoons. Figure 4–12 shows the development of rate in their sample. A steady rise in the rate of speech during the school years is evident. Kindergarteners produce, on the average, a little more than 2 syllables per second. The rate of development is steady and strong to fourth grade, when an average of 3.2 syllables per second is reached. Then there is a developmental lag between fourth and sixth grade, followed by another strong increase to 3.8 syllables per second in eighth grade. A more modest increase to 4 syllables per second occurs by sophomore year, and then, apparently, a decline during the last two years of high school. These data are of course affected by small sample size. Smoothed and interpolated data are shown in Table 4–3.

It seems odd that even in the later high-school years the children in this study did not speak at rates similar to those reported by other researchers for adults. There are three explanations for this, all of which may be true. First, it is possible that the full adult rate is not reached until after high school. It may be that a slower rate is characteristic of adolescent speech. Second, the social context of the testing situation was a school, and the test was administered by authority figures. These social elements may have resulted in the children using a more formal style of speech production, which may have slowed rate. Finally, Kowal, O'Connell, and Sabin included pauses less than 250 msec in duration, and in the older children particularly, who have shorter pauses, this may have reduced the overall

FIGURE 4-12 The development of speech fluency: the rate of speech by grade level in schoolchildren.

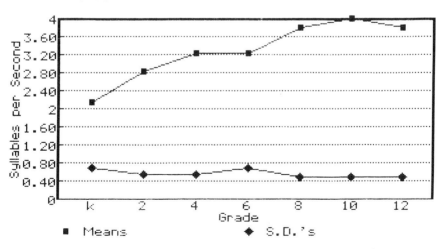

TABLE 4-3   Speech Rate in Schoolchildren in Syllables per Second

GRADE	MEAN	STANDARD DEVIATION
K	2.33	.70
1	2.56	.64
2	2.78	.58
3	2.97	.57
4	3.15	.56
5	3.28	.58
6	3.40	.59
7	3.57	.57
8	3.74	.55
9	3.83	.53
10	3.92	.52
11	3.90	.52
12	3.88	.52

figure. The "developmental lags" that are visible at sixth grade and senior year in Kowal, O'Connell, and Sabin's data most probably reflect sampling error. But these differences do not mean that Kowal, O'Connell, and Sabin's data cannot be used for clinical purposes. Indeed, the more formal testing situation they used is similar to the testing situation in a clinic.

As the mean rate of speech increases through the school years, the variability of speech rate remains about the same, and it is rather low. Tiffany (1980) has made an excellent case that adults talk nearly as fast as they can. The low variability in the rate of speech in schoolchildren, variability that remains low despite a rising central tendency, suggests that children too are probably talking about as fast as their speech mechanisms and coordinative structures will allow. Since all of the children in this sample were physiologically normal, it might be cautiously presumed that the group was also physiologically similar. It might also be that children talk at similar rates for social reasons. As with other aspects of language and speech, it is desirable to sound like one's peers.

Amster (1984) examined the rate of articulation in 128 preschool children as they spoke spontaneously to an adult. She found a clear developmental trend, even when the relation of rate to utterance length was factored out. This suggested that the increasing rate with which children speak as they grow is a result of the combined maturation of motoric and linguistic factors. Figure 4-13 shows her results for the different age groups and utterance lengths. It is clear that for the children, as for the adults, the relation between utterance length and rate is stronger at shorter than at longer lengths, suggesting an informational rather than a respiratory explanation of the effect. Amster's results seem rapid, when compared with those of Kowal, O'Connell, and Sabin (1975). The differences may be attributable to geographical or socioeconomic variation, but probably they

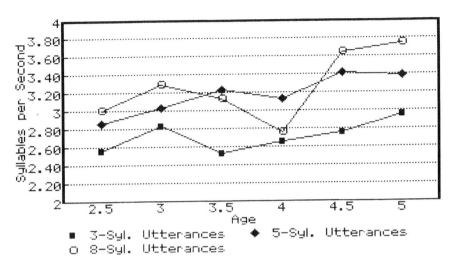

FIGURE 4-13   The development of speech fluency: the rate of speech by age and utterance length in preschool children.

reflect (1) the more formal, hence slower, speech task used by Kowal, O'Connell, and Sabin, and (2) the inclusion of more pause time in the Kowal et al. study. Amster removed all pause time.

Hutt (1985) measured the rate of twelve mothers' speech when playing with their children. The mothers were unaware of the purpose of the study. She found that boys' mothers talk faster than girls' mothers. This finding is illustrated in Figures 4–14 and 4–15. Perhaps it is more important that the relative rate, or difference between the child's and the mother's rate, was larger for the boys than for the girls, as shown in Figure 4–16. The implications of this piece of information for the sex ratio in stuttering are clear: it may well be that parents create a more demanding communicative environment for male than for female children.

The Duration of Segments

Findings

1. Segment duration becomes briefer and less variable with development (Subtelny, Worth, and Sakuda, 1966; Naeser, 1970; DiSimoni, 1974; Tassiello, 1975; Zlatin and Koenigsknecht, 1976; Gilbert and Purvis, 1977; Smith, 1978).

2. The duration of segments is shorter in longer than in shorter words (Klatt, 1973; Umeda, 1975: 1977; Darley and Spriestersbach, 1978).

3. The duration of segments is more influenced by utterance length in older than in younger children (DiSimoni, 1974).

4. The tendency for sounds in stressed syllables to be longer than those

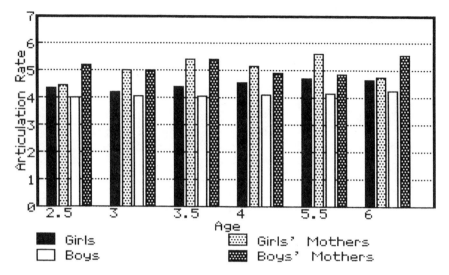

FIGURE 4-14   The development of speech fluency: the rate of speech of children and their mothers by sex.

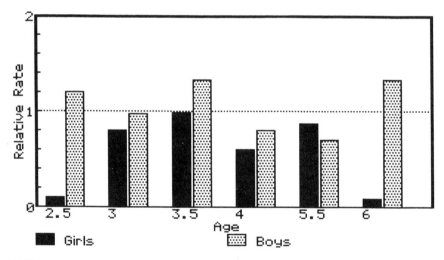

FIGURE 4-15   The development of speech fluency: the relative rate of speech for preschool children by sex.

in unstressed syllables is greater in two-year-olds than in four-year-olds, but it is not greater in four-year-olds than it is in adults (Smith, 1978).

5. The tendency for final-syllable sounds to be longer than nonfinal-syllable sounds is more pronounced in the speech of two- and four-year-olds than it is in the speech of adults (Smith, 1978).

6. Coarticulatory overlap (undershoot) increases with age (Kuehn and Tomblin, 1974; Thompson and Hixon, 1979; Kent, 1983).

Theory

An even smaller unit of speech is the *phone,* the individual segments that make up each syllable. Even though each syllable consists of nothing but the sounds in it, the duration of a syllable is determined by more than just the number of sounds it contains. First, some sounds take longer than others. In a moment, we will look at the duration of individual sounds. Second, some syllables are produced faster because of the types of phones they contain. Specifically, syllables that begin with consonants are produced more quickly than syllables that begin with vowels (MacKay, 1974). In fact, the type of sound initiating the syllable is more important in determining a syllable's duration than the number of phones in the syllable. Presumably, the ballistic release from plosive consonants and the rapid movements made in producing other consonants speeds up the speech gestures that make up the rest of the syllable. Third, speakers may overlap adjacent gestures (coarticulate) more and thus increase the number of phones per second (Amerman, Daniloff, and Moll, 1970).

There is another way to look at speech rate at the phone level. We can look not only at how many phones can be produced in a second, but at the duration of single phones. This more microscopic measure of speech rate is strongly affected by the phenomenon of coarticulation. Speakers may do two different things to increase the number of phones they produce per second—they may speak more rapidly, moving the speech mechanisms at greater velocity, or they may alter the timing with which speech gestures begin and end, increasing the amount of coarticulatory overlap between adjacent gestures. For example, a word like /pap/ requires the jaw to open and close. One way of saying /pap/ more quickly is to open the jaw more rapidly to the same point and then close it more rapidly. But the duration of /pap/ can also be shortened by initiating the closing gesture earlier in time, even before the jaw is fully opened. Some of the /a/ is sacrificed. As coarticulation becomes extensive, the quality of sounds deteriorates, and the speaker is said to "undershoot" phonemic targets. This is somewhat more true for vowels than for consonants.

There are constraints within which this decision must operate: (1) the speed of movement is limited to the speaker's physiological capacity; (2) certain sounds and certain features of sounds depend specifically on the speed of movement or on the duration of time between events—for example, consonant-vowel transitions depend on the rate with which movement occurs, and voiced-voiceless distinctions depend on the relative timing of consonantal release and voice onset; and (3) undershoot can go only so far before the loss to intelligibility is too great. However, within these constraints, speech can be speeded up either by faster speech movements or by briefer and less extensive speech gestures.

There have been few studies of phone duration and coarticulation in normal children. Kuehn and Tomblin (1974), Thompson and Hixon (1979), and Kent (1983) compared older and younger speakers and found more undershoot, that is, greater coarticulatory overlap, in older speakers. The tendency to articulate more slowly and precisely is one of the salient characteristics of childish speech. Some studies have been done on the duration of phones in children of different ages. DiSimoni (1974) asked ten children in each of three groups—three, six, and nine years of age—to produce the sound /p/ surrounded by the vowel /i/. They produced this utterance alone, and also as part of a sentence frame. The purpose was to see if the effect of utterance length on sound duration, known to occur in adults, was present in the speech of children at different ages. It was, but there were changes in central tendency and variability that occurred with development. The mean duration of /p/ declined with age, as did the standard deviation.

Tassiello (1975) asked thirty seven-year-olds and thirty five-year-olds to respond to picture stimuli and produce words beginning with /s/ in a variety of vowel environments. Because there were no differences in the duration of /s/ in different environments, she pooled the data. Figure 4–16 shows that the seven-year-olds had briefer durations of /s/ than the five-year-olds. Standard deviations for the five-year-olds were 14.11; those for the seven-year-olds were 11.07.

FIGURE 4-16   The development of speech fluency: the frequency distributions of /s/ duration in five- and seven-year-olds.

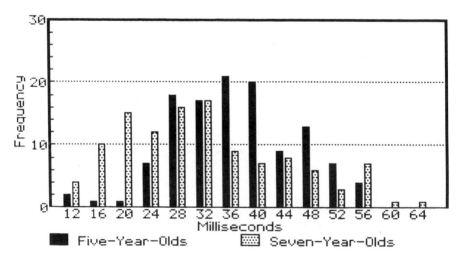

As children mature, they tend to produce briefer sounds with diminishing variability of duration. This suggests that the growing child is improving in fluency. Production becomes more rapid as well as more precise. It becomes easier for the child to speak more rapidly.

The duration of segments is briefer in certain environments—longer utterances, longer words, unstressed syllables, the beginnings of clauses, and the beginnings of syllables, to name a few—and it is interesting to see if these contextual effects are the same for children of different ages as for adults.

Smith (1978), in a study of the development of temporal patterns of English, compared the duration of vowels and consonants at the ends of syllables with those that were not at the ends of syllables. For vowels the differences between final-syllable and nonfinal-syllable sounds were as follows:

	/b/ words (msec)	/d/ words (msec)	/t/ words (msec)
Adults	118	124	70
4-yr-olds	135	123	64
2-yr-olds	159	155	70

And for consonants the differences between final-syllable and nonfinal-syllable sounds were as follows:

	Range (msec)
Adults	17–34
4-yr-olds	22–58
2-yr-olds	33–86

The tendency for final syllable speech sounds to be lengthened is evidently greater in younger than in older speakers. When the duration of vowels in stressed syllables was compared with the duration of vowels in unstressed syllables in the three age groups, the stressed vowels were longer, as follows:

	/b/ words (msec)	/d/ words (msec)	/t/ words (msec)
Adults	56	56	37
4-yr-olds	54	55	31
2-yr-olds	66	73	39

The tendency for vowels in stressed syllables to be longer than those in unstressed syllables is evidently greater in younger than in older speakers.

In both of these results, however, an interesting pattern is evident. There seem to be larger differences between the two- and four-year-olds than between the four-year-olds and the adults. This suggests that the period between two and four years is one of rapid development in the timing of speech production. Much of the information reported in previous sections supports this idea also, namely, the development of speech rate, rhythm, and continuity. This is also the time when, typically, a large minority of children show an unusual number of discontinuities in their speech (Yairi, 1981), and also when stuttering often begins (Yairi, 1982). It seems clearly to be a critical period in fluency development. During periods of rapid development of any kind, even a small lag in development may have effects that are larger than life. Language skills also are developing rapidly during the same period, and it is possible that parental expectations for children's communicative development are paced by linguistic rather than motoric factors. Parents may expect as much from children as their developing language suggests is appropriate, but this expectation may be more than the children's motoric systems can live up to.

DiSimoni (1974) measured the duration of certain consonants in the speech of older and younger children and compared the durations in longer and shorter utterances. He found that the durations were more affected by utterance length in the older than in the younger children. This is the opposite of observations made by Smith (1978). It may be that the effect of utterance length on segment duration is a different kind of contextual effect than that of stress and syllable position. I suggested earlier that the tendency to speed up rate during long utterances was a strategy used by speakers to increase the rate of information flow. If this is the case, such an effect would be expected to come later in development, as speakers try to match social expectations for information flow. However, Amster (1985) showed this effect to be present in preschool children as young as three and one-half. The other effects—final-syllable lengthening and the lengthening of vowels in stressed syllables—are a more basic part of the code, and would be expected to be acquired by children at an early age.

THE DEVELOPMENT OF SPEECH RHYTHM

Findings

1. Young children (eighteen to thirty-six months) are unable to imitate sentences lacking normal rhythm (Eilers, 1975).
2. At the one- and two-word stages of development, children typically do not produce syllable sequences with stress contrast, substituting stressed for unstressed syllables, with or without modification (Ingram, 1974).
3. "Two-year-olds tend to use far fewer reduced syllables than do adults, so that their speech rhythm has fewer syllables per foot, or more beats per utterance; in short, it sounds more syllable timed" (Allen and Hawkins, 1980, p. 231).

4. Children's productions of forms that are polysyllabic in their adult form are more likely to drop initial unstressed syllables than they are to drop unstressed syllables that follow stressed ones, for example, /weɪ/ for "away" /geɪp/ for "escape" /nænə/ for "banana" (Ingram, 1974).
5. In the babbled speech of prelinguistic infants, there is very little difference in the durations of the first and second syllables of a two-syllable "word" (Oller and Smith, 1977; Smith, 1978), but by age two the durational differences take on nearly adult values, although this latter fact has been disputed (Keating and Kubaska, 1978).
6. Children's early productions have only heavy (stressed) syllables, some accented, some not (Hawkins, 1979; Keating and Kubaska, 1978).
7. Syllables are totally reduced (deleted) by two- to three-year-olds in two phonetic environments—(1) word initial or (2) next to another light (unstressed) syllable (Hawkins, 1979).

Theory

The rhythm of speech is an important perceptual cue to our recognition of speech as meaningful stimuli. Eilers (1975) asked children eighteen to thirty-six months old to imitate sentences which had been altered in various ways. Alterations of word order and of meaningfulness produced many errors because the children were unable to use their knowledge of language structure and content to recall the sentences. When pitch and intensity were altered, but word order and meaningfulness were left intact, the children had no difficulty imitating, but when the duration of syllables was artificially increased, performance deteriorated sharply, and the experimenter found it difficult to obtain imitations at all. The presence of normal rhythms in the stimuli were important in determining whether the children would react to them as sentences.

The very first words children produce do not show as much stress contrast as in adult speech (Ingram, 1974; Allen and Hawkins, 1980). The adult rhythm of language is not as easily discerned in the speech of children in the one- and two-word stages of development. Two-syllable words containing one heavy (stressed) and one light (unstressed) syllable are typically produced as if they were spondees, with both syllables being given full vowel color and duration. The only indication of stress is in the raised fundamental frequency of the stressed syllables. Furthermore, many of the sounds in the unstressed syllable may be lost, and instead the child produces a nearby, usually adjacent, stressed syllable. Typically, a child's reduplication consists of one heavy accented syllable followed by a heavy unaccented one (Hawkins, 1979). For example, "rayray" for "raisin" or "bebe" for "Betty."

Syllables are completely reduced, or deleted, under two circumstances: when an unstressed syllable initiates a word (/weɪ/ for "away") and when there are two unstressed syllables in a row (/sʌmbəi/ for "somebody"). Sometimes, when two or more unstressed syllables occur in a row, both are deleted, and in their place the child uses one syllable, possibly containing elements of the two lost unstressed syllables in combination, or possibly just duplicating the stressed syllable. For example, "tayto" /teɪtoʊ/ for "tomato," and "pumjums" /pʌmdʒʌmz/ for "pajamas."

These latter substitutions are more characteristic of later development, and they suggest some growing awareness of the unstressed syllable, since elements of these syllables are incorporated into the child's speech. "Tayto," for example, seems like a more mature word than "maymay" for "tomato," and "pumjums" seems somewhat more sophisticated than "jamjam" because an awareness of unstressed syllables is evident, even though they are not yet produced. Later, at around the four-morpheme level of development, when some ability to produce unstressed syllables is evident, longer sequences of them, and complex combinations of stressed and unstressed syllables will still create difficulty, as in "thermoneber" for "thermometer." In this example, the rhythm is correct, although it seems reasonable to conclude that it is the complex rhythm of the word that causes the articulatory error. "Ferigerator" for "refrigerator" is another example of the same type.

Allen and Hawkins (1980) note that children produce *some* stress contrast from the beginning but do not shorten syllables for this purpose until later. They believe that children learn to reduce syllables with timing to make stress contrast more apparent, so that the stressed syllables become more salient by contrast. This is a reasonable enough explanation of the sequence of development, but it could also be that the children learn to shorten syllables, even though they can already signal stress, to increase the rate at which they communicate information. This aspect of rhythmic development has to wait, however, for the child to develop the capacity for rapid movements of the articulators that the brief, unstressed syllable requires.

Allen and Hawkins suggest as an explanation for the patterns of syllable reduction in children that their speech is trochaic, that is, it is easier for children to produce a word like "raisin" than one like "away," but they concede that this explanation doesn't account for the difficulty children have saying two unstressed syllables in a row. On the other hand, the explanation offered here, based on the fact that children lack the capacity for rapid movement, accounts for both of these observations.

These patterns of syllable reduction show that the child's ability to produce the rhythms of English are developing, but beyond that they show that stressed syllables are easier to produce. This may be because the stressed syllables, being longer, are more forgiving of the child's slow-moving speech mechanism. In other words, it may be easier for the child to produce stressed syllables because there is more time for the child to coordinate the move- ments into appropriate speech gestures. However, other explanations also seem feasible. The unstressed syllable is certainly less salient than the stressed syllable, and children may simply overlook it at first. We might expect that it would be a little later in the developmental sequence, when word endings are becoming important, that the child begins to pay more attention to unstressed syllables, and, having noticed their importance, starts to produce them. The ability to use stress contrastively to convey dif- ferences in meaning is an even later development (Atkinson-King, 1973) and seems to have less to do with fluency than with the development of linguistic knowledge.

Two other aspects of development at this stage may bear on fluency development. It is at about the same time in development, when speech rhythm is being acquired, from two to three years of age, that about one- third of children begin to produce long and frequent repetitions of parts of words (Yairi, 1981). It may be that the demand on the child's mechanism to produce speech that is appropriately rhythmic, or speech that is rapid and requires unstressing to achieve rapidity, is more than some children have the capacity for. Repetitions of parts of words could result from such an imbalance between demand and capacity.

The second aspect of development that may bear on stress is the use of hand gesture. At the one-word stage of development, gesture is an im- portant accompaniment to speech, and the gesture of pointing, produced synchronously with the utterance of an emphatic single word is the first sign that later on stressed syllables will be produced synchronously with gestures. Whether this early synchrony of gesture with speech is fortuitous or not is an interesting topic for research and discussion. In any event it may be the beginning of gestural synchrony, which seems in adult speech to assist in the easy production of long strings of syllables.

THE DEVELOPMENT OF EASE IN SPEECH

Theory

We have no direct measures of the effort children expend in the pro- duction of speech, either muscular effort or mental effort, and thus no find- ings on this topic. However, it is not an extravagant leap of speculation to suppose that the amount of time it takes a child to execute an utterance is related to the amount of muscular effort required. Arkebauer (1964) has shown that intraoral air pressure, at least, is lower in utterances that are produced at a faster rate, and this suggests that a faster rate is associated with reduced, not increased, effort in adults. But there is no information on the development of this relation in children. Similarly, one would suppose that increased activity in the speech muscles would stiffen coordinative structures and slow the velocity of movement. In this way, too, muscular effort should be less, not more, during rapid, fluent speech. The most rapid speech should be attained with a minimum of muscular activity.

It is probably not too speculative to infer from the development of syllabic rate that children learn to produce speech with less and less effort. Similarly, it does not seem too extravagant a speculation to infer that the amount of time a child takes in pausing before the execution of a sequence of speech movements reflects the extent to which the child must plan the utterance. Thus pause time, and perhaps other forms of discontinuity, seem to reflect mental effort just as speech rate seems to reflect muscular effort. It remains to be shown, however, to what extent these inferences are contaminated by other influences.

One can conclude (from data presented earlier on the location and uninterruptibility of central nervous system activity just before speech attempts) that some thought is required just before an utterance to plan its execution, but once this planning is accomplished the utterance is executed automatically. When this conclusion is put together with the data reported earlier on the length of unfilled pauses in children's speech, which tend to shorten as the child grows, it appears that younger children spend more time planning an utterance, and that the planning time decreases as the child develops. One may also conclude, from the fact that the rate of speech increases as children grow, that they acquire the ability to talk with less muscular effort.

COORDINATION

Findings

1. The maximum DDK rate increases with increased age, up to eighteen to twenty years of age (Dawson, 1929; Jenkins, 1941; Lundeen, 1950; Irwin and Becklund, 1953; Fletcher, 1972).
2. The maximum rate of repetition in a finger-tapping task increases steadily from six to nineteen years of age (Ream, 1922).
3. Reaction time decreases as children mature, a five-year-old's RT for a simple task being about twice as long as an adult's (Cratty, 1970).
4. Speech production variability decreases with age (Tingley and Allen, 1975; DiSimoni, 1972; Eguchi and Hirsch, 1969).
5. An adult level of stability of speech motor control is achieved by eight to twelve years (Kent, 1976).

Theory

It is evident without an elaborate review of these findings that the child's capacity to produce speech movements in a smooth and coordinated way increases with maturity. Development in the ability to react more quickly (Cratty, 1970), and decreasing errors in repetitive movement tasks suggest that coordination for speech (Dawson, 1929; Jenkins, 1941; Lundeen, 1950; Irwin and Becklund, 1953; Fletcher, 1972) and for nonspeech movements (Ream, 1922) increases with maturity. Decreased variability in the execution of speech movement tasks (Eguchi and Hirsch, 1969; DiSimoni, 1975; Tingley and Allen, 1975) confirm that speech coordination is also developing. However, there is little direct evidence that the development of speech motor control *depends on* the speed of reaction time or the ability to make rapid repetitive movements. It seems logical to draw the inference, but empirical confirmation would be far more satisfying.

In addition to the obvious findings, and in spite of the clear relation of these findings to the development of speech coordination in children, several additional factors need to be considered to understand this aspect of speech fluency. The ability to coordinate speech, as described earlier, depends not just on the person's ability to react and move quickly but on several additional variables.

When the coordinative structures of the speech mechanism are conceived of as mass-spring systems, several considerations for the development of coordination become evident. Children's speech structures are small. The moving parts have less mass, and the muscles that move them are short and thin by comparison with those of adults. Decreased mass will allow, indeed it will predispose, the structures to accelerate and decelerate more rapidly. In addition, the shorter and thinner muscles will, other things being equal, increase the resonant frequency of the systems, making it easier for them, perhaps even constraining them, to move at higher velocities. The most obvious example of these tendencies is in the higher fundamental frequencies of voicing that children show as a result of shorter thinner vocal folds and less voluminous vocal tract spaces.

The vocal folds act as a passive mass-spring system, and the frequency of their vibration is determined entirely by their length, mass, and springiness in response to the driving force of the breathstream. The articulatory movements of speech, the slower movements of the upper articulators, and the abductor-adductory movements of the vocal folds are not determined quite so mechanically, but depend on appropriately timed and distributed neural signals to the muscles in each coordinative structure. Some of this timing and distribution is likely to have been built into the organism as "oscillators," predispositions for certain structures to move in certain ways with certain timing relations. But some of the timing and distribution of neurological control depends on the child's developing nervous system.

Earlier I identified several variables upon which speech coordination was hypothesized to depend—the inhibition of functionally related muscles, the entrainment of anatomically distinct movements with each other, lateralization of certain functions of the brain in one hemisphere, and, perhaps as a result of lateralization, the diminution of interference of one brain function with another. For most of these variables, children are less coordinated for speech than adults.

Children seem less able to inhibit functionally related muscles; that is, they are more likely to entrain anatomically distinct but functionally related movements with each other. The ability to wink without moving the contralateral eyelid or to perform various finger, hand and limb, or tongue movements without moving other structures at the same time is not present in very young children but develops as their neurological systems mature. Lateralization of the cerebral hemispheres also develops in the young child, and interference effects may be more pronounced in children than in adults (Krashen, 1973). All of this suggests what is evident—that children's nervous systems are immature and are still developing well after speech and language are acquired. The child speaks with a mechanism that is not well coordinated neurologically.

However, even though the control systems of neurological coordination are immature and unable to send signals to the speech mechanism that are appropriately timed and distributed to produce coordinated speech movements, the child's vocal mechanism is small, reactive, and speedy. It should take only a small error of timing or distribution to have a proportionally large impact on the accuracy and timing of movements. It seems not surprising, then, that a rather large minority of children find it difficult to speak with adult fluency and show patterns of disfluency that alarm their parents.

REFERENCES

ALLEN, G., and HAWKINS, S., Phonological rhythm: definition and development, in *Child Phonology, Volume 1: Production.* New York: Academic Press, 1980.

AMSTER, B., The rate of speech in normal preschool children. Ph.D. dissertation, Temple University, Philadelphia, 1984.

ARKEBAUER, H. J., A study of intra-oral air pressure associated with the production of selected consonants. Ph.D. dissertation, State University of Iowa, Ames, 1964.

ATKINSON-KING, K., Children's acquisition of phonological stress contrasts, *Working Papers in Phonetics,* No. 25. Los Angeles; University of California, 1973.

BERNSTEIN, N., Are there constraints on childhood disfluency? *Journal of Fluency Disorders,* 6 (1981), 341–50.

BLOODSTEIN, O., and GANTWERK, B., Grammatical function in relation to stuttering in young children, *Journal of Speech and Hearing Research,* 10 (1967), 786–89.

CALDWELL, A., Linguistic competence and disfluency behavior in male and female children. Unpublished M.A. thesis, University of Tennessee, Knoxville, 1971.

COLBURN, N., Disfluency behavior and emerging linguistic structures in preschool children. Convention address, American Speech-Language-Hearing Association, 1979.

COLBURN, N., and MYSAK, E., Developmental disfluency and emerging grammar I. Disfluency characteristics in early syntactic utterances, *Journal of Speech and Hearing Research*, 25 (1982a), 414–20.

COLBURN, N., and MYSAK, eds., Developmental disfluency and emerging grammar II. Co-occurrence of disfluency with specified semantic-syntactic structures, *Journal of Speech and Hearing Research*, 25 (1982b), 421–27.

CRATTY, B., J., *Perceptual and Motor Development in Infants and Children*. London: Macmillan, 1970.

DARLEY, F., and SPRIESTERSBACH, D., *Diagnostic Methods in Speech Pathology*, 2nd ed. New York: Harper & Row, 1978.

DAVIS, D. M., The relation of repetitions in the speech of young children to certain measures of language maturity and situational factors: Part I, *Journal of Speech Disorders*, 5 (1949), 303–18.

DAVIS, D. M., The relation of repetitions in the speech of young children to certain measures of language maturity and situational factors: Part II and Part III, *Journal of Speech Disorders*, 5 (1939), 235–46.

DAWSON, L., A study of the development of the rate of articulation, *Elementary School Journal*, 29 (1929), 610–15.

DEJOY, D., and GREGORY, H., The relationship of children's disfluency to the syntax, length, and vocabulary of their sentences. Convention address, American Speech-Language-Hearing Association, 1973.

DEJOY, D., and GREGORY, H., The developmental nature of fluency in children: data from two preschool age groups. Convention address, American-Language-Hearing Association, 1975.

DISIMONI, F. G., Influence of utterance length upon bilabial closure duration of /p/ in three-, six-, and nine-year-old children, *Journal of the Acoustical Society of America*, 55 (1974), 1919–21.

EGUCHI, S., and HIRSCH, I. J., Development of speech sounds in children, *Acta Otolaryngologica*, Supplementum 257, 1969.

EILERS, R. E., Suprasegmental and grammatical control over telegraphic speech in young children, *Journal of Psycholinguistic Research*, 4 (1975), 227–39.

FLETCHER, S. G., Time-by-count measurement of diadochokinetic syllable rate, *Journal of Speech and Hearing Research*, 15 (1972), 757–62.

GILBERT, J., and PURVIS, B., Temporal constraints on consonant clusters in child speech production, *Journal of Child Language*, 4 (1977), 317–32.

GORDON, P., The effects of syntactic complexity on the occurrence of disfluencies in five-year-old children. Poster session, American Speech-Language-Hearing Association Convention, 1982.

HAWKINS, S., Temporal coordination of consonants in the speech of children: further data, *Journal of Phonetics*, 7 (1979), 235–67.

HAYNES, W., and HOOD, S., Disfluency changes in children as a function of the systematic modification of linguistic complexity, *Journal of Communication Disorders*, 11 (1978), 79–93.

HELMREICH, H., and BLOODSTEIN, O., The grammatical factor in childhood disfluency in relation to the continuity hypothesis. *Journal of Speech and Hearing Research*, 16 (1973), 731–38.

HUTT, D., The relative speech rates of mothers and their children. M.A. thesis, Temple University, Philadelphia, 1985.

INGRAM, D., Phonological rules in young children, *Journal of Child Language*, 1 (1974), 49–64.

IRWIN, J. V., and BECKLUND, O., Norms for maximum repetitive rates for certain sounds established with the sylrate, *Journal of Speech and Hearing Disorders*, 18 (1953), 149–65.

JENKINS, R. L., The rate of diadochokinetic movements of the jaw at the ages seven to maturity, *Journal of Speech Disorders*, 6 (1941), 13–22.

KEATING, P., and KUBASKA, C., Variation in the duration of words, *Journal of the Acoustical Society of America*, 63 (1978), Supplement 1, 56 (A).

KENT, R., Anatomical and neuromuscular maturation of the speech mechanism: evidence from acoustic studies, *Journal of Speech and Hearing Research*, 19 (1976), 421–47.

KENT, R. D., The segmental organization of speech, in *The Production of Speech*, ed. P. F. MacNeilage. New York: Springer-Verlag, 1983.

KLATT, D., Interaction between two factors that influence vowel duration, *Journal of the Acoustical Society of America*, 54 (1973), 1102–4.

KOWAL, S., O'CONNELL, D. C., and SABIN, E. F., Development of temporal patterning and vocal hesitations in spontaneous narratives, *Journal of Psycholinguistic Research*, 4 (1975), 195–207.

KRASHEN, S., Lateralization, language learning, and the critical period: some new evidence, *Language Learning* 23 (1973), 63–74.

KUEHN, D. P., and TOMBLIN, J. B., The use of cineradiographic techniques for the study of articulation disorders. Convention address, American Speech-Language-Hearing Association, 1974.

LUNDEEN, D. J., The relationship of diadochokinesis to various speech sounds, *Journal of Speech and Hearing Disorders*, 15 (1950), 54–59.

MACKAY, D. G., Aspects of the syntax of behavior: syllable structure and speech rate, *Quarterly Journal of Experimental Psychology*, 26 (1974), 642–57.

MALECOT, A., JOHNSTON, R., and KIZZIAR, P.-A., Syllabic rate and utterance length in French, *Phonetica*, 26 (1972), 235–51.

MUMA, J., A comparison of certain aspects of productivity and grammar in speech samples of fluent and nonfluent four-year-old children, *Dissertation Abstracts International*, 28 (1967), 2658-B.

NAESER, M., The American child's acquisition of differential vowel duration, *The Wisconsin Research and Development Center for Cognitive Learning, Technical Report #* 144, 1970.

OLLER, D., The effect of position in utterance on speech segment duration in English, *Journal of the Acoustical Society of America*, 62 (1973), 1235–37.

OLLER, D. K., and SMITH, B. L., The effect of final-syllable position on vowel duration in infant babbling, *Journal of the Acoustical Society of America*, 62 (1977), 994–97.

PORT, D., and PRESTON, M., Early apical stop production: a voice onset time analysis, *Journal of Phonetics*, 2 (1974), 195–210.

PRESTON, M., and YENI-KOMSHIAN, G., Studies on the development of stop consonants in children. *Haskins Laboratories: Status Report on Speech Research*, SR-11, 49–53, 1967.

REAM, M. J., The tapping test: a measure of motility, *Psychological Monographs*, 31 (1922), 293–319.

SILVERMAN, E-M., Word position and grammatical function in relation to preschoolers' speech disfluency, *Perceptual and Motor Skills*, 39 (1974), 267–72.

SILVERMAN, E-M., Effect of selected word attributes on preschoolers' speech disfluency: initial phoneme and length, *Journal of Speech and Hearing Research*, 18 (1975), 430–34.

SMITH, B. L., Temporal aspects of English speech production: a developmental perspective, *Journal of Phonetics*, 6 (1978), 37–67.

SODERBERG, G., The relations of stuttering to word length and word frequency, *Journal of Speech and Hearing Research*, 9 (1966), 584–89.

SODERBERG, G., Linguistic factors in stuttering. *Journal of Speech and Hearing Research*, 10 (1967), 801–10.

STARKWEATHER, C. W., Speech fluency and its development in normal children, in *Speech and Language: Advances in Basic Research and Practice* (vol. 4), ed. N. Lass. New York: Academic Press, 1981.

STARKWEATHER, C. W., Stuttering in children: an overview, *Journal of Childhood Communication Disorders*, 6 (1982), 5–14.

STARKWEATHER, C. W. Counseling the parents of young stutterers, in *Counseling in Stuttering Therapy* eds. J. Fraser-Gruss and S. Ainsworth. Memphis, Tenn.: Speech Foundation of America, 1983.

SUBTELNY, W., WORTH, J., and SAKUDA, M., Intra-oral air pressure and rate of flow during speech, *Journal of Speech and Hearing Research*, 9 (1966), 498–518.

TASSIELLO, M., Duration of /s/ in five and seven year olds. M.A. thesis, Hunter College, New York, 1975.

THOMPSON, A. E., and HIXON, T. J., Nasal air flow during normal speech production, *Cleft Palate Journal*, 16 (1979), 412–30.

TIFFANY, W. R., The effects of syllable structure on diadochokinetic and reading rates, *Journal of Speech and Hearing Research*, 23 (1980), 894–908.

TINGLEY, B., and ALLEN, G., Development of speech timing control in children, *Child Development*, 46 (1975), 434–45.

WALKER, C., and BLACK, J., The intrinsic intensity of oral phrases, *Joint Project Report No. 2*. Pensacola, Fla.: Naval Air Station, United States Naval School of Aviation Medicine, 1950.

WEXLER, K., and MYSAK, E., Disfluency characteristics of 2-, 4-, and 6-year-old males, *Journal of Fluency Disorders,* 7 (1982), 37–46.

YAIRI, E., Disfluencies of normally speaking two-year-old children, *Journal of Speech and Hearing Research,* 24 (1981), 490–95.

YAIRI, E., Longitudinal studies of disfluencies in two-year-old children, *Journal of Speech and Hearing Research,* 1982, 25, 155–60.

YAIRI, E., The onset of stuttering in two and three year old children: a preliminary report. *Journal of Speech and Hearing Research,* 48 (1983), 171–77.

ZLATIN, M., and KOENIGSKNECHT, R., Development of the voicing contrast: a comparison of voice onset time in stop perception and production, *Journal of Speech and Hearing Research,* 19 (1976), 93–111.

Stuttering:
What It Is and Is Not

INTRODUCTION

This chapter deals with the definition of stuttering. How can we recognize stuttering, and how can we reliably distinguish it from other kinds of similar behaviors, including particularly normal nonfluencies of speech? To identify stuttering, clinicians must be familiar with its characteristic behavior patterns. To make a differential diagnosis, in which stuttering is distinguished from other similar behaviors, clinicians focus on specific aspects of stuttering that distinguish it from other types of disfluencies. Behaviors that are characteristic of stuttering but not of other types of disfluency are the outer limits of the definition.

Another way to answer the question, "What is stuttering?" is to describe the different kinds of stuttering, the variations in behavior that can occur and still be considered stuttering. These permissible variations are the inner limits of the definition.

Stuttering can vary in a number of ways. First, it can be more or less severe. Second, certain categories of stuttering behavior can be identified, and these variations too are a part of the definition.

Findings

Core Behaviors

1. In the disfluencies of normal adult speakers, word repetitions make up 71 percent, phrase repetitions 17 percent, part-word repetitions 12 percent (McClay and Osgood, 1959).
2. In adult stutterers, word repetitions make up 37 percent, and part-word repetitions 63 percent of all disfluencies (Soderberg, 1962).

117

3. The syllabic repetitions that the layman identifies as stuttering (Sander, 1963) are common to all stutterers (Wingate, 1964).

4. The most characteristic stuttering behavior is repeated speech elements (Soderberg, 1967). Sounds, syllables, words, or phrases may be repeated, although sound and syllable repetitions are most characteristic. Typically, the element is repeated only two to five times (Van Riper, 1984).

5. Word repetitions may or may not be judged as stuttering. If a word is repeated more than once ("like, like, like this") it is more likely to be judged as a stuttering behavior (Curran and Hood, 1977).

6. The frequency with which disfluent behavior occurs has a bearing on whether listeners will judge the behavior to be stuttering or not. Even single-unit word repetitions (usually considered normal nonfluency) are judged to be stuttering behaviors when they occur on more than 15 percent of words (Hegde and Hartman, 1979b), and filled pauses, such as "uh," will be judged as stuttering if they occur on 20 percent of spoken words (Hegde and Hartman, 1979a).

7. The mean duration of stuttering repetitions is 1.6 seconds; the standard deviation is 3.0 seconds (Sheehan, 1974).

8. The frequency of movement in sound and syllable repetitions is usually close to the maximum diadochokinetic rate (5 to 10 per second) (Van Riper, 1984) for the speech structure involved and the age and sex of the person (Fletcher, 1972).

9. Prolongations of sounds beyond the normal duration are also common in stutterers (Van Riper, 1984).

10. The average duration of a prolongation is 0.87 seconds (SD = 0.72 seconds) (Sheehan, 1974).

11. Blockages and postural fixations of the airway occur in some stutterers. They may be located at any of the points of articulation in the vocal tract (Van Riper, 1984).

12. Tremors occur in the speech and voice muscles in some confirmed stutterers. The muscles fasciculate at frequencies of 7 to 9 per second, and the movements associated with them are usually small in amplitude for the structure involved (Van Riper, 1984).

13. The speech muscles of stutterers are abnormally active during stuttered, and to a lesser extent, during nonstuttered speech (Freeman and Ushijima, 1978; Shapiro, 1980). The muscle activity is abnormal in that it occurs in muscles that should be relaxed, such as antagonists, or at the wrong time in muscles that should be flexed.

Accessory Features

14. In addition to the core behaviors described above, stutterers also perform a great many other behaviors in attempts to postpone, interrupt,

escape from, avoid, or disguise the core behaviors. These secondary or accessory behaviors are both varied and common (Van Riper, 1984). They seem to be learned as a way of coping with the core behaviors (Wingate, 1964; Brutten and Shoemaker, 1967).

Coarticulation

15. Stuttered sounds frequently lack the appropriate transitional formant patterns (inappropriate coarticulation) (Agnello and Buxton, 1966).
16. In the repetition of a consonant, advanced stutterers use the schwa instead of the appropriate vowel, and in the prolongation of a continuant the articulators are not in the appropriate position for the sound that follows (Stromsta, 1965; Agnello & Buxton, 1966).
17. Normal speakers under DAF also lack transitional coarticulation (Rawnsley and Harris, 1954).
18. Some authors (Allen, Peters, and Williams, 1975) think that the type of coarticulation stutterers exhibit is appropriate for the whispered version of the appropriate vowel.

Individual Variability

19. There is a wide variability in behavior from stutterer to stutterer but consistency within a single stutterer, particularly when the word or sound upon which stuttering occurs is held constant (Barr, 1940; Black, 1957; Van Riper, 1984). The variability is more pronounced in the secondary than in the core behaviors.
20. In some stutterers, clusters of behaviors seem to occur in sequence (Black, 1957; Sheehan, 1974).

Severity

21. There are various ways of determining the severity of stuttering, but most authorities agree that the frequency with which the behaviors occur and their duration are factors to consider (Van Riper, 1984).
22. The severity judgments of speech-language pathologists are predictable from knowledge of the stutterer's reading rate and the number of intrasentence pauses (Prosek et al., 1979).

Theory

It ought to be said at the very beginning that the distinction between core behaviors and accessory features is somewhat artificial. It is a distinction that has a history in our field, and was originally proposed by Wingate (1964), when he noted that repetitions, prolongations, and blockages were behaviors that distinguished stuttering from other forms of disfluency. The division of stuttering behaviors into core and accessory features also suggested a relation between the two, a relation in which the accessory features were at least added on to the core behaviors. Later theorists (Brutten and Shoemaker, 1967) would suggest that the accessory features were a different kind of behavior. The distinction is artificial in the sense that all stuttering behaviors are changed as the disorder develops.

The stutterer typically begins repeating whole words and then goes on to repeat parts of words. These repetitions also change. With time, the duration of the repeated element is likely to diminish to a briefer syllable, containing a schwa instead of the original vowel, and then the rate of repetition may also change, typically becoming faster. These are developmental changes that occur *within* a core behavior. Similar changes occur in other core behaviors, and there are also patterns of development in the accessory features. These patterns of development are described more fully in the next chapter. The point being made here is that the binary categorization of behaviors may be useful, but it tends to obscure the continuous development and change that these behaviors show over time.

Probably the most important, certainly the most obvious fact about stuttering is one that is not listed above. The speech of stutterers is not as continuous, not as rapid, and not as easily produced as the speech of nonstutterers. Stutterers pause, block, and repeat and prolong elements of speech more frequently than nonstutterers. However, it is difficult to use this fact as a way to distinguish stutterers from nonstutterers because nonstutterers also hesitate, pause, and repeat elements of speech. If all kinds of disfluencies are considered together, a group of stutterers will have an average percentage of disfluent words that is higher than that of a comparable group of nonstutterers. But there would be some overlap between these two distributions. There would be some stutterers whose frequency of discontinuity was very low, lower than the most disfluent of the nonstutterers.

The same sort of finding would emerge if we compared rates of speech. The stutterers as a group would talk more slowly, perhaps much more slowly, than the group of nonstutterers. But there would be a few who talked just as fast as the average nonstutterer, and there would be some nonstutterers who were slower speakers than many of the stutterers. So neither rate nor continuity are viable ways to identify (diagnose) individual stutterers, even though a high frequency of discontinuity and a slow rate of speech are salient characteristics of the disorder.

If we could measure the effort put into speech production, we might—or might not—find a different situation, but there is no unequivocal way to measure this variable at present.

It is clear from the first few findings in the list above that repetition is a key characteristic of stuttering. In adults who stutter, repeated elements make up a large proportion of disfluencies. In normal adult speakers, the proportion is much smaller. This is illustrated in Figure 5-1. Furthermore, the length of the repeated element is a factor. In adults who stutter, short elements—sounds or syllables—tend to be repeated during disfluencies, but in adults who do not stutter, the repetitions that do occur are of larger elements—whole words and phrases. So one way to identify a stutterer is to look for a higher than normal percentage of words on which sounds and syllables are repeated. Typically, nonstutterers repeat sounds and syllables on fewer than 1 percent of spoken words. Stutterers, on the other hand, may repeat sounds and syllables on anywhere from 0 to 100 percent of spoken words. The problem in using this approach to distinguish stutterers from nonstutterers is the low end of that large range. There are a few stutterers who do not repeat sounds or syllables at all. The diagnostic net we have cast to sweep in all stutterers has allowed a small number to escape.

Adding other types of core behaviors—prolongations and blockages—to the criteria for diagnosis will reduce even more the number who get through the net, but some still escape. There are a few stutterers, in fact, who show absolutely no overt stuttering behaviors at all, who talk almost normally all or most of the time, yet who report that they are stutterers. Furthermore, on being interviewed, they will tell you that they *would* repeat, prolong, or block if they didn't do something else, perform some other behavior such as substituting for the word they are about to say another one which is "easier" for them, or by slowing down the rate at which they talk, or by tapping their fingers together silently and rhythmically and timing their speech to the rhythm, or by thinking very carefully about producing speech in a certain way, such as with longer vowels or with improved vocal resonance. This last group, those who would stutter if they didn't do something else, are sometimes known as covert stutterers. They would stut-

FIGURE 5-1   The distribution of different types of discontinuity: stutterers versus nonstutterers.

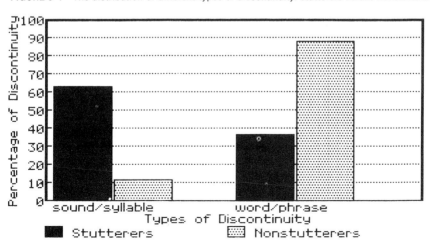

ter, but they manage to hide the stuttering or prevent it from occurring. Nearly all stutterers perform avoidance behaviors of one kind or another, but the covert stutterer is able to do it successfully. There aren't very many of these covert stutterers, but there are some. They are really stutterers, and our diagnostic net should catch them too.

Unfortunately, we have no way, short of the client's report, of verifying the presence of these successful avoidance behaviors. It would be helpful if there were some task we could ask them to do that would uncover the stuttering. Suggesting that they talk without using these techniques doesn't really work. The stutterers who avoid stuttering successfully are highly motivated to conceal the disorder and usually cannot reveal it, even when it would be clearly beneficial to the clinician performing the evaluation. We have to take their word for it. This is not really so awful, since it is hard to imagine why these people would claim to be stutterers when they were not. We can probably believe them when they say that they would actually stutter if they didn't use the avoidance behavior. This is of course not as rigorously scientific an approach as we would like, but our first duty as scientists is to be true to the validity of the phenomenon being observed. If we lack the means to examine it objectively, we cannot assume or pretend that it doesn't exist.

To some, this discussion may seem to have dwelt for too long on covert stuttering. The covert stutterer who never reveals any of the overt features—the repetitions, prolongations, and blockages that characterize the disorder—is unquestionably a rare kind of stutterer. However, I raise the matter of covert stutterers because of the implications it has for all stutterers. If some stutterers can avoid so successfully that they never repeat, prolong, or block, and if nearly all stutterers avoid stuttering as much as they can, both of which seem fair presumptions, then how are we to know from the behavior we can observe how severe stuttering in a particular individual is?

If some stutterers appear overtly normal, then many, probably most, perhaps even all stutterers, are avoiding some stutters. Also, some stutterers are probably better at avoiding than others. The frequency with which these behaviors occur, then, is a necessary, but not a sufficient, way to assess the severity—indeed not even the presence—of the disorder. Add to this the problem of situational variation, which I haven't yet described (see pp. 172–174), and it should be fully appreciated how poor a behavioral sample we get when the frequency of overt stuttering behaviors is used as a measure of severity. Still, we have little choice but to rely on what we can hear or see.

Consequently, we can define stuttering, for purposes of diagnosis, as a higher than normal frequency of part-word repetitions or prolongations or blockages, or the presence of some reported or observable avoidance behavior which the client says reduces or eliminates the repetitions, prolongations, or blockages.

Findings 7 and 10 also cast some light on the disorder. On the average, neither repetitions nor prolongations last very long. They are, in most stutterers, brief phenomena. However, the standard deviation of the repetitions, at least, makes it evident that in a few stutterers some repetitions are very long. Also, it should be pointed out that repetitions of parts of words, however brief, strike the ears of listeners with great emotional force. They are a sharp deviation from the kind of speech a listener expects to come from a speaker's mouth.

Tremors are fasciculations—very brief muscular contractions—with little or no movement of the body part the muscle normally moves. For example, the mentalis muscle plays a role in stiffening the lower lip during the production of bilabial sounds and in depressing the lip as the bilabial is completed. A stutterer showing tremors of the mentalis might be in the position of bilabial closure, attempting to say a word like "boy," while tremulous movements of the muscle can be seen. The chin quivers much the way it does when one is about to cry, but the lips remain closed. In more severe stutterers, tremors may start in one location and then spread to another. A tremor of the mentalis might spread over the chin to the platysma and the anterior belly of the digastric muscle and then on down the strap muscles of the neck. But this is extreme.

Tremors are a sign of advanced stuttering. They may also occur in very young children, but they are still a sign that the disorder is fully acquired, that the person is using great effort to talk, and that the use of excessive effort is fully habituated. Tremors can sometimes be voluntarily interrupted by larger jerking movements, provided these are out of phase with the tremor. Van Riper (1984) says that three factors are necessary for a tremor to occur: (1) a localized area of tension; (2) a postural fixation of the muscle groups involved; and (3) a sudden ballistic movement or surge of tension or air pressure.

The accessory features of stuttering are always difficult to describe because of their extreme variability from person to person. Some examples may help. A number of stutterers show behaviors that are rhythmic—tapping feet, nodding heads, tapping fingers softly together—because the existence of a regular rhythm enables them to time the onset of speech to coincide with one of the repeated elements in the rhythmic behavior. These behaviors are usually called *timers*. Timers need not be rhythmic, however. Many stutterers find that they can escape from a block by timing an attempt on a word to coincide with a slap on the thigh, a stamp of the foot, a blink of the eyes, or any movement that produces a stimulus of brief duration.

Stutterers also do many things to postpone the attempt of a word that they fear they will stutter on. Stutterers may stop, say "uh," look toward the ceiling as though lost in thought for the right word, divert their speech to side issues, inject a note of humor, or put in any kind of aside, sigh, lick their lips, say "well," or "I mean," or use any number of other tricks, to postpone the attempt on the word. Sometimes postponing the attempt avoids the stutter. Most often it does not, and to the time taken up by the stuttering itself we can add the time taken up by the behaviors designed to postpone or forestall the stutter. Most people will recognize these postponement behaviors as, for the most part, behaviors that nonstutterers use to stall for time when talking so as to think about what to say next. Stutterers use them to postpone attempts on words they anticipate stuttering because listeners accept these behaviors as normal aspects of discourse. They are inconspicuous.

Many stutterers try to hide the disorder or disguise it, pretending that it is something else. Some pretend not to have heard a question so as not to have to answer it. Some stutterers in school pretend they do not know the answer to a question, even though they know it perfectly well, because they expect to stutter in answering it. Occasionally, a stutterer will pretend to be deaf or to have some other speech disorder to hide the fact of stuttering. More typically, stutterers, having just stuttered, might try to cover their tracks by acting as though their hesitations were really a search for the word, or uncertainty over the content.

Perhaps the most common category of behaviors are forcing and struggling to get through a stuttered word. Pushing out air with vigorous abdominal contractions is the most common kind of forcing. Usually, this forcing is accompanied by simultaneous articulatory or glottal closures. The stutterer blocks off the airway at the glottis or in the mouth, tries to force through this blockage by pushing from the abdomen, but simultaneously increases the pressure at the blockage. Occasionally, a stutterer will perform an irregular respiratory pattern, such as taking a deep breath, or trying hard to breathe in some special, but not normal way.

Many stutterers, particularly young people, go to great lengths to avoid talking in situations where they feel they will stutter. Adults too are likely to talk less in situations that are difficult for them. Some stutterers go so far as to give up talking almost totally and communicate through writing or not at all. But this is a very unusual route. Speech is so efficient as a way to transmit information that it is hard to avoid it altogether, even when its efficiency is reduced by stuttering.

It is very common for a stutterer to begin to say a word, sense that stuttering is going to occur or has just begun to occur, abort the attempt on the word, and back up to an earlier point to try again. This pattern has been called "stopping and restarting." In milder stutterers, it is often a successful avoidance of stuttering. In more severe stutterers it will sometime succeed, but as often as not, the person will back up, then stutter on a word that is located earlier than the one that was originally stuttered. This may prompt a second back-up to an even earlier position, where another difficult word may be encountered and stuttered. This pattern has a certain

Kafkaesque quality. The stutterer keeps getting diverted farther and farther from the original goal and may lose sight of it altogether. Or it may seem as though the person is talking backward instead of forward.

Many stutterers learn that when they anticipate stuttering on a particular word they can substitute another word for it and not stutter. Probably this doesn't work all the time; that is, they occasionally stutter on the substitute. A great many stutterers do not use this trick because they cannot find a substitute word that signifies their communicative intent. Others try this technique for a while and come to realize that it seriously hinders their communicative effectiveness by diverting them from their original idea. But for some stutterers it is a highly effective avoidance behavior. It involves considerable effort, however, even when successful, because the job of word-retrieval is greatly increased. But beyond that, changing a word in a sentence usually involves changing other parts of the sentence, and a new construction is also required. This diverts the speaker farther from the original intention. Word-changing is a most insidious form of avoidance because when it is successful it is completely inconspicuous, and this is highly encouraging. It is also insidious because its bad effects—failure to communicate as clearly and directly as possible—are not immediately apparent to many speakers. It seems at first a small sacrifice.

Most, probably all, of the accessory features of stuttering are designed to postpone, avoid, terminate, escape from, hide, disguise, or diminish the impact of stuttering. Certainly, when these behaviors are first developed, they are used for these purposes. With continued use, many of them seem to lose their capacity to help the stutterer avoid a display of the behaviors. This loss of potency with continued use of avoidance techniques is very common and an interesting aspect of the disorder. It is not immediately clear why the effectiveness of these techniques should diminish with continued use. One of the earliest ideas about stuttering was that these tricks diminished stuttering by diverting the stutterer's attention from the disorder. They distracted the stutterer from a morbid attention to disfluency. Because of this their effectiveness depended on their novelty as stimuli. Once they became familiar that novelty was gone, and they no longer worked. But many of these tricks don't seem very novel as stimuli. Not novel enough, anyway. Who could be distracted by tapping fingers or a nodding head or a synonym? But the idea of distraction may turn out to have some merit after all. Recent research and theory in the motor control of normal behavior suggests that the amount and kind of attention that is paid to a movement has a powerful effect on the smoothness and coordination with which the movement is performed (Armson, 1986).

What is compelling about many of these tricks is that they require the stutterer to talk in a different way, to say a different word or to say the same word in a different way, altering the pattern, particularly the timing, of the movements that are made to produce the word. It may be the case that making movements that one is less accustomed to making, movements that are less automatic, promotes fluent speech. Or conversely, that stuttering is more likely to occur on a highly habituated series of speech movements and less likely to occur on less well practiced sequences. See, however, the sections on the adaptation of stuttering (pp. 196–202) for information that is almost entirely the opposite of this idea.

Most stutterers show some but not all of these avoidance behaviors. Each stutterer has his own individual pattern of stuttering. As a result, the disorder shows extreme variability from stutterer to stutterer. There is much less variability in the behaviors used by any one stutterer. A specific person, given the same word in the same speech situation, is likely to attempt the word in a similar way. There is some variation, to be sure, particularly when an attempt is made that fails. At this time, the stutterer is likely to try something different. But the point is that the variability in behavior between stutterers is far greater than that within stutterers. There is also far more variability among accessory features than there is among core behaviors. Most stutterers repeat or prolong brief elements of speech, or block. But there is no way to characterize, in a way that describes all or even most stutterers, the accessory features. They are too varied among the population of stutterers to be characterized. Many stutterers have few accessory features and simply stutter openly. Others have an elaborate armamentarium of avoidance devices.

This pattern of variability suggests, but does not demonstrate, that experience, which is highly variable from person to person, plays more of a role in the development of the accessory features than it does in the development of the core behaviors. Not that the accessory features are learned and the core behaviors are not, but that learning is more important to the form that the accessory features take than it is to the form that the core behaviors take. The form of the core behaviors, being more alike from stutterer to stutterer, seems determined to a greater extent by nonlearning, nonindividualistic events. There is, of course, a counterargument to this idea. Some things that are not learned are highly individualistic, faces for example. But the accessory features of stuttering seem learned not only because of their variability but also because of their relation to the disorder, their relation to behaviors performed by nonstutterers for similar reasons, and because of the way they are distributed in the behavioral sequence.

Another aspect of behavioral variability is the possibility of patterns of behavior. Some stutterers seem to show a characteristic sequence of behaviors. For example, a typical pattern might be to try first to say the word, sense that it would be stuttered, search for a substitute, fail to find an adequate one, take a deep breath, try again, sense that it would be stuttered again, stop for a second time, back up to the beginning of the sentence, restarting with "I mean," make a third attempt, encounter stuttering for the third time, and this time push hard to force the word out. There might be some variation from time to time, but something like this sequence of events often recurs in a stutterer. The question is: When there is a typical or characteristic sequence of behaviors, what determines the order in which the behaviors are performed?

Van Riper (1984) suggests that the least conspicuous behavior will be tried first, and if it fails, another more conspicuous one will be tried. In some cases, the sequence suggests this possibility. But sometimes there are sequences that do not seem determined by conspicuousness to the observer. Of course, it is not the observer's beliefs about conspicuousness that matter, but the stutterer's, and it is not easy to determine what those beliefs might be. Other researchers suggest that the behaviors occur according to the order in which they were learned, the most recently learned occurring last (Brutten and Shoemaker, 1967). This idea fits well with the fact, previously mentioned, that the avoidance behaviors tend to lose their potency with continued use. Stutterers might learn to use a behavior to avoid stuttering. It works for a while and becomes a habitual part of speech behavior. After a while, it is no longer effective, and another behavior is acquired that works better. But the old one is still a habit and is not discarded so easily, so the new behavior is tacked on to the old one. Soon the second one wears out and a third is added. This continues until a characteristic sequence of behaviors is acquired, the last one being the most recently acquired. Although this idea fits the available data reasonably well, there isn't any clear evidence that it is so. It is very difficult to determine the order in which behaviors are acquired by stutterers.

COARTICULATION

When children first begin to stutter they usually repeat whole words. After a while they begin to repeat parts of words—usually whole syllables in which the vowel is repeated with the same full vowel color it will have in the word when they finally say it fluently, that is, "pee, pee, pee, pee, people." After a little more development has taken place however (see pp. 137–165 for a full discussion of development), the vowel in the stuttered portion of the word changes. The schwa, or neutral vowel /ə/ is used instead of the vowel that is appropriate for the word as spoken fluently, that is, "puh, puh, puh people." This change is considered one of the danger signs that stuttering is becoming an increasingly serious problem (Walle, 1975). In the speech of a fully developed stutterer, the use of the appropriate vowel during stuttered portions of a word would be unusual. This appears to be as true for prolonged sounds as it is for repeated sounds. What does this developmental shift mean?

Those theorists who believe that stuttering is primarily a disorder of the vocal mechanism argue that the schwa, or a more neutralized schwa-like vowel, is characteristic of whispered versions of a vowel (Allen, Peters, and Williams, 1975). For these theorists, the use of the schwa represents a failure of the vocal mechanism. This explanation accounts for the fact that some stutterers use the schwa, but it doesn't account well for the fact, also well established, that the very young stutterer (or the incipient stutterer according to some, or the highly disfluent child) does not usually use the schwa. The idea that stuttering is a result of the vocal mechanism's not functioning properly would be supported by an observation of the use of the schwa in stuttering at onset, but such is not the case.

What, then, is a more complete explanation? Another characteristic of the schwa is that it is briefer in duration than the full vowel, and the movements used to make the schwa are less extensive. Thus the use of the schwa, and its intrusion into the speech of the developing stutterer, support two other theoretical ideas—that stutterers are trying to hurry through their stuttering, and that they are talking with less extensive movements. The first of these is simply a way of saying that as children begin to stutter they attempt to talk more normally. They begin to try to compensate for the fact that stuttering behaviors take up time without contributing information, and so they try in various ways to hurry through the stuttering. Shortening the vowels is one way of speeding up the process, or so it may seem. This is not to say that children using such compensatory behavior are necessarily aware of what they are doing. Such a behavior could be acquired with little awareness.

The second idea, that speech movements are restricted during schwa production, can be used in two theoretical ways. The first way is, like the idea just described, that young stutterers are learning to move their speech mechanisms less extensively to save time. The other use of the idea, however, is more explanatory. It may be that increased muscle tension makes it difficult for the stutterer's speech mechanism to move as extensively as that of the nonstutterer. In other words, the intruded schwa may not be a coping behavior, but a physiological consequence of increased tension in the speech muscles. Although more powerful as an explanation, this latter idea does not explain well why the schwa is not intruded in very early stuttering. That is, since the schwa appears after the child has been stuttering for a while, the increased muscle activity cannot be a primary cause, but is instead in some way a part of the child's reaction to the preexisting disfluency.

SEVERITY

The problem of stuttering severity has both clinical and theoretical significance. Clinically, we need to be able to assess the severity of any disorder to write a complete diagnostic report, to prioritize clients for treatment, and to plan therapeutic intervention. The theorist needs to understand the severity of stuttering because a theoretical description of the disorder should account for the variation in severity that occurs among and within stutterers.

Here a brief digression is necessary. When a theory is suggested to identify the cause or causes of stuttering, it is most compelling if it satisfies two crucial tests: (1) the theory should explain why some people become stutterers and others do not and (2) it should explain why some stutterers stutter severely while others exhibit very mild signs. Simply put, if a theorist suggests that a variable contributes to the cause of the disorder, we would be inclined to accept the theory if (1) the variable operates in stutterers more than in nonstutterers and (2) it operates more in severe stutterers than it does in milder ones. For example, if a theorist suggested that stuttering was caused by the same gene that was responsible for male baldness, we should expect to find more stutterers who were bald than nonstutterers, and we should expect that the severe stutterers were balder than the milder ones.

However, caution is warranted here. It is entirely possible that the presence of stuttering in an individual is a result of one set of variables and the severity of the disorder is determined by another set of variables. So, although a theoretical explanation that satisfies both of these tests is compelling, we should not disallow theories that fail to explain the presence of the disorder but do explain its severity. This caution is important because, as we shall see, a large number of variables seem related to the presence or absence (or the onset) of the disorder but do not seem to be related to the severity (or the development) of it. Stuttering severity, at present, seems unrelated to a number of apparently causative variables. Despite this problem for the theorists, it is still important, both for clinical and for theoretical purposes, to understand what methods validly and reliably assess stuttering severity.

There have been a number of suggestions for assessing severity, and it is not totally clear which is best. However, some judgments will help in choosing a severity measure. First, we can set aside some measures on grounds of theoretical bias. One must avoid theoretical bias in evaluating severity. A theorist who believes that stuttering is caused by the same gene that causes baldness might be tempted to say that the balder the stutterer is the more severe his stuttering is, but this would clearly be putting the cart before the horse. Brutten and Shoemaker (1967) believe that stuttering is caused, at least partially, by a stutterer's learned reactions of anxiety to speech situations. They assess severity partly according to the intensity of the person's anxiety in response to speech situations as compared with his anxiety in response to nonspeech situations. Although valid within their own framework, this measure seems too closely related to their theoretical position to be a valid measure of severity for others. We would need to know in some independent way that anxiety is related to the severity of stuttering in all cases (and we do not) before assessing severity by this means.

We can also set aside measures of severity that are related to prognosis. The word *severity* can refer to several things, and there is no reason why it cannot refer to the difficulty of treatment. This use of the word, however, muddies the waters of understanding. The concept of severity seems clearer if we restrict the word closely, using it to refer only to variations in the extent to which the disorder impairs an individual's ability to communicate. Prognosis is something quite different. A more fully developed argument for this position may be found in Starkweather (1983).

Let us define severity, then, as a measure of the extent to which a disorder impairs a person's ability to use speech for social, vocational, and educational purposes. This use of the word seems to promote better clinical and theoretical understanding. When the term is used in this way, it helps us prioritize a waiting list, and it helps us decide which of our clients is in the most trouble as a result of the disorder. A measure of severity, then, should tell us how severely impaired the speaker is as a communicator.

Stuttering is a disorder primarily because the speaker cannot produce meaningful speech as quickly or as easily as other people can. But it also has, as another important ingredient, a cosmetic factor. I refer to the fact that listeners are made uncomfortable by stuttered speech, and that they evaluate stutterers negatively because of this. This is true of any speech disorder to a certain extent, but it is true of stuttering in a more direct way (Woods and Williams, 1976). Furthermore, this cosmetic factor is an important element in the difficulty stutterers have in communicating. That is, they have difficulty communicating in part because of the impact their speech has on listeners, and this factor needs to be considered as an element of severity along with those other elements, the extra time and effort stutterers require to talk. Consequently, severity should be assessed in three ways—the rate at which meaningful speech is produced, the ease with which meaningful speech is produced, and the impact of the disorder on listeners. Satisfying these three criteria establishes the validity of a severity measure.

As with any measure, validity is the first criterion. A measure of severity must assess the severity of stuttering and not something else. But given that a measure is valid, it must also be reliable. This second criterion means that a technique for assessing severity must be one that any trained clinician can repeatedly use with the same sample of stuttered speech and get the same results, within reasonable tolerance. It also means that different clinicians should get the same results when they measure the severity of the same sample of stuttered speech. If these two criteria are met, a third one comes into play. This third criterion is simplicity. Given several ways of assessing severity, all of which are equally valid and reliable, the simplest one is the best.

Some clinicians measure total speaking time for a monologue or for a series of utterances produced in a dialogue and divide by the number of words or syllables. That is, they measure speech rate. This is elegantly simple, quite reliable, and gets to the heart of one of the main impairments in stuttering—the extra time that the stutterer takes to communicate. But this measure only indirectly gets at effort of speech production and impact on listeners. It assumes that if the stutterer takes longer to speak he must also be exerting greater effort and having greater negative impact on listeners. If those assumptions are acceptable, then speech rate is the perfect measure of severity because it is the simplest. But the assumptions are only barely tenable. Some evidence (Prosek et al., 1979) indicates that measures of speech rate and the frequency of intrasentence pauses are predictive of speech pathologists' judgments of stuttering severity. But this result, although important, only deals with a portion of the validity problem.

Other clinicians count the frequency of stuttering events and divide by the total number of words. This method is also highly reliable and elegantly simple, but it too rests on assumptions that are untenable, specifically, that any given stuttering event is equal in its contribution to severity as any other. That is, two stutterers both of whom stutter on 6 percent of their words must, according to this way of measuring severity, be equally severe. Yet in fact, one stutterer could take two or three times as long to say the same number of words. Or, one stutterer could struggle tensely through each episode, displaying highly abnormal behavior, while the other had only brief episodes of stuttering that took up little time and cost little effort. Frequency too is a poor measure. Appealing as they are because of their simplicity, neither method—frequency of stuttering events nor speech rate—satisfies the first criterion, which is that the measurement be valid.

Although there is no empirical evidence to support the idea, it seems intuitively correct to say that the validity of measuring severity is enhanced considerably if the duration of stuttering events is measured, and the amount of time taken up by stuttering behavior is calculated as a percentage of the total talking time. There is, in adopting this measure, a small sacrifice of reliability because the stuttering events are typically brief, and accurate measurement of their durations is not always easy. With practice, however, highly reliable and valid measurements can be made with a stopwatch (Amster and Starkweather, 1986). With more elaborate equipment, the measurement of these durations is even more reliably, validly, and easily done, but few clinicians have such equipment.

When measuring durations, even by stopwatch, a great advance in validity is made. In addition, and perhaps more important than satisfying the validity criterion, it becomes possible to calculate, with little further effort, the extent to which individual stuttering behaviors detract from efficiency of communication. This *differential* measurement is a great help in assigning priorities to individual behaviors as therapy targets. A hypothetical case is shown in Figure 5-2, illustrating this idea.

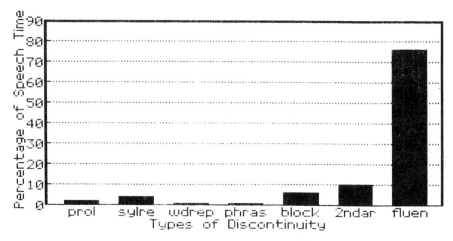

FIGURE 5-2 The distribution of speech time among fluent utterance and different types of discontinuous utterance.

The difficulty with this measure is that it assumes that the duration of a behavior is an accurate reflection of its effort and abnormality. Most of the time this is probably true, but in some stutterers it will not be true. Some stutterers will show behaviors that are relatively brief but still effortful or abnormal. For these stutterers, this method is not as valid as for others.

Another difficulty with this measure is the success with which a stutterer uses inconspicuous avoidance behaviors. If, during an assessment, a stutterer uses an avoidance behavior and the examining clinician sees and records it, then the measurement of severity is accurate, provided the duration of the avoidance behavior is the same as the duration of the behavior it was designed to avoid. But if the avoidance behavior is inconspicuous—a certain posture, a word change—or if it is very brief, such as an eyeblink, the clinician could miss it altogether or record a brief duration, and the validity of the measure would be threatened. The more avoidance a stutterer uses successfully, the less his severity will *appear* to be. Consequently, it would be useful to be able to assess the extent to which a stutterer does and can avoid stuttering, and then to inflate his severity measure by this amount.

Minifie and Cooker (1964) compared a number of different measures of severity and concluded that the one most in agreement with observer judgments was to count all syllables, including repeated ones, and divide by the number of words spoken per minute: $S/(W/M)$, where S = syllables, W = words, and M = time. This measure is somewhat easier to do than measuring the duration of stuttering events and yet it allows for that duration to have an impact, since the longer they are the slower the stutterer's speech rate will be.

This measure would not be accurate however, for a stutterer whose primary behaviors were other than repetitions. Also, it counts all behaviors as equal in severity if they occupy an equal amount of speech time, when in fact some behaviors are highly abnormal in appearance or show evidence of requiring great effort to speak but do not occupy much extra time. For a stutterer showing a pattern of brief effortful behaviors or behaviors that are brief in duration but highly abnormal in appearance, this measure would not provide a valid assessment of severity. Perhaps most important, this measure does not allow for the influence of pauses, which are an important determiner of speech rate, which may vary considerably from individual to individual, and which may or may not be related to stuttering severity.

Van Riper (1984) suggests that the following factors must be taken into account in assessing severity, although he is uncertain about how much weight should be given to each factor: percentage of words stuttered, average tension exhibited on a block, amount of tension exhibited on the block with the most severe tension, average duration of blocks, duration of the longest block, amount of avoidance behavior, and the amount of emotional involvement. These are certainly factors that enter into stuttering severity. The extremity of a stutterer's behaviors should always be noted. A stutterer who stutterers on only 1 percent of his words but stutters very badly on those may have a substantial negative impact on listeners. But, although the extremes should be noted, it is not clear, as Van Riper says, how much weight they should be given in arriving at a final measure of severity. Also, since the extremes of tension are at present quite purely a matter of judgment, the reliability of this aspect of Van Riper's severity equation is quite low.

I believe that the matter of emotional involvement is not an aspect of stuttering severity. Not that stutterers cannot be emotionally involved with their stuttering. They often are and the clinician needs to know about it, but this information does not tell very much about the extent to which communication is impaired. It may tell us the extent to which the client is disturbed, and it is surely important in determining the prognosis for recovery. The stutterer who is more emotionally involved will not respond as well to therapy modifications as the one who is calmer. So emotionality should be assessed but not considered an aspect of severity.

It is time now, having seen the nature of the behavior patterns that comprise stuttering and the elements of its severity, to ask what these facts tell us about the nature of the disorder. Different theorists would of course choose different elements and aspects to emphasize. For me, three findings seem more illuminating than the others. The first finding is the repetitiveness of stuttering. Of the core behaviors, the excessive amount of repetition, the brevity of the repeated element, and the number of times the element is repeated are what most clearly distinguish stuttering from normal nonfluencies. The second finding is the presence of excessive muscle tension in the speech mechanism. The third finding is the important role played by avoidance, certainly in the accessory features, but also perhaps in the core behaviors.

The importance of repetitiveness becomes more evident when we look at the development of stuttering. The repetitions we see in advanced stutterers—young or old—seem to grow out of repeated whole words. The child who is going to become a stutterer typically begins to show signs of unusual behavior between two and three years of age, or just when utterances longer than one word are being produced. The first sign is excessively long (perhaps ten iterations) and frequent whole-word repetitions. There are occasional exceptions to this—children who seem to begin by blocking, or whose pattern follows another course—but typically a great many long whole word repetitions are the first sign that something unusual is going on.

Many of the children who show this first sign recover spontaneously, probably 30 to 50 percent (see pp. 143–147), but those who do not recover spontaneously follow a course of development in which the repeated elements become shorter and shorter. The repeated whole words become repeated parts of words, and the speed of the repetition rate increases. Even though the repeated elements change, repetitiveness continues to be a behavioral feature of the disorder for most children and adults. Some few, as we have already seen, learn patterns of behavior that successfully avoid repetitiveness, but even in these stutterers, it is repetitiveness of speech elements that is being avoided. What is important to understand about repetitiveness is that it is an element of stuttering from the very beginning of the disorder, and it remains an element of the disorder, even if it is avoided or disguised.

At the time excessive whole word repetitions usually appear, children are still learning to combine words, and normal children learn to do this wonderfully well, developing the motoric skill to string together a great many words in the right order. The ability to put words together develops with great speed between the ages of two and four. This linguistic skill would not be possible without the earlier or concurrent development of the motor skill that enables children at this age to string together long sequences of different syllables. Developing children are genetically well equipped to acquire language and equally well equipped to develop the motor skill that the use of language depends on. Not only do children develop the ability to put long strings of words together, they learn to do this with great speed and ease, hardly any thought being devoted to the process. Children learn, in other words, to be fluent.

It should be stated clearly that we do not know why some young children begin at this stage to repeat whole words excessively, typically at the beginnings of sentences. These children, who are the ones at risk for developing stuttering, are not rare—perhaps as many as 30 percent of two-to three-year-olds show excessive repetitions (Yairi, 1983)—but neither can it be said that they are showing normal speech behavior. They are showing a pattern of discontinuity that occurs with some frequency in children of that age. The important point is that many children, indeed most children, do not show this pattern of discontinuity.

Why then do some? We don't know, but it may be that somehow the ability to string words together and to habitualize that process goes awry. The difference is that in the children who are at risk for stuttering the same word is repeated just as automatically and easily as a string of different words. It may be that the same mechanism which fosters the stringing together of different words also facilitates the stringing together of repetitions of the same word. Normally, long strings of the same word would be rejected by the mechanism and separated from the proclivity to string words together. But in stutterers, the editorial mechanism that says in effect: "No, no, the words have to be different words to be strung together automatically," doesn't function properly, and children not only learn to produce long strings of repeated whole words but learn to do so automatically. From this point, the rest of the development of stuttering follows from these children's attempts not to repeat elements of speech; not to do what their mechanism has already developed the ability to do automatically.

For whatever reason some children show the tendency to repeat words excessively, it is clear that repetitiveness is a characteristic of stuttering that is associated with its onset. With development, repetitiveness either declines or remains stable; it does not increase. The other two important aspects of stuttering behavior, tension and avoidance, are just the opposite. They are typically not present, at least they don't seem to be, at the onset of the disorder. And with continued development of stuttering, as we shall soon see, there is a tendency for muscle tension and avoidance to increase. But that is a matter that should be discussed in the next chapter, after the sad story of stuttering development has been told more fully.

REFERENCES

AGNELLO, J., and BUXTON, M., Effects of resonance and time in stutterers' and nonstutterers' speech under delayed auditory feedback. NIMH, HEW Project No. 11067–01, 1966.

ALLEN, G., PETERS, R. W., and WILLIAMS, C. L., Spectrographic study of fluent and stuttered speech. Convention address, American Speech-Language-Hearing Association, 1975.

AMSTER, B., The development of speech rate in normal preschool children. Ph.D. dissertation, Temple University, Philadelphia, 1984.

AMSTER, B., and STARKWEATHER, C., The development of speech rate in normal preschool children. Unpublished manuscript, Temple University, Philadelphia, 1986.

ARMSON, J., Recent research on the motor control of normal movements. Unpublished manuscript, Temple University, Philadelphia, 1986.

BARR, H., A quantitative study of specific phenomena observed in stuttering, *Journal of Speech Disorders,* 5 (1940), 277–80.

BRUTTEN, E. J., and SHOEMAKER, D. J., *The Modification of Stuttering.* Englewood Cliffs, N.J.: Prentice-Hall, 1967.

BLACK, D. C., A study of the consistency of sequences of stuttering behavior. M.A. thesis, University of Pittsburgh, Pittsburgh, 1957.

CURRAN, M. F., and HOOD, S. B., Listener ratings of severity for specific disfluency types in children, *Journal of Fluency Disorders*, 2 (1977), 87–97.

FLETCHER, S., Time-by-count measurement of diadochokinetic syllable rate, *Journal of Speech and Hearing Research*, 15 (1972), 757–62.

FREEMAN, F., and USHIJIMA, T., Laryngeal muscle activity during stuttering, *Journal of Speech and Hearing Research*, 21 (1978), 538–62.

HEGDE, M. N., and HARTMAN, D. E., Factors affecting judgments of fluency: I. Interjections, *Journal of Fluency Disorders*, 4 (1979a), 1–11.

HEGDE, M. N., and HARTMAN, D. E., Factors affecting judgments of fluency: II. Word repetitions, *Journal of Fluency Disorders*, 4 (1979b), 13–22.

McCLAY, H., and OSGOOD, E. I., Hesitation phenomena in spontaneous English speech, *Word*, 15 (1959), 19–44.

MINIFIE, F., and COOKER, H., A disfluency index, *Journal of Speech and Hearing Disorders*, 29 (1964), 189–93.

PROSEK, R., WALDEN, B., MONTGOMERY, A., and SCHWARTZ, D., Some correlates of stuttering severity judgments, *Journal of Fluency Disorders*, 4, 1979, 215–22.

RAWNSLEY, Qa. F., and HARRIS, J. D., Comparative analysis of normal speech and speech with delayed sidetone by means of sound spectrographs, Bureau of Medical Research Project NM003–04.56.03, 1954.

SANDER, E., Frequency of syllable repetition and stutterer judgment. *Journal of Speech and Hearing Disorders*, 28 (1963), 19–30.

SODERBERG, G., What is average stuttering? *Journal of Speech and Hearing Disorders*, 28 (1962), 85–86.

SHAPIRO, A., An electromyographic analysis of the fluent and disfluent utterance of several types of stutterers, *Journal of Fluency Disorders*, 5 (1980), 203–31.

SHEEHAN, J. G., Stuttering behavior: a phonetic analysis, *Journal of Communication Disorders*, 7 (1974), 193–212.

STARKWEATHER, C. W., *Speech and Language: Principles and Processes of Behavior Change*. Englewood Cliffs, N.J.: Prentice-Hall, 1983.

VAN RIPER, C., *The Nature of Stuttering*, 2nd ed. Englewood Cliffs, N.J.: Prentice-Hall, 1984.

WALLE, G., *The Prevention of Stuttering* (film). Memphis, Tenn. Speech Foundation of America, 1975.

WINGATE, M. E., A standard definition of stuttering, *Journal of Speech and Hearing Disorders*, 29 (1964), 484–89.

WOODS, C. L., and WILLIAMS, D. E., Traits attributed to stuttering and normally fluent males, *Journal of Speech and Hearing Research*, 19 (1976), 267–78.

YAIRI, E., The onset of stuttering in two and three year old children: a preliminary report, *Journal of Speech and Hearing Disorders*, 48 (1983), 171–77.

The Onset
and Development
of Stuttering

INTRODUCTION

Information about the onset and development of stuttering has the potential of telling us much about the nature of the disorder. Specifically, one would hope that a clear understanding of how the disorder begins, of the circumstances surrounding its onset, would be useful in understanding its cause. This promise, as we shall see, is only partially fulfilled. But there is more. Stuttering is a disorder which changes, often rapidly, in its early stages. This process, which is the development of stuttering from its beginning to a more advanced state, can teach us about the factors that affect stutterers and shape their behavior into its "final" form. The quotation marks around "final" are to signal that the disorder really never stops developing, although it usually stabilizes for periods of time. In this chapter also, we will learn something of the genetics of stuttering, the familial patterns of the disorder, and information that is essential to an understanding of it. We will also learn something of the learning processes that are involved, or may be involved, and we shall try to understand better how the genetically transmitted component differs from the learned component.

This chapter also presents a tangential discussion of the distribution of stuttering in the general population, the percentages of people who stutter, from which the risk of stuttering can be derived. In addition, there are certain populations in whom the risk of acquiring the disorder is greater than in others, and these facts also shed some light on the nature of the problem. Somewhat less revealing but nonetheless interesting is the fact that certain populations that might be expected to have more stutterers among them than the norm, do not.

ONSET

Findings

1. Most stuttering begins between the onset of speech and puberty—median age of onset is four years (Andrews and Harris, 1964). Figure 6-1 illustrates the range and the average age of onset.
2. The disfluencies of preschool children who stutter are primarily whole-word repetitions and interjections, and these behaviors are also common in the disfluencies of children judged to be "highly disfluent but not stuttering" (Westby, 1979). Although repetition of whole words is most common, part-word repetitions and other signs of more advanced stuttering also occur in the speech of very young (down to age two) children (Yairi, 1981).
3. In children, onset is typically gradual. Often there is nothing unusual in the circumstances at the time of onset: no shock, fright, illness, or injury (Van Riper, 1971). This last idea is of course not a finding, but the absence of one. Yet it has the force of a finding because one would suppose that if there were any systematic pattern of environmental events at the time of stuttering onset, it would show itself in any review of the recollections of parents. There is no systematic pattern, but many parents report that there was a source of emotional tension in the household at or around the time of onset—the death or illness of a family member, marital discord, the absence of the parents, or the child's illness or entry into a new school. Nearly as many, however, report that nothing unusual was happening.

FIGURE 6-1   The onset of stuttering in seven studies.

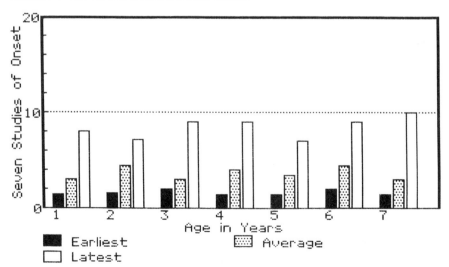

Theory

Parents often ask their speech clinicians a number of questions about the onset of stuttering. Usually parents, from their highly personal motivation, are interested in the same important questions as theorists trying to understand the nature of the disorder. Some of these important questions are: "How does stuttering begin?" "Is there something unusual about the circumstances under which it begins?" Parents want to know if they did anything wrong. "What characteristics does the disorder have at onset?" "Why does one child begin to stutter while another does not?" "Is it genetic or environmental?" These are just a few questions about the onset of stuttering. There are many more, most of them unanswered. We know less about the onset of stuttering than about any other aspect of it. As we shall shortly see, one important question is whether stuttering indeed has an "onset."

In this chapter I will try to provide clinicians with answers for a few of these questions, but be forewarned: the answers do not come easily. First, there is the problem of recovering information from parents. Because onset is gradual in most cases, parental concern is often low at first, and the child's speech behavior has been unusual for a while before the parents overcome their natural tendency to deny the problem and take the child for professional evaluation. Typically there is then another very long delay before the child sees a speech pathologist. This occurs because of what I like to call "the sociology of nonreferral."

Most parents first take their child to a pediatrician, who tells them that the child's stuttering is normal and will be outgrown. It might be noted that the pediatrician has virtually no reason for making this assumption, other than the spontaneous recovery figures, which are questionable, and little information or understanding, certainly less than a speech pathologist (Russell, Mastriano, and Reath, 1978), on which to base it. Pediatricians are actually taught to make this recommendation. Yet, if it were true that all children outgrow it, there would be no stuttering.

The parents, of course, believe the pediatrician and do little about the problem for a considerable period of time, often a year or more, during which the disorder, when it persists, becomes considerably more severe and the prognosis worse (Gottwald and Starkweather, 1985). By the time the speech clinician, who is trained in the close observation of speech and language behavior, sees the child and makes the diagnosis, the child is often struggling hard to talk and is already a confirmed stutterer. By this time also the parents have forgotten a good deal of the information concerned with onset. When one considers that the disorder is easily preventable if treated early (Gottwald and Starkweather, 1984), it seems that much stuttering is caused by the advice given out by misinformed pediatricians.

Another reason it is hard to answer parents' questions about stuttering onset is the difficulty of defining precisely what is meant by the word *stuttering*. Our field has traditionally excluded from the definition of the disorder the pattern of behavior (easy whole-word repetitions) out of which stuttering most typically develops. So deciding when a child began to stutter is a matter of deciding at what point his speech behavior changed enough in a certain direction to fit the definition. It seems that the tail is wagging the dog. We would do better to allow the observed behavior to determine the definition. In this text, the onset of the disorder is described as a sequence of development, which begins with relatively benign behavior and becomes, through its development, a stuttering problem. It seems foolish to think of its onset as the point when it becomes a problem. It's like trying to decide when a puppy becomes a dog. Stuttering can and should be diagnosed when the first signs of unusual fluency behavior appear, however benign they may seem to be in the beginning. A simple criterion for *abnormal* is more than two percent of words that are repeated, wholly or in part, more than twice. That criterion is a little stringent and might catch a few children who are not really going to stutter. Consequently, it is a good idea to add one more criterion—that the child's parents be concerned about his speech. When there is tension in the home, it seems to add to the severity of the problem, making the child's disfluencies larger, more frequent, and more abnormally filled with tension.

For all of these reasons, it is difficult to provide satisfying answers to the questions parents, or theorists for that matter, ask about the onset of stuttering.

DEVELOPMENT

Findings

1. There is a tendency for the amount and frequency of disfluency in normal speakers to decrease with age during the second year of life (Yairi, 1981), and presumably throughout the preschool period. During the school years, there is a continued, but slight, decrease in the frequency of disfluency in normal children when all types of disfluency are considered together (Kowal, O'Connell, and Sabin, 1975).
2. Stuttering changes over time. The pace of this change is highly variable, and the course of development is also variable, but some common characteristics are identifiable as trends of development in young stutterers (Bloodstein, 1960).
3. There is a tendency for the disfluencies of stuttering children to fragment briefer and briefer units of speech (Bloodstein, 1960) and for the rate of repetition to increase (Walle, 1975; Van Riper, 1984).
4. There is a tendency for the amount of tension and forcing to increase (Bloodstein, 1960).
5. Early stuttering is likely to be episodic over time. With development, this changes to fluctuations in severity over time (Bloodstein, 1960).

6. Early stuttering is as likely to occur in one circumstance as in any other, but with continued development it tends to become associated with specific speaking situations (Bloodstein, 1960).
7. There is a tendency for children who stutter to recover spontaneously (Sheehan and Martyn, 1970; Ingham, 1985).
8. Females are more likely to recover than males (Andrews et al., 1983).
9. Stutterers are late in passing speech milestones (Andrews et al., 1983).
10. Parents and other adults are likely to talk more rapidly to stuttering children than to nonstuttering children (Meyers and Freeman, 1985b).
11. Reductions of parental speech rate are significantly correlated with the extent of improvement in children's stuttering during treatment (Starkweather and Gottwald, 1984).
12. Parents and other adults are more likely to interrupt a stuttering than a nonstuttering child during disfluent speech (Meyers and Freeman, 1985a).
13. When stuttering begins in the adult, it usually does so suddenly and is often associated with a traumatic event. It may be preceded by a period of mutism (Freund, 1966).
14. Children may also have traumatic onset, the mute period being reported in some of these cases also (Van Riper, 1971).
15. Adult onset may also follow physiological trauma (head injury) (Peacher and Harris, 1946).
16. A few cases of stuttering following brain injury have been reported in detail. The site of lesion has varied (Van Riper, 1984). Diffuse brain injury has also been reported as a precursor to stuttering behaviors (Helm, Butler, and Benson, 1978).
17. Stuttering has occasionally been reported as a sequel to aphasia (Head, 1926; McKnight, 1963; Eisenson, 1947; Nielson, 1942; Helm, Butler, and Benson, 1978).
18. A few cases have been reported in which remission of stuttering has followed brain surgery performed for other purposes (Guillaume, Mazars and Mazars, 1957; Jones, 1966).

Theory

Bloodstein's landmark study (1960) on the development of stuttering uncovered a number of patterns which are revealing about the nature of the disorder. The commonest course of development is as follows: the first behavior noticed as abnormal is excessive repetitions of whole words or brief phrases at the initiation of clauses. "Excessive" means two things: (1) the word or phrase is repeated more times than is considered normal—not just "Mommy, Mommy, can I go out?" but "Mommy, Mommy, Mommy, Mommy, Mommy, Mommy, Mommy, can I go out?"; and (2) the repetitions occur on too many words, not just 1 or 2 percent of words spoken, but as many as 10 percent or more. It should be noted that these whole-word and phrase repetitions, although frequent and long, are produced without muscular tension, and there is typically no sign that the child is trying to terminate them, indeed, from the parents' perspective, such children seem unaware that their speech behavior is unusual.

This pattern may last for a very brief or a very long time. In a large number of children—probably half (Ingham, 1985), but perhaps as many as 80 percent (Sheehan and Martyn, 1970) of those whose parents noticed excessive repetitions—the repetitive behavior will spontaneously stop after a week or two. It may then start up again at a later time or not. It may come and go several times before finally disappearing.

Although the percentage of spontaneous recovery is reasonably high, it is not high enough to recommend that early stuttering is something parents should ignore. At least 20 percent, and perhaps as many as 50 percent of children whose parents notice excessively repetitive speech behavior will go on to become fully developed, chronic stutterers. Some of these will also recover, but not without the memory of a childhood largely spent forestalling and avoiding ridicule, shame, and guilt. And a few unfortunate souls will go on to be chronic adult stutterers, with a self-image stamped "Caution. Stutterer inside. Speak with caution."

It is uncertain why early infantile stuttering sometimes changes in such a sinister direction. Nor is it known why in other cases there is a spontaneous recovery. But there is a model of stuttering development that seems descriptive of events. In this model, the capacities for fluent speech—the motoric, cognitive, and linquistic skills that make easy speech possible for most children—interact with demands for fluency placed on the child by the external communicative environment and by the child himself. As the capacity for fluency grows, the expectations of parents and of the child as well also increase. Very young children are expected to be hesitant and stumbling in speech. Older children are expected to produce more words more quickly and more easily. In this way, capacities and demands for fluency are simultaneously increasing. If the environment demands more fluency than the child can produce, stuttering will begin. Whether the stuttering will continue or remediate depends on whether a growing capacity to produce fluent speech can catch up with the world's accelerating demands.

The "Demands and Capacities Model" of stuttering development (see pp. 75–78 or Gottwald and Starkweather, 1984) is simply a descriptive model, a way of saying that there are some children who recover spontaneously, some who become confirmed stutterers but later are able to develop new fluency habits, and still others who never recover. The model also suggests that there are both inherent and environmental factors at work and that both sets of factors change over time with development. The point of the model is to show some of the relations between different sets of factors. It is desirable to do this so that researchers interested in one factor or another may eventually be able to establish what effect a change in that factor will have on the probability that a child will or will not outgrow stuttering. Importantly, the model does not assume that the variables determining whether a child will become a stutterer are necessarily the same as those contributing to the development of stuttering.

Another idea properly belongs to the model of stuttering development. It has already been said that the environment makes demands on children and that those demands change as a function of children's development. But this environment is composed of the behavior of people, and people respond most to the behavior of other people. Consequently, an important reason for changes in the communicative environment surrounding disfluent children is their behavior. This idea, that the disfluency itself causes certain patterns of behavioral change in the speech of those who talk to such children, can be attributed to research by Meyers and Freeman (1985a; 1985b). These studies have shown that adults tend to talk more rapidly when talking to children who stutter and to interrupt them more often, the interruption occurring during the child's discontinuities. In another study, Starkweather and Gottwald (1984) found it possible to predict the extent of a child's recovery in a prevention program from the extent of reduction in the parents' speech rate. A lesser but still significant predictor was the child's own rate of speaking.

These studies suggest that whether the pattern of excessively repetitive but easy speech will change deleteriously or not and whether the change will be rapid or slow, depends at least in part on the communicative environment. If the environment is one of time pressure, such as would come from rapidly paced turn-taking, rapid parental speech rate, or a rushed household, the relaxed whole-word or phrase repetitions may be shortened so that only a portion of each word is repeated—"Mommy, Mommy, Mommy," becomes "Mo-Mo-Mommy." Perhaps the stuttering child begins to sense that repeated elements take up time without contributing information, and tries to shorten the duration of the repeated element by cutting it off. See pp. 147–148 for some information that supports this idea.

If the communicative environment is demanding of children's abilities to formulate language (Wall and Myers, 1984; Starkweather and Gordon, 1983), such as might occur if the parents use adult vocabulary or syntax, or if children are simply unusually bright and advanced linguistically, such children may find that the simultaneous demands of language formulation and motor planning for the execution of coordinated speech are too much for the capacity of their young central nervous systems, so that hesitant and discontinuous speech occurs more often. Under these circumstances, the discontinuities would be likely to occur at points in the utterance when language formulation or word-finding is taking place—at clause boundaries and before lexical items of infrequent usage.

If the communicative environment is demanding of cognitive behavior in connection with speech, as might happen if there is frequent questioning by significant others, or demands for speech performance, children's speech may be more hesitant or discontinuous. In this case, the discontinuities would probably occur primarily under those speech circumstances that are pragmatically similar to demand speech situations, that is, such children will be likely to exhibit discontinuities when the demanding circumstances are present.

Finally, if the communicative environment includes negative reactions to disfluency, then children may try very hard not to stutter, and these attempts not to stutter may include using extra force of airflow, increased rate of speech during stuttering "to get past it," more muscular force in articulatory or glottal movements, or simply avoidance of the words and situations in which word repetition is anticipated. In this case the muscular tension, struggle, and avoidance would occur more often in the presence of those individuals who demonstrate the negative reactions. Soon, however, the negative evaluations that are present in the external environment become internalized, and the children react to discontinuities with the same attitudes they have seen demonstrated by significant others.

Under any combination of these circumstances, the period of relaxed whole word repetitions may last only for a very brief time. If, on the other hand, the communicative environment is less demanding of fluency, the period of relaxed whole-word repetitions may be extended for a year or more. And during this extended period of time, some children may develop their capacity for speech coordination enough so that the excessively repeated whole words drop out of the picture.

Two other characteristics of stuttering should be mentioned—the change from episodic to chronic stuttering, and the tendency for stuttering to become specific to certain situations. Early stuttering comes and goes. Periods of disfluency are followed by periods of fluency. In some children the periods of fluency tend to lengthen and the disfluent periods shorten and finally disappear. In others, the reverse occurs and stuttering persists. Usually, however, there is not enough time and insufficiently documented observations to reach a prognostic conclusion on the basis of changing episodes. Nevertheless, when parents report long periods of fluent speech interrupted by brief periods of stuttering, the clinician should feel comfortable about telling the parents that such a report is a good sign that the disorder is in a relatively early stage.

The second characteristic is also a sign of the extent to which stuttering has developed. If the parents report that a child only stutters when talking to certain people, or only in certain situations, it suggests a more advanced stage of development than if the child is as likely to stutter when talking to anyone or in any situation. It is important to distinguish "situation" and "listener" from periods of tension or excitement. All children speak more disfluently during periods of tension—when moving or changing schools, when their parents divorce, or after the death of a family member. And all children speak more disfluently during periods of excitement. When parents come home from work and the house is suddenly full of energy, at a birthday party, around holidays, or when rough-housing—these are all times of excitement. Speaking under conditions of excitement is probably the most potent evoker of disfluent speech, even more than periods of stress. It is often helpful to counsel parents to keep the excitement level down. If all behaviors are being performed with extra energy, speech will also be produced with extra energy and effort, and disfluent speech may result. But these ad hoc periods—excitement and tension—are not the same as the episodes of disfluency, which are weekly or fortnightly periods during which children stutter in many circumstances as compared with a similarly long period when there is no stuttering at all.

PATTERNS OF DEVELOPMENT

Let us now examine more closely the typical changes that occur when stuttering develops. Bear in mind that this is only the most typical picture. There is substantial variation from child to child. Bear in mind also that these developmental changes occur in very young children, typically younger than four and many of them only two or three years of age. Typically, when it is first noticed that the child's fluency is abnormal, the presenting behavior is excessive amounts of whole-word repetitions. The first change from this behavior is a truncation of the repeated element from whole words to parts of words. The child stops saying "But, but, but, but, but I don't want to," and begins to say "Buh, buh, buh, buh, buh, but I don't want to." The repeated element may be shortened further to "b-b-b-b-but" as the schwa is substituted for the vowel in the word during the repetition. Note that the final complete word, when produced fluently, contains the correct vowel. An attempt to shorten the repeated element even further may be responsible for the insertion of the glottal stop /ʔ/ after each schwa during the repetition in some children.

It is evident that one characteristic of the typical course of development is a progressive truncation of the repeated elements (Bloodstein, 1960). What is of course less clear is what motivates this change. A reasonable speculation is that such children are trying to hurry through the stuttering, which is after all not helping to achieve their communicative intention. The speculation seems warranted for several reasons: (1) adult stutterers often report desiring to keep the stuttering episode as brief as possible; (2) there is evidence that stuttering children are likely to be under time pressure because adults are likely to talk faster to stuttering than to nonstuttering children (Meyers and Freeman, 1985b); (3) reductions in parental rate of speaking and other sources of time pressure are often followed by reductions in children's disfluency (Starkweather and Gottwald, 1984); and (4) adult stutterers are more fluent when they speak more slowly (Adams, Lewis, and Besozzi, 1973). Under time pressure to communicate, speech that wastes time will naturally be avoided if possible.

The next change in the most typical course of development is the use of one or more behaviors that indicate there is tension in the larynx. Three behaviors are common—prolonged vowels with pitch rise, broken words, and increased loudness. The first of these—prolonged vowels with pitch rise—have been described as siren-like. The child tries to say "May I have some?" and the vowel in "may" is prolonged—"Maaaaaaaaay I. . . . " and as the vowel is sounded, the pitch of the voice rises slowly and steadily from three to five tones. The rise continues as long as the vowel is prolonged so that an extensive pitch change will occur if the child has a very long vowel prolongation.

Another symptom of increased tension in the larynx is increased vocal loudness. This can be associated with prolonged vowels in just the same way as pitch rise is, that is, the voice becomes increasingly loud as the vowel is prolonged, but in some cases I have seen, a louder than normal voice was used on whole sentences or in whole situations where stuttering occurred. It looked, in these cases, as if the children had acquired a habit of increasing airflow—pushing harder and talking louder—thus raising the loudness of the voice in circumstances where stuttering was likely. It should be noted that these descriptions are taken from the records of very young (2:5–4:1) children.

Increased vocal tension also shows itself as broken words—"My na-ame is Chu-uck"—in which the vowel is begun, then cut off abruptly by a tight closure of the glottis, then reinitiated. The tension of the tightly shut glottis is evident both from the abrupt termination of the voice and from the quality of the subsequent reinitiation of the vowel.

It is quite common for laryngeal tension to accompany truncated and speeded up repetition. When this happens, there will be either a repetition with pitch rise—/mamamamamamamamami/—or a repetition in which each repeated element is terminated by a glottal stop—/maʔmaʔmaʔmaʔmaʔ mami/. Chronic hoarse, harsh, or breathy voices are common, and vocal nodules occur from time to time. Some children begin to prolong conso-nants as well as vowels at this time, saying words like "Sssssee my bear?" It has been suggested (Conture, 1984) that these prolongations may occur as the child tries to stabilize an oscillating speech mechanism; that is, the example above would have been preceded developmentally by sentences like "Suh, suh, see my bear?" Another possibility is that consonantal prolongations represent a continued attempt to shorten the stuttering episode even fur-ther by dropping the vowel out altogether.

After this appear forcing and struggle—trying to get the word out by using the abdominal muscles to apply force against the air in the lungs, or by squeezing at the glottis, or by the application of extra force at any of the points of oral articulation. Abdominal pressure is usually accompanied by laryngeal squeezing (otherwise there would be an expulsion of air). This combination—a tightly valved larynx and increased abdominal pressure—represents the Valsalva maneuver, which is a reflexive behavior engaged during defecation, childbirth, and the lifting of heavy weights. Some stutterers have reported a simultaneous tightening of the rectal muscles, which is also part of the full reflex (Parry, 1984).

Blocks, both laryngeal and oral, in which the child's speech production comes to a complete halt, and the vocal tract is immobilized and closed at the larynx or one of the points of oral articulation, also occur at this time. These blocks are also a truncation of the stuttered element, but they are tense.

When forcing and struggle are located at one of the points of articulation they may also be or may become accompanied by facial contortions and other more external signs of the struggle within. Just as tension in the intrinsic laryngeal muscles is usually accompanied by visible tension of the strap muscles of the neck, so too the relatively invisible tension of the tongue-tip and tongueback or the more obvious bilabial tension may be accompanied by larger external tensions of the face. Bilabial forcing is likely to be accompanied by tension of the mentalis, orbicularis oris, and quadratus labii inferior and superior. Excessive muscular tension during tongue elevation is likely to be accompanied by extra muscle activity in the masseter and the pterygoids. These facial and neck tensions, in advanced stutterers, can be widespread tremors and shaking of the affected parts. Sometimes the tension seems to radiate from the lips or jaw to more distal parts of the face and neck.

At this stage of development, the stutterer is of course often just stuck, unable to speak, and some tricks for getting started may be learned—timers such as slapping the table, nodding, blinking, or stamping. Very young stutterers may use very peculiar starters, reflecting their immature knowledge and awareness of the speaking process. For example, one two-and-a-half-year-old girl would press the palm of her hand against her cheek and slide it forward in an attempt to squeeze the word out of her mouth as if it were toothpaste that wouldn't come out of the tube. The older stuttering children (five to six years of age) learn to use the same starters that nonstutterers use—"well," "let me see," "I mean," and the ubiquitous "um." In the stutterer, however, these words are likely to be spoken with more tension, and they may change in form through habitual use. As an example of the latter phenomenon, an adult stutterer I knew had learned to use "uh" as a starter. He used it whenever he felt he was getting stuck on a word. Since he had the most difficulty with plosive sounds, he produced many sentences like "C- uh, -an I t-uh -alk to you?" In time, however, the intruded "uh" changed its shape to resemble a slightly prolonged /l/, so that the same sentence sounded like "Clllan I tlllalk to you?" Intelligibility, not usually a problem in stuttering, was affected. Another stutterer got into the habit of using "for example," as a starter. By the time he was an adult, he preceded any word on which he expected to stutter with a prolonged /ffff/.

Children who stutter are not likely to use a sophisticated phrase, such as "for example," as a starter. Instead their starters usually involve physical effort—stamping, and just pushing with abdominal force are probably the most common. Although their tricks and starters reflect an unsophisticated knowledge of speech and language, they are, when they perform behaviors like these, as advanced in their stuttering development as the adult who bounces his head three times to initiate a hard word.

Finally, the more elaborate secondary features develop, those designed to avoid stuttering, such as changing words, hiding stuttering by pretending a hesitation or repetition was something else, postponing the attempt on the word, diverting attention from disfluency, or avoiding talking altogether. In the beginning, these tricks are usually effective. The timers and the starters (see pp. 123–127 for a more detailed description) help the stutterer get started; the avoidance devices are successful in avoiding or escaping from more primary stuttering behaviors; the postponers postpone. But after repeated use two things happen. The behaviors gradually lose their effectiveness, and they change in form. Both changes are insidious.

Many stutterers are advised to take a deep breath before they try to talk. At first, this advice pays off. The stutterers stop, take a deep breath, and then try the word again and find it easier to say. They then begin to take a deep breath every time they begin to stutter or think they will stutter. They have found the answer. But soon the behavior becomes habitual and automatic. Without even thinking, the deep breath is taken at the first thought that the following word is going to be hard to say fluently. And as the behavior becomes automatized, its effectiveness begins to diminish. The deep breath is taken and the word is stuttered anyway. Naturally, the stutterer tries again, usually with an even deeper breath. This somewhat new behavior may work and continue for a while, but then it too loses its effectiveness. And soon an even deeper breath, and so on. In time, the shoulders may be elevated, the head thrown back, and the arms moved outward away from the rib cage to allow for a fuller expansion. When this too is habituated, it loses its effectiveness, and the stutterer is left with a bizarre, almost seizure-like behavior with which speech is occasionally initiated.

This pattern, in which behaviors start out being effective as avoiders, starters, and so on, gradually lose their effectiveness as they become habituated, and then grow into bizarre behaviors with no evident purpose, is common for many different kinds of stuttering behaviors. It is the last, most disruptive, course of development. It leads to behavior patterns that are so strange, so apparently purposeless, that stutterers who reach this stage may be mistaken for epileptics. In several cases, stutterers in this stage were stopped by the police for routine checks and later attacked and injured by the police, who misinterpreted their violent, jerky movements as aggressive acts.

Although patterns of development are highly individual, three elements seem to be present in most if not all cases, excluding those that involve head injury or emotional trauma. First, the discontinuous behavior—the pauses, repetitions, prolongations, and broken words that take up time but do not convey information—become truncated. This change seems most attributable to time pressure, either from an environment that is demanding of time or from the child's own sense that there is only so much time in which to talk. The second element that is almost always present as stuttering develops is an increase in the amount of effort—muscular tension in the vocal tract—that is used to talk. The third element is the increased use of behaviors designed to avoid or hide stuttering.

Like the truncated discontinuities, the increase in muscle tension that occurs as stuttering develops is probably attributable to stutterers' reactions to their difficulty in talking. The extra time taken up by excessive repetition, the reactions of significant others to excessive repetition, and a number of other things that seem to contribute to stuttering's growth and development are factors which would be likely to cause stutterers' to inject greater force and effort into their speech attempts. Their attempts to make the mechanism move faster to overcome the time taken up by noninformational repetitiveness, their struggle to inhibit the repetitiveness, to stop its onward rush, to hide it from others, to avoid its occurring in the first place, are all efforts that would be likely to introduce muscle tension into the speech mechanism. There are, perhaps, other explanations of increased muscle tension, but it seems simplest to ascribe this aspect of the disorder to the stutterers' reactions to their own speech and their efforts to normalize their speech behavior.

Avoidance is also important in the development of the disorder. Many of those who repeat whole words excessively manage to grow into normal speakers. Those who do not are the ones who react to the repetitiveness in their speech with struggle, forcing, tension, and avoidance—responses that are all motivated by a too intense aversion to disfluency, to repetitiveness, or to dead air. Not only do they react in this avoidant way, they incorporate this reaction into their habitual talking pattern. Some do this very quickly and become tense, struggling speakers within a few weeks or even days. Others go on producing whole words repetitively for quite a long time with no apparent reaction of avoidance and struggle. But those who will end up with fully developed stuttering are in most cases motivated, I believe, by an intense aversion to the repetitiveness in their speech. Where does this intense aversion come from?

A common pattern of parental reactions to disfluency is for the parents to show visible signs of discomfort when their child is stuttering. They are made uncomfortable by the stuttering because clearly something is wrong with their child. The pain parents feel with this knowledge is acute. Each time the child stutters this pain returns, and each parent reacts to it in a different way. Many avert their gaze. They just can't look at the child while the stuttering is occurring. Others turn completely away. One mother said, "I try to find something to do in the refrigerator." Perhaps most parents simply stiffen and wait out the momentary blockage. Many hold their breaths. When the child finally gets the word out, they relax noticeably, start breathing again, and sit back in their chairs a little bit, or resume the normal body movements that listeners typically perform when someone is talking to them. And this is the point.

Communicative behavior is dyadic. The speaker and the listener are simultaneously engaged. While the speaker talks, the listener moves to the cadence of the speaker's speech rhythm; nods, movements of arms and legs, indeed the whole body sends a continuous signal that information is being received. This communicative dance is a little different when the listener is a parent and the speaker is a child, but it still occurs. When the speaker breaks the usual rhythm of utterance by repeating words or phrases or by stuttering with struggle and tension, the listener's rhythm changes too. Information is not being received, and the sounds that are being produced do not have the cadence of continuous speech. So the listener's nonverbal behavior changes too, and it changes in ways that reflect the discomfort stuttering produces. This discomfort is present in anyone who listens to stuttering, but the level of discomfort is highest in parents. Stuttering children immediately see the effect that their stuttering behavior has on their parents. They see their parents' reactions. The parents are uncomfortable; they are hurt; they are afraid. The children naturally take on these same attitudes.

The process is not much different from the way children acquire an attitude toward anything. If a child's parents are afraid of dogs and cower when dogs appear or avoid situations in which there are likely to be dogs, the child will quickly learn to do the same thing. Parents who show their enthusiasm for music or art are likely to have children who share their enthusiasms. So it is not surprising that children who stutter acquire attitudes toward their stuttering that are the same as the attitudes their parents display in their nonverbal reactions each time the child stutters.

The course of development just described begins with repeated whole words and phrases that are at first produced without a struggle. There is another, less common, course of development that begins with a sudden and dramatic change in speaking behavior—these individuals were previously fluent—and seems more likely to be associated with emotional trauma or disturbing events, often associated in some way with talking. For example, in one case a five-year-old girl was left with an unfamiliar babysitter while the parents went away for a week's vacation. It was the child's first separation from her parents. The babysitter was a middle-aged woman whom the mother described as a "nonstop talker." During the vacation the parents called several times, and both the babysitter and the daughter reported that everything was all right, although the little girl seemed sad. When the parents returned, the daughter tried to greet them and blocked laryngeally in attempting to talk during a moment of intense emotion. She continued to block when initiating utterances for several months. The mother, a speech pathologist, devised a therapy plan based on singing, and the blocking gradually disappeared.

In another case, one of five-year-old twin brothers was hospitalized with a serious respiratory illness, while the other twin stayed home. During the separation, both twins began to block laryngeally. The behaviors proliferated into full-blown stuttering over the next few months, and persisted until the twins were eighteen years old, at which time the twin who was hospitalized recovered. The other twin continued to stutter into adult life.

It often seems that when stuttering begins in clear association with emotional trauma the traumatic event has some connection with speaking. In the case of the twins just described, the hospitalized twin had a respiratory illness which may have made it difficult for him to speak. In the previous case, the babysitter had a peculiar talking pattern.

A third case illustrates a more obvious connection between the emotional trauma and the stuttering behaviors that developed. A seven-year-old French boy and his mother were driving in Paris when they had an accident. The boy was not injured, but the mother's larynx was damaged as she was thrown against the steering wheel. She was treated surgically, but failed to regain full use of her larynx. As a result, her voice was rough and hoarse, and she developed a habit of speaking on inhalation, which she did with the same poor vocal quality her exhaled voice had. The boy visited his mother in the hospital as she recovered from surgery and when she first begin to speak in her new and very different voice, the boy began to stutter. What was most compelling about the boy's stuttering pattern was that it involved the frequent use of speaking on inhalation as a trick to avoid stuttering on words that he expected to be difficult.

Although the cases described above are cases of emotional trauma, stuttering can also begin with head injury or stroke. In these cases too, the symptoms appear in their final form almost at once. There is little if any development. Often too, in cases of cerebral trauma, there is a period of mutism after the trauma, Then, when the person first tries to speak, the stuttering behaviors are fully developed.

It should be noted that stuttering of nontraumatic origin is almost exclusively a disorder of childhood. We ought perhaps to call it "developmental" stuttering. Stuttering of traumatic origin seems to occur with equal frequency in adults and in children. One fact seems curious. Stuttering that begins with emotional trauma is nearly identical in its characteristics to stuttering that begins with head injury. One simple explanation is that it is the emotional shock of having a head injury that produces the stuttering, but several studies have associated specific types of cerebral lesions, specifically diffuse injury throughout the brain, as predictive of stuttering behavior, and this suggests that it is indeed the injury to the brain that causes the symptoms, not an emotional shock.

On the other hand, it isn't really clear how a severe emotional shock can affect the brain. There may be longlasting changes in brain physiology following such events. The picture is also obscured by the fact that at this time we lack a comprehensive analysis of the fluency behavior of the brain injured. It might be that the disfluency behaviors of the brain injured are only superficially like the behaviors of individuals whose stuttering developed without trauma. It is perhaps the most conservative route at present to consider developmental (garden variety) stuttering as a different kind of disorder than stuttering that begins with cortical injury or emotional trauma.

However, the fact that there is such a thing as a stuttering or stuttering-like behavior pattern that develops following injury to the brain or severe emotional shock has theoretical importance. It lays open the possibility that the more common type of stuttering is also caused by some difference in the structure or organization of the brains of stutterers. Doubtless this brain aberration, if it exists, would be of lesser magnitude, an aberration which, except for the stuttering pattern it produces, would be within normal limits. It is possible that young children begin to stutter because of some difference in their brains, although there is not much suggestion as to what this difference might be.

INCIDENCE AND PREVALENCE

Findings

1. Estimates on the percentage of the general population that stutter vary but seem to center around 0.7 to 1.0 percent (Milisen, 1957).
2. The risk of ever stuttering is estimated variably: mean = 4.2 percent, median = 4.9 percent (Andrews et al., 1983).
3. Stuttering has been observed in all societies in which it has been investigated (Van Riper, 1984; Frank, 1970). Cross-cultural comparisons have not been made with scientific rigor.
4. Stuttering is more common among children less than twelve years of age (1.0 percent) than among adults (0.8 percent) (Andrews and Harris, 1964). There may be a kind of critical period for stuttering acquisition, corresponding to the later stages of the language acquisition

period (five to seven years), when speech and language production are becoming habituated and automatized (Andrews and Harris, 1964).

5. Stuttering is more common among males than among females (Hull and Timmons, 1969, and many others). Ratios vary from 3.1:1 to 10:1.

6. During the second year of life, females are as disfluent as males. (Yairi, 1981), but clinical populations of the same age contain more males than females (Gottwald and Starkweather, 1984).

7. Stuttering is three times more common in the families of stutterers than in the families of nonstutterers (Wepman, 1939; West, Nelson, and Berry, 1939; Johnson, 1961; Records, Kidd, and Kidd, 1976).

8. A high prevalence of stuttering has been theorized to be associated with diglossia (Ralston, 1976).

9. There may be a slightly higher prevalence among lower socioeconomic groups than among higher ones (Morgenstern, 1956).

10. Stuttering occurs only rarely among the deaf (Backus, 1938; Harms and Malone, 1939).

11. Stuttering may be more prevalent among the retarded, in particular among children with Down's syndrome (Gens, 1951; Gottseleben, 1955; Schlanger and Gottsleben, 1957; Edson, 1964).

Theory

The first three findings demonstrate that stuttering is widespread. In addition to having been found in all societies, even primitive ones, it should be noted that there are references to stuttering in ancient literature as well (Van Riper, 1984), which at least indicates that the disorder has been a problem for our highly communicative species for a very long time. It is not a modern phenomenon.

It might also be noted that nothing that even resembles stuttering has been found in the communicative behaviors of other species, but of course, ours is the only species that uses language and speech to communicate with. Still, if stuttering were a simple mechanical problem, one might expect to find it in the complex sequences of birdsong or whale songs. Interestingly, one of the early attempts to teach a chimpanzee human language was the Kelloggs' raising of Vicki as if she were a human baby. Vicki learned to say two or three words—*papa* and *cup* were demonstrated—but she produced these words with great difficulty and strain, and many a speech clinician has thought, on seeing the film of the Kelloggs' work, that Vicki's speech resembled that of a human stutterer.

There was a great deal of interest in the 1930s and 1940s in the prevalence of stuttering among primitive societies. Wendell Johnson, from his semantogenic point of view, believed that the presence of stuttering in a society should depend on the language the society had available to them for describing it. This idea led to a number of investigations of native American tribes, and in one at least, the Bannock-Shoshone then located in Idaho, no stuttering was observed. The investigator in that instance made one of the classic errors of research and concluded that the absence of information was significant, and that the "Indians had no word for it." A later investigation by Frank (1970), however, showed that the tribe had hidden their stutterers from the investigator so as not to be blamed for the problem.

Although it appears that stuttering is present in all societies, its prevalence in different societies varies to a certain extent. Ralston (1976), in her investigations of the people of Nevis in the British West Indies, found stuttering in about 5 percent of the population, which is remarkably higher than usual. She believed that the reason for this high percentage was the fact that the language of Nevis was divided into two distinct social dialects, a high form used for school and business, and a familiar form used for friendly and familiar interactions. This pattern, which is common in many societies, is called *diglossia*. Her theory was that the additional stress of having to decide which form to use, particularly in ambiguous social situations, increased the likelihood of stuttering.

Although the theory is interesting, there are two alternative explanations that make it difficult for us to accept the linguistic one without question. As is always the case in comparisons of one culture with another, there are nonlinguistic cultural differences as well. There are, for example, dietary differences. We don't have any reason to believe that stuttering is caused by a dietary deficiency, but neither can we rule out the possibility that the high percentage of stuttering in Nevis is caused by some unknown variation in the local diet. An even more likely alternative explanation is based on genetics. As a subsequent section of this chapter shows, there is a known genetic component to stuttering. Nevis, or any culture for that matter, is genetically as well as culturally distinct from other societies. That is, on the whole, Nevisians tend to marry other Nevisians so that the flow of genetic material into and out of the society is relatively small. As a result, there is a distinct gene pool that is as characteristic of the society as its culture. Indeed, this restricted gene pool may influence the culture in many ways. So it may be that stuttering occurs more often in Nevis simply because genes bearing the factor that predisposes individuals to stuttering also occur more often among Nevisians. And of course the same may be said of any society where the percentage of stutterers is higher, or lower, than in other societies.

This kind of argument can also be made for the fact that stuttering is more prevalent among lower socioeconomic groups (Morgenstern, 1956). There is a tendency for individuals of similar socioeconomic status to marry, and so here too there may be a restricted gene pool. There are also dietary differences, and indeed there may be significant cultural differences that accompany lower educational levels and lower income levels. The explanation that comes most quickly to mind, however, is the additional stress of daily living that poverty creates, and it is indeed a possibility that the presence of stress in family life predisposes the children of lower socio-economic groups toward stuttering.

Three groups show an unusually high proportion of stuttering—males, the families of stutterers, and children. The high incidence of stuttering in the families of stutterers reflects the genetic component of the disorder, at least partly, and is discussed in a subsequent section of this chapter.

More interesting from a theoretical point of view is the finding that stuttering is more common in children. Of course, this finding results from the observations, already described, that (1) stuttering typically begins in childhood and (2) that a high proportion of children recover from the disorder. However, a close look at the data presented by Andrews and Harris (1964) reveals the possibility of a kind of critical period for stuttering. In this landmark study, 1,000 children were followed for an extended period of time. The onset and course of many health problems, among them stuttering, were observed and recorded. Most of the children began to stutter when they were quite young, before they entered school. A few began to stutter when they were older. Of those who began to stutter during the preschool period, a good many recovered before they reached the age of six and one-half. Similarly, stuttering that began later, after the age of seven, was also typically brief in its duration. The children who became chronic stutterers, however, were all stuttering between the ages of five and one-half and six and one-half. In other words, a child who begins stuttering during the preschool period has a reasonable chance, about 50 percent, of recovering soon. The same is true of a child who begins stuttering later, after age seven. But if a child begins stuttering at a young age, and the problem persists into the five and one-half to six and one-half year range, there is a good chance that it will become a chronic disorder. It looks as though there is a critical period, somewhere between age five and age seven, during which the patterns of speech become automated or habituated so firmly that it is difficult later to change them. And if stuttering is present during this period of time, it too will be difficult to change later on.

The finding that stuttering is much more prevalent among males than among females is also of great theoretical interest, but it has proven to be difficult to explain. Of course, the genetic studies (see pp. 160–162) have made it evident that the genetic component of the disorder is sex-linked, and it seems possible, on this basis, that the sex ratio is at least partially determined by genetic factors.

The observation made by Yairi (1981) that there were just as many females as male stutterers among children in the third year of life suggested to a number of theorists that the sex ratio is a result of differential recovery rates among boys and girls. Girls, perhaps because their language skills develop at an earlier age, are more likely to recover. Also, as will be seen in the subsequent section, there is a genetic component to the recovery from stuttering, and this fact lends weight to the argument that the sex ratio is a matter of differential recovery. In the Stuttering Prevention Clinic at Temple University, we have observed at this writing forty families of pre-school-age stutterers. Most of the children were boys. But this is not a random sample of stuttering children. The parents who seek clinical help are those whose children are in the most trouble, either because their stuttering is worse or because it has already persisted long enough to worry the parents, so our observations should not be given much weight.

Other explanations of the sex ratio have been offered. Many of the earlier theorists, who looked at stuttering as a problem resulting from emotional stress, felt that boys were subjected to greater pressure for excellence of performance or were stressed in other ways. This seems to be a weak argument. There are certainly many societies where there is only a small difference in parents' expectations of performance, and it seems that there is not as much of this difference in the United States as formerly. Girls too are under great pressure to perform well in a number of different ways.

A few theorists have suggested that the different patterns of maturation in boys and girls may be responsible for the sex ratio. Others have noted that there are differences between the sexes in cerebral lateralization, specifically with regard to the development of brain organization, and that this might be at the heart of the sex ratio. A few have noted the connection of cerebral lateralization to language development and related this either to the incidence of stuttering or to the likelihood of recovery from stuttering.

There are still many explanations of the sex ratio, and it remains one of the more intriguing findings about stuttering. It is a finding that a solid theory of stuttering will have to account for. None yet has offered a completely convincing explanation of the sex ratio. Even the genetic explanations, which come closest to explaining it, have not provided information specifically related to sex in a way that predicts the ratio. The very low incidence of stuttering among the deaf is discussed elsewhere in this text (see pp. 244–245).

The higher incidence of stuttering among the retarded, particularly among Down's syndrome children, presents, as many findings do, a variety of explanations. First, the finding that it is Down's syndrome children in particular who are likely to be stutterers may confirm the genetic factor, because Down's syndrome is a genetically determined condition. Stuttering, however, is not a necessary part of the syndrome. Other explanations for the higher prevalence of stuttering among the retarded range from the additional stress experienced by this population to the greater likelihood of brain injury. But a stronger argument, in my opinion, is that the retarded are slower in developing speech and language. As a result of this delay in development, the critical period (see p. 157) during which their speech patterns are being habituated occurs later and may be extended. Because it occurs later, there is more opportunity for stuttering to have begun, and consequently a greater possibility that it will be present during the critical period of habituation. In addition, the slower development of the retarded may also extend the critical period itself, which will also increase the probability that a child will be stuttering when this critical period comes to a close. Information that would confirm this notion would come from a study on the recovery rates of retarded stutterers, but this study has yet to be done.

GENETIC STUDIES AND LEARNING THEORY

Findings

1. Stuttering is found 90 percent of the time in both twins of monozygotic twin pairs but only 25 percent of the time in both twins of dizygotic twin pairs (Nelson, Hunter, and Walter, 1945; Howie, 1981). The risk to a monozygotic co-twin is 77 percent.

2. There is a predisposition to acquire stuttering which is genetically transmitted (Records, Kidd, and Kidd, 1976). Among relatives of stutterers, the incidence of stuttering is 14 percent (Kidd et al., 1981). The risk to relatives varies by sex of relative and sex of proband (Andrews et al., 1983). Severity (frequency of stuttering) is not related to familial patterns (Kidd et al., 1980).

3. Among the adult relatives of stuttering females, 18 percent stutter; among the adult relatives of stuttering males, 13 percent stutter (Kidd et al., 1980). Of these relatives 51 percent recover spontaneously, 66 percent of females and 46 percent of males. The difference is primarily attributable to relatives who are the same sex as the stutterer, brothers of male stutterers being three times as likely to persist as recover, while sisters of female stutterers are twice as likely to persist as recover (Seider, Gladstein, and Kidd, 1983). Furthermore, 48 percent of right-handed males among stuttering relatives of stutterers recover spontaneously, while only 35 percent of left-handed relatives recover. This is not a significant difference. But when left-handed and right-handed stuttering female relatives of stutterers are compared, the right-handed stutterers recover 69 percent of the time, while the left-handed ones recover only 20 percent of the time, and this *is* a significant difference (Seider, Gladstein, and Kidd, 1983).

4. Disfluencies may be experimentally induced in both stutterers and nonstutterers through the use of avoidance conditioning (Hutchinson and MacKay, 1973).

5. In some stutterers, stuttering behaviors may be increased with positive

reinforcement (Costello and Felsensfeld, 1979), although it is more common for them to be decreased (Starkweather and Lucker, 1978).
6. The effects of punishment are complex. Some authors have reported simple reductions in stuttering following punishment (Martin and Siegel, 1966a; Martin and Siegel, 1966b; Martin and Siegel, 1969; Siegel, 1970). Others have suggested that some stuttering behaviors increase while others decrease under punishment (Brutten and Shoemaker, 1967; Webster, 1968; Martin, Brookshire, and Siegel, 1964). Others have noted that stimuli not usually considered aversive, such as unemotional words (e.g., "tree") are as effective in reducing the frequency of stuttering as the more typical aversive stimuli (Cooper, Cady, and Robbins, 1970). Strongly aversive stimuli may be less effective as punishers of stuttering than mildly aversive stimuli (Starkweather, 1970).

NATURE VERSUS NURTURE

Theory

There is a predisposition to acquire stuttering, which is genetically based. This conclusion follows from the first finding from the genetic studies. Given one twin who stutters, the probability that the other one will also stutter is sharply different in monozygotic than in dizygotic twins. If it is assumed that the only difference between monozygotic and dizygotic twins is that monozygotic twins share identical genetic material while dizygotic twins share genetic material to the same extent as nontwin siblings, then the conclusion that genetic inheritance plays a major role in stuttering is inescapable.

One should be just a little cautious, however, about assuming that it is only the similarity of genetic material that differs between monozygotic and dizygotic twins. This caution derives from the fact that an individual's environment is determined in an important way by the individual. Consequently, monozygotic twins, being genetically alike, are likely to shape their environments more similarly than dizygotic twins. So it is reasonable to consider the conclusion somewhat inflated; that is, the sharp difference in the probability of concordant (sharing the same trait, i.e., stuttering) twins between monozygotic and dizygotic twins may not all be attributable to genetics. Some of it may be attributable to more similar environments in monozygotic twins. However, this caution does not seem sufficient to overrule the very large difference in probability that the data suggest, and so it seems correct to conclude that there is a genetic predisposition to stutter.

Two other points need to be made about the genetically based predisposition to stutter. First, not all monozygotic twin pairs are concordant.

At least 10 percent of them are discordant, and this suggests that the environment plays some role in determining whether both or only one of the twins are stuttering at the time of the observation (Andrews et al., 1983). Second, the role of the environment need not be to determine who will begin to stutter and who will not. It could be that the environment plays its role by affecting either the likelihood of recovery or the severity of the disorder. We shall see that severity and recovery appear to be variables independent of the probability of being a stutterer.

This second point—that the predisposition to stutter is independent of stuttering severity—shows itself in the literature in several ways. In the genetic studies of Kidd and his colleagues (1980) this finding is apparent. The likelihood that a relative of a stutterer will also stutter depends on the sex of the relative and the sex of the stutterer, and it depends on the closeness of their relationship. But Kidd was unable to predict the severity of the relative's stuttering from knowledge of the severity of the proband's stuttering. This suggests that the variables determining severity may not be the same as the variables determining whether a person will be a stutterer, and it is a suggestion confirmed by other related observations in other areas of the literature. Were it not for the confirmation, the idea would not be easily derived from Kidd's observations alone, for he measured severity in the crude but reliable way that researchers usually do, by counting the frequency with which stuttering behaviors of all types occur, a measure of severity that ignores several important elements of severity (see pp. 128–133). However, the observation is confirmed, and so the conclusion seems warranted.

Sex is a major predictor of stuttering. From five to ten times as many males stutter as females (Andrews et al., 1983), but sex seems to determine the probability of recovery, not the probability of onset. This conclusion is derivable from Yairi's observation (1981) that at very early ages (two to two and one-half years) the sex ratio is 50–50. It only seems to appear in children who are of school age. Also, in the genetic studies, Kidd and associates (1980) observed a significant difference between the sexes in the recovery rates of stuttering relatives of stutterers. It seems that girls are just as likely as boys to show the early symptoms of stuttering but have a better chance of recovering from the disorder. The difference in recovery rate is strongest at preschool ages, although it persists into the school years. But by the time children are 7 or 8 years old, a clear sex ratio is already evident. This implies of course not only that girls are more likely to recover, but that stuttering is much more amenable to remission during the preschool years. This is particularly true for girls, but it is also true for boys. Consequently, early intervention and prevention of the disorder from developing further should be a major effort of speech clinicians.

Another conclusion that can be derived from the genetic literature is that handedness seems related to recovery. In the study by Seider and associates (1983), right-handed males were 1 1/3 times as likely to recover as left-handed males, but right-handed females were almost 3 1/2 times more likely to recover as left-handed ones. Clearly the tendency to recover from stuttering is related both to sex and to handedness.

One hypothesis that has been offered for the different recovery rates of females is their tendency to develop language and speech skills at earlier ages than boys (Andrews et al., 1983). This idea is compelling and should be investigated further, but it is too early to conclude that the faster development of speech and language skills in girls is related to their faster recovery. First, it is not really a well-derived finding that girls acquire language at earlier ages than boys. There are some differences between the sexes in language development, but the old adage that girls are earlier developers while the boys catch up later is not clearly established. Second, the clear involvement of handedness in recovery from stuttering suggests that recovery may be more related to some aspect of brain organization for neuromotor coordination than to language development per se. Language development is itself probably affected by brain growth and organization. Thus the involvement of language in stuttering may be tangential rather than causative.

So the genetic literature leads to the conclusion that there is a predisposition to stutter. This predisposition may be related to stuttering onset, that is, it may be a genetic predisposition that causes some children to produce excessive amounts of nonstruggled repetitive speech around two to three years of age. That is a possibility. But the evidence on recovery in families suggests that there is a genetically based predisposition to recover from stuttering, because recovery rates in the families of stutterers are predictable. Thus the finding that monozygotic twins are more likely to be concordant than dizygotic twins may result from the finding that monozygotic twins are more likely to share the same probability of recovery than dizygotic twins, making concordance for stuttering more likely. This explanation is made somewhat more plausible by the fact that recovery rates are sex-linked.

In spite of the wealth of information we have about stuttering in children, we are still unable to answer the parents' most important question—"Why did my child begin to stutter?"—with any assurance of being right. We can say that there is a genetic factor involved, but we do not know whether this factor determines which young children will have excessively repetitive speech or whether it determines which children will recover from a period of repetitiousness without becoming chronic stutterers. More important, however, is the vagueness of the term *genetic predisposition*. The knowledge that genetics plays some role in stuttering has been an important contribution to our understanding, but it does not give a very specific answer to the parents' question. So it is still important to answer "We don't know yet."

It is also important to be aware that the fact of a genetic predisposition to acquire or retain a pattern of behavior does not diminish the role of the environment. Given the predisposition, the environment shapes the behavior. Considering that *behavior* is another term for physiological activity, it should come as no surprise that genetics plays a role in determining a behavior pattern. But so too does the environment. What we need to know is what aspects of the behavior pattern are genetically related and what aspects are environmentally related.

So what do we know? We do not know why some young children show excessively repetitive speech while others do not. It could be that this early behavior is genetically determined, but there is insufficient evidence to reach that conclusion. It could also be that communicative time pressure, emotional levels in the home, or a sense of insecurity in the child causes this behavior. But there is also insufficient evidence to reach that conclusion. Some parents report emotional tensions in the home of one sort or another, but there is no systematic pattern to these accounts, and many parents, probably most, report that nothing unusual occurred during the time when the child gradually began to talk with excessive repetitions. This is not evidence. It is the absence of evidence, and unreliable besides.

We know a little more about what causes some children to begin to struggle in their speaking. The evidence from interactive studies (Meyers and Freeman, 1985b) suggests that adults are likely to talk more rapidly to children whose speech is repetitive, and clinical studies (Starkweather and Gottwald, 1984) suggest that reductions in the parents' and the child's speech rate are predictive of recovery. This information, however, is only indirectly suggestive. We can't say with certainty that the rate of parents' speech causes the child to begin to struggle. Probably, there are many other causes. Parental interruptions, nonverbal reactions to stuttering, high-level language and vocabulary, stress in the household, and insecurity in the child have also been suggested as possible causes for the child beginning to struggle with speaking. But there is insufficient evidence yet to be sure. So it seems reasonable to conclude that, given excessively repetitive speech, a child's chances of developing into a chronic stutterer depend, at least partially, on the communicative environment surrounding that child.

This raises the question of learning. If the environment plays a role in the disorder's development, what learning process is involved? It seems clear that avoidance conditioning, at least, is involved. In this type of learning, a person performs a behavior to forestall the occurrence of an aversive or noxious stimulus. The use of secondary devices, such as stallers, timers, and so on, seems clearly to be this kind of behavior. But a good case can be made that the earlier signs of struggle and forcing—more rapid repetitions, intruded schwa, laryngeal tension, and respiratory pushing—are also behaviors that the child performs to hurry through the time-consuming but noninformation-bearing periods of disfluency. This idea is derived from the typical developmental pattern of increasingly effortful speech production. It is not derived from the more rigorously controlled experiments on the effects of punishment and reinforcement on stuttering. These studies have relevance to the clinical management of stuttering, but they do not provide very useful information about the learning processes that may be responsible for stuttering development or onset.

It has been suggested (Shames and Sherrick, 1963) that stuttering behaviors may develop through instrumental conditioning. Specifically, Shames and Sherrick (1963) believed that repetitive speech would attract the attention of parents or others, and that this attention would reinforce the behavior. Then, as the parents grew more accustomed to the repetitions in the child's speech, they might pay attention only to those behaviors that were more abnormal. In this way a pattern of differential reinforcement would cause the child's speech to become progressively abnormal.

This course of development is similar to the learning process that causes some institutionalized children to learn to injure themselves to gain attention from overworked or disinterested staff members. As an explanation for stuttering, however, this idea seems counterintuitive on two grounds. One, there is no evidence that the parents of stuttering children are inattentive. For a person to learn to perform a behavior that is painful, aversive, or even effortful to gain attention it is necessary that they be unable to gain attention by the more ordinary and less aversive means of displaying affection, showing off, and so on. Second, the developed stutterer has a strong tendency to hide or disguise his disorder. Most stutterers will go out of their way to hide their stuttering, or at least postpone its discovery by others. It seems unlikely that such an attitude would develop toward a behavior that was originally learned as an attention-getting device.

Learning may play a role in the development of the young stutterer's attitude toward disfluency. *Attitude* may be defined as the tendency either to approach or avoid a stimulus. If stutterers try hard not to stutter, forcing and struggling their way through episodes of disfluency, then it is fair to say that they have a negative attitude toward the behavior. Where do they acquire such an attitude? A reasonable guess is that they learn attitudes toward disfluency from the same source and in the same way that they learn attitudes toward everything else.

How do children acquire such tendencies to avoid or approach? Occasionally, they may discover the utility or reinforcement value of a stimulus on their own and develop a positive attitude toward it, or they may encounter an aversive stimulus on their own and learn to avoid it. But most often, young children adopt the attitudes of significant others with little or no direct exposure to the thing itself. They do this through the learning process known as modeling or *vicarious conditioning* (Bandura, 1969; Starkweather, 1983). In this process the child sees a parent, or some other knowledgeable adult, reacting to a stimulus, and as a result of the observation the child acquires a tendency to react in the same way. Parents who are afraid of dogs may try to model confidence when they encounter dogs in the child's presence, but it is hard to control the nonverbal signs of fear and aversion—the hesitant rhythm, the brief facial grimace, and the forced smile betray the underlying emotion.

In the Stuttering Prevention Clinic at Temple University, I have been struck many times by the similarity of children's attitudes to those of their parents. If parents look away whenever their child is disfluent, the child is likely to develop a pattern of breaking eye contact during disfluency. If parents stiffen during the child's disfluency, the child will develop a tense body posture during stuttering. If parents pretend that nothing is happening when the child stutters, the child will deny the problem or believe that listeners don't realize it is occurring. If, on the other hand, parents are openly willing to talk about the child's disfluency, the child will not hesitate to perform it and will show less struggle and avoidance. These clinical observations suggest that modeling is the learning process by which children acquire attitudes toward their disfluency.

REFERENCES

ADAMS, M. R., LEWIS, J. I., and BESOZZI, T. E., The effect of reduced reading rate on stuttering frequency, *Journal of Speech and Hearing Research*, 16 (1973), 572–78.

ANDREWS, G., and HARRIS, M., *The Syndrome of Stuttering*. London: Heinemann, 1964.

ANDREWS, G., HOWIE, P. M., DOZSA, M., and GUITAR, B., Stuttering: speech pattern characteristics under fluency inducing conditions, *Journal of Speech and Hearing Research*, 25 (1982), 208–16.

ANDREWS, G., CRAIG, A., FEYER, A.-M., HODDINOTT, S., HOWIE, P., and NEILSON, M., Stuttering: a review of research findings and theories circa 1982, *Journal of Speech and Hearing Disorders*, 48 (1983), 226–46.

BACKUS, O., Incidence of stuttering among the deaf, *Annals of Otology, Rhinology, and Laryngology*, (1938), 632–35.

BANDURA, A., *Principles of Behavior Modification*. New York: Holt, Rinehart & Winston, 1969.

BLOODSTEIN, O., The development of stuttering. I. Changes in nine basic features, *Journal of Speech and Hearing Disorders*, 25 (1960), 219–37.

BRUTTEN E. J., and SHOEMAKER, D. J., *The Modification of Stuttering*. Englewood Cliffs, N.J.: Prentice-Hall, 1967.

CONTURE, E., Symposium address. Annual Diamond Conference, Temple University, Philadelphia, 1984.

COOPER, E. B., CADY, B. B., and ROBBINS, G. J., The effect of the verbal stimulus words "right," "wrong," and "tree" on the disfluency rates of stutterers and nonstutterers, *Journal of Speech and Hearing Research*, 13 (1970), 239–44.

COSTELLO, J., and FELSENSFELD, S., Positive reinforcement of stuttering in young children. Convention address, *American Speech and Hearing Association*, 1979.

EDSON, S. K., The incidence of certain types of nonfluencies among a group of institutionalized mongoloid and nonmongoloid children. M.A. thesis, University of Kansas, Lawrence, 1964.

EISENSON, J., Aphasics: observations and tentative conclusions, *Journal of Speech and Hearing Disorders*, 12 (1947), 290–92.

FRANK, A., Tsatsanugint: the Bannock-Shoshone Indians did have a word for "it." Convention address, *American Speech and Hearing Association*, 1970.

FREUND, H. *Psychopathology and the Problems of Stuttering.* Springfield, Ill.: Charles C Thomas, 1966.

FROESCHELS, E., *Selected Papers (1940–64).* Amsterdam: North Holland, 1964.

GENS, G. W., The speech pathologist looks at the mentally deficient child, *Training School Bulletin,* 48 (1951), 19–27.

GOTTSLEBEN, R. H., The incidence of stuttering in a group of mongoloids. *Training School Bulletin,* 51 (1955), 209–18.

GOTTWALD, S., and STARKWEATHER, C. W., Stuttering prevention: rationale and method. Short Course, American Speech and Hearing Association, 1984.

GOTTWALD, S., and STARKWEATHER, C. W., The prognosis of stuttering. Miniseminar, American Speech and Hearing Association, 1985.

GUILLAUME, J., MAZARS, G., and MAZARS, Y., Epileptic mediation in certain types of stammering, *Revue Neurologique,* 94 (1957), 59–62.

HARMS, M. A., and MALONE, J. Y., The relationship of hearing acuity to stammering, *Journal of Speech Disorders,* 4 (1939), 363–70.

HEAD, H., *Aphasia and Kindred Disorders of Speech.* London: Macmillan, 1926.

HELM, N. A., BUTLER, R. B., and BENSON, F. B., Acquired stuttering: differential characteristics. Convention address, American Speech and Hearing Association, 1978.

HOWIE, P. M., Concordance for stuttering in monozygotic and dizygotic twin pairs, *Journal of Speech and Hearing Research,* 24 (1981), 317–21.

HULL, F. M., and TIMMONS, R. J., *National Speech and Hearing Survey.* United States Office of Education, Project No. 5–0978, Grant #32–15–0050–5010 (1969).

HUTCHINSON, E. C., and MacKAY, G. R., Conditioning speech nonfluencies through the use of an aversive stimulus, *Folia Phonatrica,* 25 (1973), 373–82.

INGHAM, R., Assessment of stuttering in children, in *Stuttering Therapy: Prevention and Early Intervention,* J. Gruss ed., Memphis, Tenn.: Speech Foundation of America, 1985.

JOHNSON, W., *The Onset of Stuttering.* Minneapolis: University of Minnesota Press, 1961.

JONES, R. K., Observations on stammering after localized cerebral injury, *Journal of Neurology and Neurosurgery,* 29 (1966), 192–95.

KIDD, K., Genetic models of stuttering, *Journal of Fluency Disorders,* 5 (1980), 187–201.

KIDD, K., HEIMBUCH, R., RECORDS, M., OEHLERT, G., and WEBSTER, R., Familial stuttering patterns are not related to one measure of severity, *Journal of Speech and Hearing Research,* 23 (1980), 539–45.

KOWAL, S., O'CONNELL, D. C., and SABIN, E. F., Development of temporal patterning and vocal hesitations in spontaneous narratives, *Journal of Psycholinguistic Research,* 4 (1975), 195–207.

MARTIN, R. R., BROOKSHIRE, R. H., and SIEGEL, G. M., The Effect of Response Contingent Punishment on Various Behaviors Emitted During a "Moment of Stuttering." Unpublished manuscript, University of Minnesota, Minneapolis, 1964.

MARTIN, R. R., and SIEGEL, G. M., The effects of response-contingent shock on stuttering, *Journal of Speech and Hearing Research,* 9, (1966a), 340–52.

MARTIN, R. R., and SIEGEL, G. M., The effects of simultaneously punishing stuttering and rewarding fluency, *Journal of Speech and Hearing Research,* 9 (1966b), 466–75.

MARTIN, R. R., and SIEGEL, G. M., The effects of a neutral stimulus (buzzer) on motor responses and disfluencies in normal speakers, *Journal of Speech and Hearing Research,* 12 (1969), 179–84.

McKNIGHT, R. V., A self-analysis of a case of reading, writing, and speaking disability, *Archives of Speech,* 1 (1963), 251–54.

MEYERS, S. C., and FREEMAN, F., Interruptions as a variable in stuttering and disfluency, *Journal of Speech and Hearing Research,* 28 (1985a), 428–35.

MEYERS, S. C., and FREEMAN, F. J., Mother and child's speech rates as a variable in stuttering and disfluency, *Journal of Speech and Hearing Research,* 28 (1985), 436–44.

MILISEN, R., Methods of evaluations and diagnosis of speech disorders, in *Handbook of Speech Pathology,* ed. L. E. Travis. New York: Appleton-Century-Crofts, 1957.

MORGENSTERN, J. J., Socio-economic factors in stuttering, *Journal of Speech and Hearing Disorders,* 21 (1956), 25–33.

NELSON, S. E., HUNTER, N., and WALTER, M., Stuttering in twin types, *Journal of Speech Disorders,* 10 (1945), 335–43.

NIELSON, J. M., Epitome of agnosia, apraxia, and aphasia with proposed physiologic-anatomic nomenclature, *Journal of Speech and Hearing Disorders,* 7 (1942), 105-41.

PARRY, W., Stuttering and the Valsalva Mechanism: An Hypothesis in Need of Investigation. Unpublished manuscript, 214 Upland Rd., Merion, Pa., 1984.

PEACHER, W. C., and HARRIS, W. E., Speech disorders in World War II. Stuttering, *Journal of Speech Disorders,* 11 (1946), 303-08.

RALSTON, L., Stammering: a possible result of language interference in a bidialectal community, Nevis, West Indies. Paper presented to the Society for Caribbean Linguistics, Turkeyen, Guyana, 1976.

RECORDS, M. A., KIDD, K. K., and KIDD, J. R., Stuttering among relatives of stutterers. Convention address, American Speech and Hearing Association, 1976.

RUSSELL, L. H., MASTRIANO, B., and REATH, J., The pediatrician's view of speech pathology and audiology. Convention address, American Speech and Hearing Association, San Francisco, 1978.

SCHLANGER, B. B., and GOTTSLEBEN, R. H., Analysis of speech defects among the institutionalized mentally retarded, *Journal of Speech and Hearing Disorders,* 22 (1957), 98-103.

SCHUBERT, O. W., The incidence rate of stuttering in a matched group of institutionalized mentally retarded. Convention address, American Association for Mental Deficiencies, 1966.

SEIDER, R., GLADSTEIN, K. L., and KIDD, K. K., Recovery and persistence of stuttering among relatives of stutterers, *Journal of Speech and Hearing Disorders,* 48 (1983), 402-409.

SHAMES, G., and SHERRICK, C., A discussion of nonfluency and stuttering as operant behavior, *Journal of Speech and Hearing Disorders,* 28 (1963), 3-18.

SHEEHAN, J. G., and MARTYN, M. M., Spontaneous recovery from stuttering, *Journal of Speech and Hearing Research,* 9 (1970), 279-89.

SIEGEL, G. M., Punishment, stuttering, and disfluency, *Journal of Speech and Hearing Research,* 13 (1970), 677-714.

STARKWEATHER, C. W., The simple, main, and interactive effects of contingent and noncontingent shock of high and low intensities on stuttering repetitions. Ph.D. dissertation, Southern Illinois University, Carbondale, 1970.

STARKWEATHER, C., W., Eclectic learning theory and stuttering therapy, *Communicative Disorders, An Audio Journal for Continuing Education,* 2 (1977), No. 8 (in cassette form).

STARKWEATHER, C. W., *Speech and Language: Principles and Processes of Behavior Change.* Englewood Cliffs, N.J.: Prentice-Hall, 1983.

STARKWEATHER, C. W., and LUCKER, J., Tokens for stuttering, *Journal of Fluency Disorders,* 3 (1978), 167-80.

STARKWEATHER, C. W., and GORDON, P., Stuttering: the language connection. Short course, American Speech and Hearing Association, 1983.

STARKWEATHER, C. W., and GOTTWALD, S., Parents' speech and children's fluency. Convention address, American Speech and Hearing Association, 1984.

VAN HORN, H., Comparative incidence of stuttering after twenty years, *Western Michigan University Journal of Speech Therapy,* 3 (1966), 6-7.

VAN RIPER, C., *Speech Correction: Principles and Methods,* 5th ed. Englewood Cliffs, N.J.: Prentice-Hall, 1971.

VAN RIPER, C., *The Nature of Stuttering,* 3rd ed. Englewood Cliffs, N.J.: Prentice-Hall, 1984.

WALL, M., and MEYERS, F., *Language Based Therapy for Stutterers.* Baltimore: University Park Press, 1984.

WALLE, G., *Prevention of Stuttering* (film). Memphis, Tenn.: Speech Foundation of America, 1975.

WEBSTER, L. M., A cinematic analysis of the effects of contingent stimulation on stuttering and associated behaviors. Ph.D. dissertation, Southern Illinois University, Carbondale, 1968.

WEPMAN, J. M., Familial incidence in stammering, *Journal of Speech Disorders,* 4 (1939), 199-204.

WEST R., NELSON, S., and BERRY, M., The heredity of stuttering, *Quarterly Journal of Speech,* 25 (1939), 23-30.

WESTBY, C. E., Language performance of stuttering and nonstuttering children, *Journal of Communication Disorders,* 12 (1979), 133-45.

YAIRI, E., Disfluencies of normally speaking two-year-old children, *Journal of Speech and Hearing Research,* 24 (1981), 490-95.

The Variability
of Stuttering

♦ *Theoretical implications of these other fluency-enhancing effects*

♦ *Experimental findings on effects on stuttering of saying the same words repeatedly (adaptation effect)*

♦ *Theoretical implications of adaptation effect*

♦ *Experimental findings on stutterers' ability to predict the words on which they will stutter*

♦ *Theoretical implications of expectancy effect*

INTRODUCTION

One of the oddest things about stuttering is its variability. It is sometimes present, at other times absent, sometimes severe, at other times mild. The reasons for these variations are often obscure. I have already mentioned how different the symptoms may appear in different stutterers. This is one kind of variability. But another kind, which is the subject of this chapter, presents some of the most challenging information for theorists. Laypeople too are often puzzled by it. They do not understand why people who stutter cannot control their speech yet have no difficulty singing a song or talking to themselves. Even clinicians can be misled. Many clinicians don't understand why stutterers who have been taught to speak in a special way—with exaggerated voicing or at a slower tempo for example—and who show no stuttering when they talk that way, are still dissatisfied with their speech. Parents too are frustrated by the way their child stutters when they go to visit a certain relative and then speaks perfectly well as soon as they leave. When we add to this variability the fact, described in the preceding chapter, that in children the disorder often comes and goes in episodes, the picture becomes most confusing for the parents. Researchers, however, have been able to identify many of the specific circumstances under which stuttering varies, and in many instances can predict or even control the severity of the symptoms under experimental circumstances, although it is not clear, even in these instances, why the variation occurs.

It might be noted at the outset that most of the findings described below have been derived by manipulating circumstances and observing changes in the frequency with which stuttering behaviors occur. But, as we have already seen, the frequency of stuttering is an imperfect, really only a partial, measure of the disorder's severity. Consequently, the information presented below probably underestimates the real variability of stuttering.

Another idea to bear in mind is that variability may also be present in the frequency, and perhaps in the severity, of normal discontinuities— those pauses, hesitations, interjections, and revisions that even fluent speakers have in their speech. Knowledge that stuttering varies under a certain condition is much less impressive; it tells us less about the disorder if the same condition also causes the same kind of variation in the discontinuities of normal speakers.

SITUATIONAL VARIABILITY

Findings

1. Most stutterers in whom the disorder is well developed stutter more in certain speaking situations, although the nature of these difficult situations seems to be an individual matter (Brutten and Shoemaker, 1967; Andrews et al., 1983).
2. Normal discontinuities decrease in situations rated by the speaker as demanding excellence in speech (Broen and Siegel, 1972). In stutterers, the situation is more complicated. Some stutterers are more fluent in circumstances demanding excellence in speech, but many are less fluent under these conditions.
3. Stuttering behaviors occur more frequently in the presence of "difficult" listeners (Berwick, 1939). Most stutterers, but not all, report that some listeners are difficult to talk to (Van Riper, 1982).
4. Most stutterers stutter less when by themselves (Bloodstein, 1950), but they are not totally fluent (Quinn, 1971).
5. Both normal discontinuities and stuttering occur more often in stressful than in nonstressful situations (Dixon, 1947; Bloodstein, 1950; Mahl, 1956).

Theory

It is evident that stuttering varies according to the stutterer's speech situation. It is equally clear that situations that are difficult for one stutterer will not necessarily be difficult for another. Probably too, situational variability is a feature of advanced, not of early stuttering. This pattern certainly suggests as a first hypothesis that a learning process is responsible for situational variability.

Perhaps the most explicit theory of situational variation has been described by Brutten and Shoemaker (1967). They suggest that the negative emotional reaction of the stutterer to situations in which stuttering has occurred in the past evokes further occurrences of the behavior. With continued experience, a hierarchy of difficult situations develops, formed by the stutterer's experiences with the disorder. This theory explains why each stutterer's set of difficult situations is different, and it explains why situational variability develops in more advanced stutterers, who presumably have had more experience with the disorder. It also explains a common, but not universal, clinical observation that difficulty talking in one situation can appear to spread to similar situations according to the extent that the situations are similar.

Most stutterers report a set of situations in which they stutter more than in others, and it is certainly common for this set of situations to share a number of themes. For example, one stutterer had difficulty buying certain things, making long distance telephone calls, and talking to the bus driver on certain bus routes. This made no sense to him at all until, in therapy, it became obvious that his difficulty was in saying numbers. When he had to buy something and specify the quantity, or give the long distance operator the number he was calling, or tell the bus driver a street number, his stuttering was more severe than at other times. Many stutterers report other themes—difficulty talking to authority figures, asking questions, talking to a group of listeners, when trying to make a point, or when talking to children. Some themes are very common. Many stutterers find the telephone a formidable barrier to fluent speech. Most find a group of listeners more difficult to talk to than a single listener. Ordering food in a restaurant is also a common difficult situation. But none of these is universal. There are stutterers who find talking on the phone much easier than talking face to face. And it should also be noted that there are advanced stutterers who stutter equally in all situations.

Situational themes, when they are present, may result from the association of common stimulus items in thematically similar situations. If, however, situational variability were purely a matter of conditioning, then the themes that develop should be arbitrary. We should see stutterers who find difficulty speaking in situations linked by any conceivable theme. For example, we ought to see stutterers who report difficulty talking to red-headed people or people wearing hats or blue clothing, or tall people, since these are elements of the stimulus situation that are often shared from one speech situation to the next. Commonly present, they should commonly form the link of association between situations. But, in fact, stutterers do not report such arbitrary themes. Instead, their themes usually reflect social variations, usually where language pragmatics would dictate the use of different forms. For example, many stutterers report stuttering more severely when talking to authority figures. A few report difficulty talking to subordinates. None report difficulty talking to people with blue eyes. This may be because we use different language forms, a different tempo, and even slightly different phonological rules when talking to people who have different status than we do, but we do not alter the way we talk when speaking to people who have different eye or hair color.

We know that semantics, syntax, prosody, and even phonology vary somewhat from one social situation to the next. Perhaps the fluency of normal speech also varies. We know that discontinuities in the speech of nonstutterers occur with greater frequency at certain linguistic locations—on longer words and less frequently used words and at clause boundaries. When a more microscopic aspect of fluency—the duration of speech sounds—was observed by Umeda (1975; 1977), she found that speech sound duration also varied with the length and frequency of words and by position in the sentence. Perhaps if researchers were to measure the fluency of nonstutterers with more sensitivity they would find that other measures of fluency, such as speech rate and coarticulation, vary with the social situation. Even the grosser measure of normal fluency, the continuity of speech, may vary under different social circumstances.

One of the most intriguing differences between stutterers and nonstutterers is in response to situations that demand excellence in speech. Nonstutterers, when faced with a job interview or meeting an important person, or any situation when immediate impressions are important, or when speaking in public to an audience, are usually able to speak well. Occasionally, the reverse occurs—just when you want to make a good impression, you find yourself stumbling and hesitating. Some stutterers also find that when it is important for them to exercise control over their stuttering behaviors they can do so for a period of time. But they find it difficult to control stuttering for very long. Many, perhaps most, stutterers report exactly the opposite—the situation that demands excellence in speech only makes their speech worse. The harder they try to speak well, the more they struggle and force. The more they think about not stuttering, the more they stutter.

These findings and clinical observations suggest that speakers vary in the extent to which they can consciously control the fluency of their speech. The normal, and doubtless the superior, speakers have good control. When they need to they can inhibit themselves from stumbling or hesitating, usually by slowing down a little and being careful about how they form words and sounds. This control can usually be exerted even in the face of an increased tendency to pause and hesitate that the anxiety of the situation may create. The stutterer, on the other hand, is likely to have less control. Some have enough so that when it is necessary they can temporarily inhibit themselves from stuttering, usually by slowing down and being careful to form sounds smoothly. It is easier to do this when the situation is less anxious, but some stutterers can exert control even under anxiety-provoking conditions. But most stutterers lack enough control over their speech production to diminish the frequency and severity of their stuttering behaviors, and typically when the situation makes them anxious it is even harder to control.

LINGUISTIC VARIABILITY

Findings

1. Longer words, whether measured by number of syllables or by number of letters, are stuttered more often than shorter ones (Milisen, 1938; Brown and Moren, 1942; Hejna, 1955; Soderberg, 1966; Schlesinger, 1966).
2. Normal discontinuities also occur more often on longer than on shorter words, and the effect of length is more pronounced on normal discontinuities than on stutterings (Silverman, 1972).
3. Adults stutter lexical words more often than function words (Johnson and Brown, 1935; Brown, 1938; Hahn, 1942; Hejna, 1955).
4. Children stutter conjunctions and pronouns more than nouns and interjections (Bloodstein and Gantwerk, 1967).
5. Normal hesitations in adults are more likely to occur on lexical words (Goldman-Eisler, 1958; McClay and Osgood, 1959; Blankenship, 1964).
6. Prolongations in stutterers occur with nearly equal frequency on both lexical and function words (Soderberg, 1966).
7. Both normal discontinuities and stutterings tend to occur on the same word types (Silverman and Williams, 1967; Soderberg, 1967).
8. Stuttering occurs more readily on less frequently used words but only when the sentences are syntactically more simple (Ronson, 1976).
9. There is more stuttering on consonants than on vowels (Brown, 1938; Hahn, 1942; Quarrington, Conway, and Siegel, 1962; Taylor, 1966).
10. The duration and intensity of the sounds may be inversely related to the frequency with which stuttering occurs on them (Fairbanks, 1937).
11. Stuttering occurs much more often on stressed than on unstressed syllables (Froeschels, 1961; Van Riper, 1982).
12. Stuttering occurs most often on the first sound of a word (Andrews et al., 1983).
13. Words positioned early in a sentence are more likely to be stuttered than words positioned later (Brown, 1938; Hejna, 1955; Quarrington, Conway, and Siegel, 1962; Conway and Quarrington, 1963; Bloodstein and Gantwerk, 1967).
14. Stuttering occurs most often at points of high information loading (Taylor, 1966).
15. When word length is held constant, information load is not correlated with stuttering frequency (Lanyon, 1970).
16. Nonstuttering four-year-old children are more disfluent on the initial words of utterances than at other points (E-M. Silverman, 1974).
17. More stuttering occurs on words toward the beginning of long sentences than occurs on the same words when they are at the beginning of shorter sentences (Tornick and Bloodstein, 1976; Jayaram, 1984).

18. In preschool children, stuttering is more likely to occur at the begin-ning of utterances and at major clause boundaries (Wall, 1977).

19. The loci of disfluencies in normal speakers are the same as those for stutterings with the exception that there is no tendency for normal disfluencies to occur on words positioned early in the sentence (Sil-verman and Williams, 1967).

20. Propositional speech yields more stuttering than nonsense material (Eisenson and Horowitz, 1945; Bloodstein, 1950).

21. Emotionally loaded material yields more stuttering than neutral ma-terial (Bardrick and Sheehan, 1956).

22. Stuttering is more likely to occur at locations where language for-mulation is occuring (Starkweather and Gordon, 1983).

Theory

Let us look first at the properties of words that are likely to be stut-tered (findings 1 through 8). Early researchers were interested in the fact that many stutterers reported finding certain words more difficult to say fluently than others. Some stutterers do not report this pattern, but most do. It was quickly evident that the pattern of "feared," or "Jonah" words, as they were called, was an individual one, each stutterer reporting a dif-ferent set of words that were hard to say fluently. However, the early re-searchers thought they perceived some common threads, properties of words that made them likely to appear on any stutterer's list of "Jonah" words, and believed that these common threads might reveal something worthwhile about the nature of the disorder.

In some of the early investigations, samples of speech were obtained by having a group of stutterers read written material out loud, or in a few cases, by having them speak spontaneously on a given subject. The words that the subjects stuttered on were then examined for certain properties and compared with words that were not stuttered. This method often over-looked the way in which the property in question was distributed in the language, and some of the results may have reflected this distribution rather than the property itself.

Other researchers used word lists or sentence frames to present words. This method better controlled the words' properties, but the speech pro-duced by the stutterers as they read lists of words was probably different from the speech they used in conversation. A few researchers used correl-ative techniques to see if a particular word property increased the proba-bility of the word being stuttered beyond the probability of its occurrence in the language. This method allowed for the distribution of different types of words in the language and still permitted the use of naturally produced speech samples, but the use of correlation restricted the conclusions to statements of prediction rather than statements of causation, which was less than the researchers' intentions.

These early investigations into word properties were hampered by the fact that language is not just a random assortment or linear concatenation of words but a hierarchically structured series of events in which the probability of occurrence of a certain word, or class of words, is determined by the structure and by the semantic intention of the person who formulates the language. The word lists avoid this problem but do so by using speech samples that are not representative of natural language.

Most of these early investigations into the properties of stuttered words were paralleled by investigations into the properties of words on which the discontinuities of normal speakers occurred. In each case, it was found that the same properties characterized normally nonfluent and stuttered words. Somewhat later, investigators began to examine the location of stuttering in sentences and documented the fact that stuttering is most likely to occur at the beginnings of sentences and at major clause boundaries. This finding, which also turned out not to be true of normal nonfluencies, marked the end of the early era of word-bound linguistic investigation and the beginning of a new look at the effect of language variables on the probability of stuttering, a topic covered in more detail in a later section (see pp. 251–255).

The linguistic location of stuttering in sentences was easier to investigate than word properties, but the two are intimately connected, because certain types of words are likely to occur in certain positions. Studies on sentence position, however, were not without flaw. Most of them failed to account for differences in speech timing, specifically the rate of articulation, which was later discovered to vary with various word properties and with sentence position (Umeda, 1975; 1977).

Findings 1 through 7 present information regarding word properties. In adults, longer, less frequently used words serving a lexical or naming function are more likely to be stuttered than shorter, more frequently used words serving structural functions. It seemed likely from the beginning that these findings were interrelated, because lexical words tend to be longer and less frequently used than function words, but it was never made very clear which of these three properties was the one that really made the difference. Then, when it was reported that the normal discontinuities of nonstutterers are also distributed in the same way, word properties seemed much less important to an understanding of stuttering than previously supposed.

However, the similar linguistic distribution of stuttering and normal discontinuities strengthened one major theoretical idea—that stuttering behaviors develop from normal discontinuities. Of course, stuttering typically develops in children, and children's normal discontinuities are likely to be different in form from adults, but the idea of continuity of development between normal discontinuities and stuttering was nonetheless more tenable in light of the similar distribution of the two types of behavior in adult speech.

Two findings bearing on development strengthened the idea of a continuity of development between normal discontinuities and stuttering behaviors. The first of these findings, that children, unlike adults, stutter more on pronouns and conjunctions than on lexical words (Bloodstein and Gantwerk, 1967), seemed at first to mean that children's stuttering was distributed differently from that of adults. A closer look at the distribution of children's stuttering (Wall, 1977), however, made it evident that clause boundaries were the location most likely to be stuttered, and that the pronouns and conjunctions that children usually stuttered were simply "and" and "I," the words most often used by children to initiate clauses and sentences. In other words, the stutterings of children were distributed the same way as the stutterings of adults; it was the words children used that were distributed differently. The fact that children stuttered on different kinds of words than adults did not, after all, detract from the argument that stuttering develops from normal discontinuities.

The second finding, that prolongations are distributed somewhat differently than repetitions, also added strength to the argument that stuttering develops out of normal discontinuities because prolongations seem to develop a little later than repetitions and may be a kind of coping behavior. If prolongations are used differently than repetitions, they might be expected to be distributed in a different way.

In the end, it seemed evident that stuttering and normal discontinuities are distributed in the same way with one exception—the beginnings of sentences, where stuttering behaviors but not normal discontinuities are likely to be found. This one difference, however, seems important. There are several types of normal discontinuities—filled pauses, false starts (revisions), parenthetical remarks, repetitions—that are likely to occur within a sentence but at a major clause boundary for the same reason. Adults begin sentences before knowing exactly what the endings are going to be. Usually, the rest of the sentence, which is partially predictable (redundant) from the first, is easily produced. The words are found, the syntax formulated. But sometimes the sentence so blithely undertaken leads to an idea that should not be uttered, or a grammatical solecism, or an untenable rhetorical position. Sometimes too a key word in the second clause cannot be easily found. For these reasons there is likely to be a pause, hesitation, revision, or parenthetical remark at an internal clause boundary.

In stuttering, however, the major problem is not the completion of the sentence as much as it is the initiation of it. Stutterers have trouble getting started. They have found the words, formulated the sentence (at least the first part, as nonstutterers have), but they cannot get their vocal tracts to initiate the first sounds of the sentence smoothly. This difference in the distribution of stutterings and normal nonfluencies seems to strengthen arguments that although stuttering may develop from normal discontinuities, it is in adults a very different kind of behavior, a disruption not of the language system, of word-finding and sentence formulation as normal discontinuities are, but a disruption of motor speech production.

Ronson's study (1976), in which it was determined that the word frequency effect depended on certain types of sentence structure, cast major doubt on the validity of the old investigations into the properties of words, in which linguistic structure was ignored. Ronson's study set the stage for a new series of linguistic investigations, which looked at stuttering in relation to the properties of whole sentences, and to the syntactic, semantic, and pragmatic aspects of language, rather than to the properties of words.

In addition to certain words, many stutterers report having difficulty with specific sounds. Again, the pattern tends to be individual, with one stutterer reporting one set of difficult sounds, while another stutterer is likely to report a different set. Again, investigators were interested in the possibility that there were some common threads, or a probabilistic trend, in these patterns. It was quickly learned that if a large group of stutterers was sampled, there was a tendency for consonants to be stuttered more often than vowels, and Fairbanks (1937) quickly extended this observation to the more general notion that sounds that were brief in duration and low in intensity were more likely to be stuttered.

This was another way of saying that it was either the brevity of the sound or its low intensity that was responsible for its increased likelihood of being produced disfluently. Two theoretical notions are supported by this idea—that stuttering is in some way an auditory perception problem and that it is in some way a problem of the motor execution of speech sounds. Both of these theoretical ideas will recur in my discussion.

Finding 11, that stuttering occurs more readily on stressed than on unstressed syllables, is an important finding, as Wingate (1976) has pointed out. It is important because it has great predictive power—stuttering almost never occurs on a destressed syllable unless it is the first syllable of a word. But the fact is also important because the production of stress is physiologically clear. The stressed syllable is produced with a slightly higher fundamental frequency of voice, with a slightly more intense voice, and it is slightly longer than a destressed syllable. Any one of these differences could be responsible for the finding. On the other hand, auditory perception theorists found it somewhat difficult to account for the fact that syllables that are more easily perceived are more likely to be stuttered if they argued at the same time that speech sounds that are briefer and therefore more difficult to perceive are also more likely to be stuttered.

But the finding about stress is also important because it flies in the face of some of the motor control arguments. Wingate (1976) argued on the basis of the fluency enhancement literature (see below) that stuttering was less likely to occur when vowels were prolonged or accentuated. But this argument founders on the finding that the vowels in stressed syllables are clearly both prolonged and accentuated. It is in other words a little difficult to reconcile finding 9 with finding 11.

One explanation seems to work for both of these observations. When young children are first beginning to stutter, a typical way in which they attempt to cope with what they perceive to be difficulty in speaking is to try harder, to push harder. In so doing they simultaneously heighten glottal closure and press with abdominal muscles to increase the flow of air. These are the same maneuvers one uses to increase vocal loudness, but if the balance of vocal fold tension and subglottal air pressure is a little off, the vocal folds, instead of vibrating, remain tightly shut, sealing off the lower airway and allowing pressure to build up below the glottis. If this pattern of blockage becomes incorporated into children's speech, it may gradually develop into other types of stuttering behaviors. Consonants might be more difficult to produce than vowels because the rapidly changing intraoral air pressure that occurs with consonantal release requires a rapid adjustment in glottal tension in order to allow the vocal folds to vibrate. Failure to achieve this optimal vocal fold tension might result in the folds shutting momentarily, causing a glottal blockage that lasts for a moment. It lasts only for a moment because an attempt to reinitiate the consonant will alter the intraoral air pressure in the right direction and permit, momentarily, a vibration of the folds, but again the rapid change that occurs with consonantal release can start the whole process going again.

In other words, the consonants, because they are accompanied by rapid changes in air pressure, make it more difficult than the vowels for the glottal tension to maintain optimal adjustment to subglottal air pressure. Difficulty in maintaining optimal vocal fold tension would be most likely to occur when subglottal air pressure was high, as when the child is trying to force the air out, or on other occasions when subglottal air pressure surges, as in the case of stressed syllables. What is particularly hard for the stutterer to do is to maintain an appropriate glottal tension adjustment (GTA) during the combination of rapid oral movements and increased subglottal air pressure. Findings 12 and 13 are also explained by GTA because the adjustment is most difficult to make when airflow is initiated. Once the vocal folds are vibrating, their own properties of elasticity and mass tend to perpetuate the vibration. It is harder to achieve GTA from scratch. The idea that GTA can be difficult for stutterers to maintain during oral movements and the more general concept of the influence of oral movements on air pressure changes at the glottis should be attributed to Adams (1975). Much of Conture's work (Conture, McCall, and Brewer, 1977) also has dealt with glottal changes during stuttering and supports this idea.

A more detailed discussion of the role of the vocal mechanism in stuttering is presented in Chapter 9.

Finding 14 is of course an attempted explanation of the findings as well as a finding itself. It is true enough that when the information loadings of different points in a sentence are determined by the transitional probabilities technique,[1] stuttering is found to be more likely at those locations where the information loading is high. But is it the information loading itself that is the culprit? High information loading is likely to be located toward the beginnings of sentences and clauses, places where language formulation and breathing, also implicated in the precipitation of stuttering behaviors, also occur. Language formulation is discussed later (see pp. 251–255), but the initiation of airflow has already been described as a point where GTA might be difficult to achieve. So the tendency for stuttering to occur early in the sentence or at clause boundaries or at points of high information loading may be related either to language formulation or to difficulty in maintaining GTA during airflow initiation.

Another explanation of the tendency for stuttering to occur on stressed syllables, and one that resolves the theoretical issue from the motor control point of view, has to do with the precision of articulation. Syllabic stress, like the stressed words of a sentence, are produced not only louder, longer, and higher, but also more intelligibly (Hunnicut, 1985). For intelligibility to be increased, the normal variability allowed to the gestures of speech sound production is reduced, and articulation becomes more precise. The targets are constrained within a narrower range of speech movements. This is most obviously seen in the full vowel color that stressed syllables have when compared to unstressed ones, but the requirement for precision on stressed words and syllables, and presumably at other points of high information loading, is present for consonants as well as vowels. There is a natural trading relation between the velocity of movement and the precision of movement required to achieve a target.

So it makes sense that stutterers, if they are lacking in oral and vocal motor coordination, would be likely to stutter at points in the utterance where there was a linguistic demand for either high velocity of movement or precision of articulatory gesture. Stressed syllables and words may be produced more slowly, but they have high requirements for precision as well. Indeed, we may slow down at these locations to achieve the required precision. The beginnings of sentences, where of all locations stuttering is most likely to occur, require both high velocities and precision of move-

---

[1]A group of people are asked to guess one by one the words of a sentence known to another person. The number of guesses it takes to identify each word (more than twenty to thirty may be considered infinity) measures the transitional probability, or information load, of that particular word.

ment. It should be noted, however, that even though reduced speech motor coordination explains the linguistic locations of stuttering, this does not necessarily mean that stuttering is caused by reduced speech motor coordination. It is equally likely that the reduced speech motor coordination is caused by stuttering, specifically by the increased background muscle tonus that is present in the speech muscles of stutterers.

Lanyon's failure to find a correlation between information loading and stuttering when word frequency is held constant (1970) is often given the weight of a finding because of the corresponding observation that the correlation between information load and stuttering is significant when word frequency is not held constant. But it should not be given this importance. To decide that word length determines the effect, a comparison between the two correlations should be made, and it should be shown that the two correlations are significantly different under the two circumstances. Finding a significant correlation under one circumstance and not finding it under another does not demonstrate the invalidity of the significant correlation.

Why should propositional as compared to nonsense material and emotionally loaded as compared to emotionally neutral material be more evocative of stuttering behavior? Zimmermann (1980) pointed out that when the speech mechanism moves, the muscles that control movement perform their brief flexions and relaxations against a variable background of muscle tension.

When this background tension level is high, it has a number of effects—it stiffens the mechanism overall, making movement a little more difficult and a little less smooth, and it makes the muscle more reactive, likely to contract to even brief or weak stimulation. In other words, when the background tension is high, it doesn't take much to make the muscles contract and the structure begin to move, and when it moves, it will require greater effort to overcome stiffness, and move more slowly and less smoothly. These are characteristics that are descriptive of stuttered speech. The background tension level is affected by a number of factors, and the emotional level of the speaker is one. Positive excitement, incidentally, has as much of an effect as anxiety. So, when trying to speak about topics that are more meaningful or emotionally loaded, the background tension level may be raised. This would affect not only the glottis, but all the moving parts of the vocal tract, making it more difficult for them to achieve smooth easy movement.

The finding that stuttering is more likely to occur at locations where language formulation is occurring has two implications. First, as we have already noted, these points are also characterized by motoric differences, which could be the reason for the increased likelihood of stuttering. But, in addition to this possibility, the fact that cognitive activity to formulate language is also occurring cannot help the stutterer. At the least, it diverts the stutterer's attention from the task of controlling an unruly speech mechanism. It may also raise what might be called "motoric uncertainty." Speakers are less sure about their communicative intention at these points, because they are formulating language, so they are also less sure about the words they will use and consequently less sure about the movements and gestures they will make to produce those words.

FLUENCY ENHANCEMENT

Perhaps the most puzzling thing about stuttering is the fact that it can often be made to diminish or even disappear under certain specific types of stimulation. This effect is known as *fluency enhancement*. There are several types of fluency-enhancing stimuli: masking noise, rhythmic stimulation, delayed auditory feedback, singing, and a few others. Some theorists have attempted to find a common pattern in these various fluency-enhancing conditions, notably Wingate (1969; 1976) who believed that they all resulted in stutterers talking with accentuated vowels, and Sheehan (1970) who believed, along with a number of others, that these conditions distracted stutterers from morbid attention to their speaking difficulties. Neither of these two attempts to unify the fluency enhancement literature has been entirely successful, although both positions unify much disparate information.

The Masking Effect

Findings

1. Stutterers speak more fluently under conditions of masking noise (Shane, 1955; Cherry and Sayers, 1956).
2. The effect of masking noise on stuttering is greater with greater intensity of masking (Cherry and Sayers, 1956; Maraist and Hutton, 1957; Stromsta, 1958; Ham and Steer, 1967; Adams and Hutchinson, 1974).
3. The masking effect has been found to be more effective with lower frequency of masking (Stromsta, 1967), but a more recent study suggests that frequency is not a determining factor (Conture, 1974b).
4. Both the frequency and the duration of stuttering are reduced by masking (Murray, 1969).
5. Continuous masking is more effective in reducing stuttering than random or intermittent masking (Murray, 1969).
6. The effect of masking noise on stutterers is not attributable to anxiety changes (Adams and Moore, 1972).
7. Fluency is also improved when masking is removed contingent on the initiation of voicing or when the masking occurs only during the silent intervals (Sutton and Chase, 1961; Webster and Dorman, 1970).

8. There is an inverse relationship between vocal intensity and stuttering frequency when reading under masking noise (Adams and Hutchinson, 1974), but see also finding 9.

9. The masking effect occurs even when stutterers speak in a voice of normal loudness; in fact the greatest effect occurs when the difference in intensity between the voice and the masking noise is greatest (Garber and Martin, 1977), but see also finding 8.

10. The speech of nonstutterers is also changed—louder, higher pitch, slower rate, longer vowels—by masking noise (Wingate, 1970).

11. Stuttering is found only rarely among the congenitally deaf and often disappears with the onset of adventitious deafness (Backus, 1938; Harms and Malone, 1939; Wingate, 1970).

Theory

The effect of masking noise on stutterers is well established, although there are some stutterers who do not respond to it with complete fluency. But most stutterers are affected by the condition, at least to the point of having less severe, that is briefer and less effortful, stuttering behaviors. Probably a more noticeable effect would be seen if a more sensitive measure of severity were used than the frequency with which behaviors occur, specifically a measure that accounted for the duration of behaviors. In other words, masking is probably more effective as a fluency enhancer than the reported effects suggest.

The masking noise has to be bilateral and loud for the effect to occur. It seems not to be simply a distraction; masking is more effective when the stutterer does not hear himself at all. There are a number of possible explanations, but two basic ideas. One idea is that the stutterer speaks more fluently because he cannot hear himself. From this position one can predict that the extent to which stuttering is diminished depends on the loudness of the noise relative to the speaker's vocal intensity. Garber and Martin's experiment (1977) confirms this prediction.

The other basic idea is that the masking effect changes the way in which the speaker talks, and it is the change in speech production that is responsible for the effect. The motor control theories of stuttering would predict that the extent to which fluency is enhanced by masking noise is correlated with the extent of speech changes produced by masking. These changes are the well-known Lombard effect, in which vocal loudness and vocal pitch are increased while speech rate is reduced. Adams and Hutchinson's experiment (1974) seems to confirm the prediction for vocal intensity, although Garber and Martin's (1977) deconfirms it.

There have been no similar studies on rate. Martin and associates' study (1984) looked at rate and stuttering frequency simultaneously under conditions of masking noise but did not attempt to assess speech rate independent of stuttering. Naturally, when a person's frequency of stuttering is decreased by masking noise or any other condition, the absence of stuttering behaviors tends to increase the number of words that the subject can say in a given period of time. Rate of speech, as measured by words per minute, increases. And yet the person may in fact be talking (moving the speech mechanism) more slowly. Probably the only way to deal with this phenomenon is to measure the amount of time occupied by stuttering behaviors during the control condition and subtract the appropriate amount of time for the decreased number of disfluencies, so that the final rate measure is adjusted for the change in fluency. The technical difficulty of this method may have discouraged some researchers.

Another interesting aspect of the masking effect is that it seems to continue for a brief while after the masking noise has been removed. This has been demonstrated in two quite different ways. In the Webster and Dorman study (1970), the effect lasted for a few seconds after the noise was removed. This may be attributed to the slight extension of the Lombard effect that we have all experienced when the background noise to our own speech was suddenly removed. In Martin and associates' study (1984), it influenced the frequency of stuttering in an amplified sidetone condition that was presented 2 minutes later but without influencing the frequency of stuttering during non-sidetone periods that were interspersed throughout the experiment. This was clearly not the delayed Lombard effect. Somehow, the noise condition made subsequent conditions of amplified sidetone fluency-enhancing. It is not clear why this effect occurred. There is much more to be learned about the masking effect on stuttering.

Delayed Auditory Feedback (DAF)

Findings

1. DAF disrupts the speech of normal speakers, causing them to prolong syllables, speak more loudly, and sometimes repeat the sounds at the ends of words (Rawnsley and Harris, 1954).
2. The effects of DAF on normal speakers are more pronounced in children than in adults (Goldfarb and Braunstein, 1958; MacKay, 1968; Buxton, 1969), although children younger than two years show a reversal of the effects—shorter vowels, softer intensity (Belmore et al., 1973).
3. The effects of DAF on normal speakers are more pronounced in men than in women (Bachrach, 1964; Mahaffey and Stromsta, 1965), although Timmons (1971) found that sex differences disappeared when conditions were randomized, indicating that women adapt to DAF more easily than men.
4. The DAF effect on normal speakers is greater in right than in left ears (Abbs and Smith, 1970).
5. The behavioral disturbances produced by DAF in normal speakers are

substantially different from stuttering along several dimensions (Neeley, 1961; Wingate, 1970).

6. Stutterers are more fluent under DAF (Chase, Sutton, and Rapin, 1961; Bohr, 1963; Zerneri, 1966; Soderberg, 1968).

7. The optimal delay time for fluency enhancement in stutterers is 0.05 seconds (Lotzman, 1961).

8. Long-term improvement with DAF has been reported (Siegenthaler and Brubaker, 1957; Adamczyk, 1959; Goldiamond, Atkinson, and Bilger, 1962; Goldiamond, 1965; Gross and Nathanson, 1966).

9. Stutterers do not react to DAF differently than nonstutterers (Stark and Pierce, 1970).

10. Delayed auditory feedback is neither more nor less effective than masking noise in the enhancement of fluency (Stephen and Haggard, 1980).

Theory

The fluency-enhancing effects of DAF on stuttering are strong. Typically, the stutterer, after some initial discomfort caused by the disruption of ordinary speech feedback mechanisms, begins to speak at a slow rate, with prolonged vowels, and with the odd rhythm that is characteristic of this speaking condition. And typically, stuttering behaviors dramatically disappear. When the DAF condition is terminated, the stuttering behaviors recur, although in some stutterers some fluency enhancement continues, usually only for a short time. The speech of stutterers under DAF is the same as the speech of nonstutterers; that is, the rate is slower, the vowels are prolonged, the rhythm is odd, and there are fewer discontinuities.

When DAF was first discovered by Lee (1951), it was called "artificial stuttering," because it produced, in addition to the slowed rate and prolonged vowels, a tendency in some subjects to repeat the sounds of speech. However, under DAF speakers are likely to repeat sounds at the ends of words and phrases in an echo-like pattern. The feedback at one's ears signals that speech production is not as far along as it really is, and as a result, speakers hold back on ending a sequence of speech gestures. This prolongs the vowels. If speakers have terminated a sequence of movements, the signal feeds information back to them that the sequence should not have been terminated yet, so they take up the syllable again in the middle of the vowel and terminate it again. This pattern leads to the repetition of final consonants. Lee (1951) heard the prolonged vowels and repeated consonants and dubbed DAF "artificial stuttering." In fact, however, the speech of normal speakers under DAF is very different from stuttered speech. The repetitions in DAF speech tend to be at the end rather than the beginning of units, and the prolongations tend to be of vowels, not of initial sounds.

Findings 2 and 3 should not be given much attention. That children are more disrupted by DAF simply reflects the fact that they are less able to respond to the condition with the kind of cool control that adults typically can exercise. The apparent reversal of the effect in very young children is an artifact of the reticence these children show under any unusual speaking circumstance. The sex difference has already been shown to be unreal.

One factor that complicates the DAF effect is the uncertain role of auditory feedback in speech production in normal speakers. Feedback has been a long-standing component of speech production, a part of the model and considered an essential aspect of speech (Denes and Pinson, 1963). And of course we can and do hear ourselves talking. The question is: do we act on this information as we talk; that is, do we use the information our ears provide to modify our speech output as we go along?

Borden (1979) reviewed the literature on feedback processes in normal speakers carefully and critically and concluded that feedback may be necessary in the acquisition of speech production skills, but appears to be relatively unimportant in the ongoing speech production of adults. This is not to say, however, that disturbances in feedback do not alter speech. It does suggest, however, that if auditory feedback plays little or no role in speech production in adults, then it is unlikely that a disorder of speech production, such as stuttering, can be caused by a faulty auditory system that disturbs the speaker's feedback system. This argument is diminished however by the fact that (1) feedback is apparently more important in childhood, when stuttering typically begins, than in adulthood and (2) disturbances in feedback can disrupt speech even though normal feedback is not much used in speech production.

The fluency-enhancing effects of DAF have been attributed to distraction (Sheehan, 1970), slowed rate (Starkweather, 1978), and prolonged vowels (Wingate, 1976). Van Riper (1982) thought that the effect was caused by the condition forcing speakers to abandon their usual reliance on auditory feedback in favor of other feedback systems, such as proprioception. This position would not be tenable if Borden's conclusions about the role of feedback in normal speech production are correct. There is no question that DAF is highly distracting, even disturbing. Nor is there any question that it alters the usual feedback processes, whatever they may be. It also slows rate and prolongs vowels. But it remains uncertain why DAF has its fluency-enhancing effect. Is it because it changes the way stutterers talk (and several dimensions of speech may be considered) or because it changes what they hear when they are talking? Of the latter possibilities, it remains uncertain whether it is a kind of distraction effect, in which the stutterer's attention is diverted in some way, or a difference in the way speech is monitored.

More recent research has begun to compare the effects of different fluency-enhancing conditions. Stephen and Haggard (1980) looked at the differential contribution of masking noise and temporal delay under DAF. They asked eleven stutterers and matched controls to read aloud under a number of different conditions of auditory feedback. They systematically manipulated these conditions so as to be able to compare continuous and speech-contingent feedback, delayed and synchronous feedback, and various spectral characteristics of the feedback signal. All of the conditions in which feedback was altered or masked facilitated fluency by reducing the frequency of discontinuities as compared to conditions in which feedback was not altered. There were, however, no significant differences among the different conditions of altered feedback in the number of discontinuities or in the rate of speech. The authors consequently concluded that their study provided no evidence to support the idea that perceptual interference operates to produce stuttering. Instead, the nonspecific effects they found suggested to them that stuttering is reduced when "the presence of noise, possibly on an intermittent basis, acts as a distractor or cognitive device reducing the relative awareness of the stutterer's own disfluent speech" (p. 537).

Although there is evidence to suggest that simple distractors do not ameliorate stuttering (Beech and Fransella, 1968), it still seems possible that stimuli that make it difficult for stutterers to listen to themselves may ameliorate stuttering. The simple distractors used in Beech and Fransella's work had little of the power to distract the subjects from their speech that DAF and masking have. The whole concept of distraction or "a cognitive device reducing the relative awareness of the stutterer's own disfluent speech" seems deserving of a second, more tolerant look. Fluency-enhancing conditions could direct stutterers' attention away from their stuttering, away from speech production (not just stuttering), or it could be that these conditions direct stutterers attention toward speech production by altering it, and thus enhancing control. It would be useful for researchers to explore different types of distractions. Armson (1986) has recently reviewed the motor control literature. She found, among other things, a fact which has escaped our attention for a while: the amount and kind of attention a person focuses on a specific movement influences the coordination of the movement. Too much attention of the wrong sort can impair smooth and efficient movement.

Rhythmic Stimulation

Findings

1. Stutterers speak more fluently when timing the onset of words or syllables with a rhythmic signal, such as a metronome (Johnson and Rosen, 1937; Barber, 1939; 1940; VanDantzig, 1940; Bloodstein, 1950; Greenberg, 1970).

2. An irregular rhythm is less effective than a regular one (Meyer and Mair, 1963; Fransella and Beech, 1965; Fransella, 1967).

3. The effect of rhythmic stimulation may be partly due to the slowed rate of speech that this condition induces (Conture, 1974a), but some investigations suggest that there is an effect independent of rate (Fransella and Beech, 1965).

4. Any signal that informs a stutterer when to begin an utterance will enhance fluency (Beech and Fransella, 1968).

5. Nonstutterers also become more fluent when pacing their speech to a metronome, and the effect is proportionately just as great as with stutterers (Silverman, 1971).

6. Rhythmic stimulation does not seem to affect vocal intensity although it does slow down rate as it reduces stuttering frequency (Conture and Metz, 1982).

Theory

When stutterers are asked to talk so that each syllable is produced simultaneously with a regular rhythm such as that produced by a metronome, stuttering is typically reduced. The effect is a strong one, not unlike that of DAF in the success with which fluency is enhanced. Speech is drastically altered in both stutterers and nonstutterers by timing syllables to coincide with a rhythmic stimulus. Several types of changes are evident. Usually, speech is slowed by syllable timing, but because the tempo of speech production is under the control of the stimulus, it is possible to ask subjects to speak in syllable-timed speech that is as rapid as uncontrolled speech. When this is done a substantial fluency enhancement remains, suggesting that although some of the effect may be attributed to slowed rate, some of it is attributed to another element, the rhythm itself perhaps, or the use of the stimuli to time the onset of the syllable.

It is still unclear, however, why speaking in time to a rhythm should enhance fluency, either in normals or in stutterers. Under ordinary conditions, the rhythm of speech is irregular; a stressed syllable is followed by a brief run of unstressed syllables. There is a partial tendency in the direction of isochrony, that is, a tendency for the run of unstressed syllables to be produced more rapidly when the run is longer than when it is shorter, as if the speaker were trying to achieve a more regular rhythm in which there would be equal intervals between stressed syllables. But in fact, speakers do not achieve isochrony. The intervals between stressed syllables are not equal. Perhaps, however, the tendency speakers show in the direction of isochrony suggests that a more regular rhythm supports speech production. Perhaps it is easier in some way to produce speech sounds if it can be done in a more regular rhythm.

Another effect of rhythmic stimulation is a reduction in stress contrast. When speaking one syllable at a time, equal stress is placed on all syllables. This reduces the necessity of making the small surges of subglottal air pressure that produce stressed syllables (Minifie, Hixon, and Williams, 1973) and in this way simplifies the task of producing syllables. This simplification simultaneously reduces the requirements for maintaining optimal GTA, since the folds do not have to be readjusted for tension with each brief surge in subglottal air pressure. Because this explanation suggests that fluency is enhanced when motor speech production is simplified, it supports the theory that stuttering is a disorder of speech motor control. A good test of this interpretation would be to monitor abdominal muscle activity under conditions of rhythmic stimulation and see if stuttering reduction was correlated with the reduction in abdominal muscle activity.

Odds and Ends

Findings

1. When a stutterer speaks in unison with another speaker (choral speech), he is usually fluent, even if the other speaker is also a stutterer (Johnson and Rosen, 1937). The effect occurs even if the stutterer increases his rate of speech to match that of the model (Adams and Ramig, 1980).
2. A stutterer can usually say fluently a word that another speaker has just said (shadowing) (Cherry and Sayers, 1956; Cherry, Sayers, and Marland, 1956; Cherry, 1957; Sergeant, 1961).
3. Stutterers rarely stutter when they sing (Fletcher, 1928; Johnson and Rosen, 1937; Bloodstein, 1950; Klemm, 1966; Wingate, 1969).
4. Stutterers are more fluent when they read more slowly (1 word per second) than at their normal rate (Adams, Lewis, and Besozzi, 1973). They reduce rate both by slowing the rate of articulatory movements and by injecting pause time into the utterance (Healey and Adams, 1981).
5. Stutterers are more fluent when they speak in a voice that is pitched higher than usual, perhaps because when talking at a higher pitch they slow the rate of speech production (Ramig and Adams, 1980).
6. Stuttering is reduced when stutterers time hand gestures or other body movements to coincide with the production of stressed syllables or of words on which stuttering is expected to occur. In normal speakers, hand gestures tend to coincide with the production of stressed syllables (Condon and Ogston, 1966; Duchan, Oliva, and Lindner, 1979).
7. Some stutterers speak more fluently when they adopt a foreign or regional dialect or when they play a role (Sheehan, 1970).

Theory

The reduction of stuttering during choral speaking and during shadowing should be seen, most probably, as the same phenomenon. When a stutterer is given a model to follow, either simultaneously as in choral speech or with a slight delay as in shadowing, stuttering is reduced. This is a strong fluency-enhancing effect, like masking noise, DAF, and rhythmic stimulation, producing a marked reduction, and often a complete removal, of stuttering behaviors as long as the condition lasts. The effect appears not to be attributable to rate reduction, since, as Adams and Ramig (1980) discovered, when the stutterer is asked to speak in chorus with a tape recording, he will speed up to match the model and yet still show a fluency-enhancing effect. Although it is not clear just why choral speech enhances fluency, it is interesting from a theoretical point of view because the task of speaking in chorus or of shadowing is perceptually more difficult. There is an additional complex speech signal that must be processed rapidly for the information to be used. This suggests that stuttering is not a result of faulty perception. It is, conversely, intuitively correct to suppose that the motor task of speech production is simplified if the other speaker's timing decision can be used. Of course, it is not at all clear that this is why choral speaking enhances fluency, although alternative suggestions seem weak by comparison. Wingate (1976) suggests that vowels are prolonged in choral speech, which is probably true in most types of choral speech, but in the Adams and Ramig experiment described above, vowels were probably not prolonged, because speech rate was not decreased.

The effect of singing as a fluency-enhancement condition always seems to puzzle laypeople the most, and it is a strong effect. But in fact sung speech combines elements from a number of other conditions known to enhance fluency—the rhythm of the song provides a kind of support, perhaps like the support provided by rhythmic stimulation or choral speech. In addition, the vowels in sung speech are greatly prolonged relative to the consonants, and the rate of speech production is slowed. Furthermore, the lyrics of the song are preformulated and often well known to the singer. When Healey, Mallard, and Adams (1976) asked stutterers to sing a familiar song with unfamiliar words, they found the condition to be fluency-enhancing but less so than when the words were known. Perhaps important also is the fact that the words of a song are not self-formulated and are not used to communicate in the same way as formulated speech.

Healey and Adams (1981) were interested to see what changes in speaking occurred when subjects, both stutterers and nonstutterers, were asked to read slowly. They wanted to find out if the fluency-enhancing effect occurred because subjects injected pause time between words or whether they actually moved their vocal tracts more slowly, a distinction with important implications for motor and timing theories of stuttering. They asked ten normally speaking children, ten normally speaking adults, ten stuttering children, and ten stuttering adults to say two sentences which were matched for number of phonemes, number of syllables, number of words, and number of continuants.

The two sentences were "Pass the sauce to me," and "Sis took the cake out." In one condition, the subjects were asked to say the sentence at "half speed." Four measures were made: (1) consonant duration, (2) vowel duration, (3) duration of "interword silent intervals," and (4) utterance duration. Although there was a wide range across subjects in the degree to which they increased utterance duration, all groups and individuals slowed down when asked to speak at "half speed," even though their interpretation of this instruction must have varied.

There was a strong tendency for all subjects to use a combination of both strategies of rate reduction—slowing down the speed of movements during speech and pausing between words. However, extended pause durations contributed more to the overall decrease in rate than vowel or consonant duration. Healey and Adams' results (1981) suggest nevertheless that speakers slow down the most where they can inject the most time without altering the information-bearing characteristics of language. Their results seem to show that stutterers follow the same pattern. It is unfortunate that the authors of this study did not attempt to find and compare the correlations between injected pause time and fluency enhancement and between slowed articulatory rate and fluency enhancement. A comparison of the two correlations would have answered the question more explicitly.

Ramig and Adams (1980) studied a related topic—altered pitch. When asked to speak in a voice that is pitched either higher or lower than usual, stutterers tend to stutter less. This is not as strong a fluency enhancement condition as some others, because many stutterers do not show the effect, but it is nonetheless interesting. One of the ways in which altered pitch could enhance fluency is by slowing rate. Ramig and Adams set out to test this hypothesis and at the same time to see which of the two rate reduction strategies that Healey and Adams (1981) had identified would be used. They asked a group of nine stuttering children and matched controls to read an 87 syllable passage. Another group of nine stuttering adults and matched controls read another passage, 80 syllables long. Vowels located between two voiceless fricatives in the words *fish, sauce, sis,* and *fuss,* were analyzed. There were three speaking conditions—normal, high-pitched, and low-pitched— the altered pitch conditions being achieved through instructions. Utterances judged to contain stuttering were discarded. Ramig and Adams found that reading rate (stuttered words removed) was reduced in the conditions of altered pitch when compared with normally pitched voice. It may be that a speaker slows down when asked to talk in an unusual way, possibly because of the extra demands on motor planning that an alteration of normal speaking require.

To see which strategy of rate reduction was used, Ramig and Adams compared the vowel and pause durations in the normal conditions with the vowel and pause durations in the pitch-altered conditions. First, there were no differences between stutterers and nonstutterers in the strategy used to change rate. There were, however, some minor differences between adults and children. Of the children, 61 percent increased vowel duration, but only to a nonsignificant degree. All of the children increased pause duration, and significantly so. Of the adults, 59 percent increased vowel duration, whereas 81 percent increased pause duration. Both types of rate change were significant. So children seemed more inclined to pause and less inclined to lengthen vowel duration than adults.

Bearing in mind that these changes in rate occurred indirectly, following instructions to alter pitch, these results might be taken to mean that when an unusual way of talking is requested, some additional motor-planning time is needed. Adults are more likely to achieve it by combining pause and vowel durations, whereas children are more likely to achieve it by stopping completely for a moment from time to time. The results also suggest that fluency enhancement may occur indirectly as a result of the changes in rate or timing that an unusual way of talking seems to create. These results do not necessarily contradict any of the various distraction hypotheses. It could be that talking in an unusual way directs the stutterer's attention to speech or away from stuttering, or both. It is possible that rate reduction is an incidental by-product. A study is needed in which the correlation is determined between stuttering frequency and (1) the amount of rate change and (2) a measure (if one can be devised) of the stutterer's focused attention on speech. A high correlation would demonstrate that the concomitance was not coincidental.

Adams and Ramig (1980) studied another condition known to reduce stuttering—choral reading—to see what kind of changes accompanied changes in fluency. They had a speaker record a reading passage, and then asked the stutterers and controls to read along with the playback. In another condition the subjects read the passage by themselves. Vocal sound pressure level (SPL), the continuity of phonation, and vowel duration were all measured. There were no differences in vocal SPL or in the continuity of phonation between the two kinds of reading conditions, either for the stutterers or the control group. There were differences in vowel duration, however. The nonstutterers, as a group, lengthened their vowels as they slowed down to match the tape-recorded speaker's somewhat slower speech rate. The stutterers, slower in reading by themselves, shortened their vowels as they speeded up their rate to match the same speaker, this despite increased fluency in the choral-reading condition.

This finding calls to mind the fact that metronome pacing also seems to enhance fluency without slowing down the rate of speech (Beech and Fransella, 1968). Because choral reading and paced speech both control the rate and rhythm of speech externally, it may be that such conditions do not require slowed rate to achieve their effect. In contrast, conditions in which the rate and rhythm are not under external control, such as whispering, masked speech, and pitch alteration, require the stutterer to slow down and thus ameliorate stuttering.

This suggests a two-pronged explanation of fluency enhancement in which stuttering is relieved by conditions that either (1) remove from the stutterer the need to plan the rhythm of an utterance or (2) slow speech so that additional planning time is available. Such an explanation has been given (Starkweather, 1982). According to this explanation, DAF would be doubly effective, because it does impose external control over rhythm, specifically by slowing rate. Singing also typically slows rate and imposes an external rhythm. Theoretically, a test of this explanation could be made in sung speech by having stutterers sing songs that were faster and slower than their normal rate. I'm not sure if a song that fast can be found, or if found, if it can be sung, but the explanation suggests that singing would enhance fluency even at very fast rates. The familiarity of the lyrics, the changes in vocal SPL, and alterations in the relative duration of consonants and vowels might also be factors that would have to be controlled in such a test.

Another effect has not been included in most discussions of fluency enhancement. Every clinician has seen stutterers who have developed the habit of using a simultaneous hand or foot gesture, or an eyeblink, to begin a syllable on which they expect to stutter. By performing the gesture simultaneously with the syllable, the fluency of the syllable is enhanced. In normal speakers, certain types of gestures are typically performed in synchrony with stressed syllables of the utterance (Condon and Ogston, 1966; Duchan, Oliva, and Lindner, 1979). Although normal speakers may have the feeling that these simultaneous hand gestures do make it easier for them to talk, there is as yet little experimental evidence that motor speech production is enhanced by synchronous gestures, although it may be. Further investigation of the relation between speech fluency (in the broad sense defined in this paper) and gestural facilitation of speech may prove fruitful.

The apparent fluency-enhancing effects of synchronous hand gesturing seem to occur because the gesture supports the rhythmic structure of speech. That there is a rhythm to speech is indisputable, but its role in speech production is a subject of discussion. Martin (1979) believes that the existence of a rule-determined rhythmic structure implies that decisions about timing (relative accent) are made early in the production sequence. This idea is supported by analysis of slips of the tongue (Boomer and Laver, 1968), which suggest that timing decisions precede other motor speech decisions, laying down a kind of rhythmic template on which the other details of motor speech are elaborated. Because it is determined early, the rhythmic structure of speech results in a sense of momentum, a feeling that once we have started an utterance it almost goes by itself and requires some effort to abort (Ladefoged, Silverstine, and Papcun, 1973).

Martin's description of stress contrast suggests that this sense of momentum may come from the relation between accented and unaccented syllables. He states that "accented syllables are the primary targets of ballistic movements, and . . . intervening unaccented syllables are produced by 'secondary' articulatory gestures 'en route' to the target syllables" (Martin, 1979, p. 500). The rhythmic structure thus facilitates rapid, fluent speech by predetermining the temporal locations of specific units, namely accented syllables. Indeed, the perception of accent depends at least partly on temporal context and relative timing, not just on the characteristics of the accented syllables themselves (Martin, 1979).

Speech rhythm has been assessed in previous studies primarily with regard to its uses for the listener, as in Martin's theoretical paper. But it should also be considered that the enhanced expectancy of temporal targets provided by the rhythm is an aid to producing as well as perceiving fluent speech.

Foreknowledge of temporal locations provided by a conventionally shared rhythmic structure could aid in decoding language by preadjusting the listener's perceptual mechanism. If the listener is prepared in advance, or preset, to hear only stressed syllables at a particular temporal location, one decoding decision has already been made, at least partially, and the series of decisions that comprise decoding is thus shortened. Thus, rhythm may speed up the decoding process, enabling the speaker to talk at a faster rate without losing intelligibility.

This use of rhythm seems to make sense when the premise that we speak as fast as possible is accepted. Evidence in support of this premise comes from a review of normal fluency (Starkweather, 1981) which examined a number of experiments that supported a relation between rate and the level of uncertainty. If rate is slowed at points of uncertainty, as the evidence suggests, then it is effective transmission of information that is the criterion determining how quickly we talk.

Furthermore, a close correspondence between the normal rate of speech (13.5 phones per second) and measures of the maximum speed of movement of the speech mechanism, such as diadochokinetic rate (DDK), was observed by Tiffany (1980). The correspondence is also compelling between normal speech rate and reaction time. Netsell and Daniel (1974) found that reaction time for lip closure to an external stimulus was approximately 200 msec, corresponding to 5 movements per second. Of course, there may be more than 1 movement per syllable, but the correspondence between this finding and the average syllabic rate of approximately 5 syllables per second (Miller, 1951) is compelling.

There is another way of looking at this close correspondence between maximum rate for DDK and reaction time with normal speech rate, and that is that we talk even faster than we can move. Not really, of course, but it may be that something about speech makes it easier to produce at faster rates than nonspeech movements, as in reaction time studies or noncommunicative movements of the speech mechanism as in DDK rates. The element that allows for faster movement in actual speech could be the rhythmic structure discussed above. It could also be that in connected speech there is more opportunity for coarticulatory overlap. This latter possibility is intriguing for two reasons. Extensive coarticulatory overlap diminishes vowel formant frequencies and, in general, there is a loss of intelligibility as the rate of speech increases (Gay, 1978). This loss may be minimized by the fact that speech rhythm aids the decoder, and of course it is also minimized by the natural redundancy of language. Therefore two elements are present in connected, self-formulated speech—redundancy and rhythm—that could make it possible to speak more rapidly. These elements are not present in DDK or reaction time tasks. Consequently, normal speakers are able to "talk faster than they can move." This may not be so for stutterers.

ADAPTATION

Findings

1. Stuttering decreases with repeated speaking of the same or similar material (Johnson and Knott, 1937; Sheehan, 1951; Wischner, 1952; Newman, 1954; Leutenegger, 1957; Rousey, 1958).
2. The disfluencies of normal speakers also decrease with repeated speaking of the same or similar material (Brutten, 1963b; Silverman, 1970a, 1970b).
3. Stuttering decreases just as readily when the repeated readings are fluent (choral) speech as when they are disfluent (Frank and Bloodstein, 1971).
4. Adaptation also occurs with repeated utterance of single words on which stuttering has occurred, but with further repetition of the same word, stuttering will return, leading to alternating periods of fluency and stuttering (Silverman and Williams, 1971).
5. After adaptation has occurred, a rest period will result in a spontaneous recovery of stuttering nearly to the original level (Johnson and Knott, 1937).

6. There is a tendency for the same words of a passage to be stuttered in repeated readings (the consistency effect) (Johnson and Knott, 1937).
7. There is a tendency for stuttering to occur on words adjacent to words previously stuttered (Brutten and Shoemaker, 1967). There have been

failures to demonstrate the adjacency effect (Wong and Bloodstein, 1977).

8. Anxiety does not systematically decrease during an adaptation sequence, although it is correlated with the frequency of stuttering on the first trial (Gray and Brutten, 1965).

9. The adaptation effect is specific not only to the words spoken but to the speech gestures used in producing them—whispered adaptation is independent of voiced adaptation (Bruce and Adams, 1978).

Theory

The adaptation and consistency effects are in many ways more interesting historically than theoretically. At one time, the fact that stuttering showed adaptation and consistency was given great theoretical importance. This emphasis arose because of the similarity in shape of the adaptation curve to the curves shown during the extinction of learned responses. In an extinction curve, there is an early rapid reduction in the frequency with which the behavior occurs, then a gradual flattening until the base rate of performance is reached. A similar pattern is evident when stutterers are asked to read a passage out loud repeatedly. They stutter a great deal less on the second reading than on the first, somewhat less on the third reading than the second, and a bit less on the fourth reading than on the third. By the fifth reading, the decrease in stuttering frequency is quite small. With continued repeated readings, a plateau is reached and there is no further reduction. Given a rest period, there is a spontaneous recovery much like that seen following a rest period after the extinction of a learned response. This sequence of events is illustrated in Figure 7-1. Early theorists were impressed by the similarity between adaptation and learning curves and

FIGURE 7-1 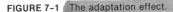 The adaptation effect.

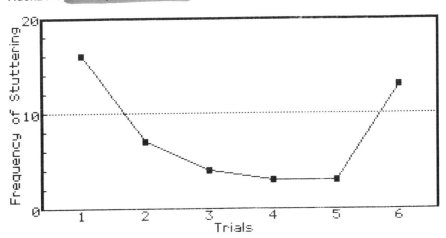

reasoned that stuttering was a learned behavior which was extinguished during adaptation and then spontaneously recovered after a rest period.

Because the prevailing theories of the day were that stuttering was a learned response based on fear and anxiety, theorists reasoned that with increased familiarity, the fear of stuttering or of the speech situation diminished and as a result stuttering decreased. Experiments suggested, however, that anxiety had little effect on adaptation. Gray and Brutten (1965) monitored the anxiety level of subjects during an adaptation sequence and found no clear relationship between the reduction in stuttering frequency and fluctuations in arousal level during an adaptation sequence except that stutterers with high arousal levels tended to show more stuttering on the first trial. After the first trial there was no relationship between these two variables. Evidently, the decrease in stuttering that occurred with repeated reading had little to do with reductions in anxiety.

The early finding that nonstutterers also showed a reduction in the number of discontinuities with repeated readings of the same material was perhaps not given as much importance as it deserved. It was, to be sure, interpreted as suggesting that stuttering and normal discontinuities were related developmentally—the familiar continuity hypothesis—but the possibility that the adaptation effect might occur with other behaviors, or be something other than the extinction of a learned behavior, was not fully appreciated.

The learning theory explanation of adaptation was attractive not only because it explained the shape of the adaptation curve—by itself not a very compelling reason for accepting the learning theory explanation—but also because it explained so well the other part of adaptation, the consistency effect. When a stutterer is asked to read a passage repeatedly, there is a tendency for certain words to be stuttered on each reading, in spite of the concurrent adaptation of stuttering on other words. These consistently stuttered words are individually specific and share no common characteristics. This combination of facts led theorists to conclude that the words that showed this consistency effect had greater habit strength than other words in the passage that extinguished more easily. This idea led to the prediction that if the passages were read many more than the usual five times, even the consistently stuttered words would eventually lose their ability to elicit stuttering and adapt out. However, attempts to achieve zero frequency stuttering through long periods of adaptation did not succeed.

The learning theory explanation of the adaptation effect also predicted that words not previously stuttered would acquire the capacity to elicit stuttering by continued association with words that were consistently stuttered. There were several ways such an association could occur, but the simplest idea was that words adjacent to stuttered words would be more likely to be stuttered on subsequent readings. This idea came to be called the "adjacency effect." Some evidence of its occurrence was reported (Brutten and Shoemaker, 1967), but other investigators failed to confirm the idea.

Two other ideas were invoked in the 1970s. The first was that adaptation occurred because of stimulus habituation. Stimulus habituation is a common phenomenon: the tendency for a stimulus of any kind to lose its stimulus value with repeated presentation. One example is familiar to anyone who has had a clock that strikes the hour. After a while, you don't hear it strike because you become so habituated to the sound. Our central nervous systems are adept at tuning out redundancy. If a person is asked to perform any task repeatedly, the nature of performance is likely to change as stimuli that elicit various aspects of the performance become habituated. For the stutterer in an adaptation sequence, stimulus habituation would gradually diminish all reactions—not just fears—to words, sounds, and the speaking situation. In addition, reactions to the occurrence of stuttering would also diminish. This last part of the idea was perhaps the most important element, since, according to Johnsonian theory, much of the stutterer's behavior consists of reactions to stuttering and attempts to minimize it.

This idea predicted that more adaptation would occur with repeated readings that included stuttering than would occur with repeated fluent readings, and to test the prediction, Frank and Bloodstein (1971) asked stutterers to read a passage in chorus with other stutterers four times and then to read the passage alone. They compared the frequency of stuttering on the fifth reading following four choral readings with the fifth reading following four nonchoral readings and found that the extent of adaptation was not much different. Apparently, one needn't stutter during adaptation to show the gain in fluency. This study may not have caused the demise of the stimulus habituation idea, since it dealt only with the reactions-to-stuttering part of it, but it caused grave injury when combined with failures of the adjacency effect and other tests of the extinction of word fears hypothesis. Almost by default, the "practice effect" was left as an explanation of the adaptation effect.

This idea was that adaptation occurred because the stutterer was able to "practice" specific motor sequences, an explanation related to motor control theories that developed somewhat later. The idea was probably slow to develop because of an inherent problem in the explanation. If stutterers could adapt out their stuttering behaviors through motor practice, why didn't the common use of speech for everyday communicative purposes provide enough practice to do the same thing? True, some stutterers are extremely reticent and get little practice, but there are also many who talk a great deal. Of course, the difference is that in the adaptation sequence the person says the same words, repeats the same speech gestures and motions, over and over again without much rest between readings, whereas in the communicative uses of speech the same motions and speech gestures are said too infrequently to avoid the recovery of any adaptation effect that might occur.

One prediction from the motor practice effect is that an adaptation sequence in which individual words are said repeatedly would diminish stuttering more rapidly than one in which the practice on individual words was distributed. To test the idea Dancer (1966) had stutterers read a passage five times in a standard adaptation sequence and then had them read each word in the passage five times. A greater adaptation effect occurred when the practice was distributed more closely.

The practice effect interpretation of adaptation was confirmed in another way by Bruce and Adams (1978), who looked at the effect of whispering on adaptation. They asked stutterers to read a passage five times. On the second, third, and fourth trials, the speakers had to whisper. The whispering resulted in less adaptation than reading out loud. Bruce and Adams concluded that adaptation occurred only if the behaviors practiced were the same ones tested later. Even a small alteration in the behavior practiced diminishes the effect. But how does motor practice temporarily facilitate fluency? The answer to this more basic question is not clear. Any movement repeatedly performed becomes temporarily easier to do, and this seems to be the kind of change that is occurring. It is a motor effect, most likely, not a perceptual or a learning-based phenomenon. But beyond that, it tells us little about the nature of stuttering.

So in the end the scorecard shows several wins for the practice effect interpretation of adaptation and several losses for the stimulus habituation and learning theory interpretations.

EXPECTANCY

Findings

1. The ability to predict the words on which stuttering will occur varies from 0 to 100 percent (Knott, Johnson, and Webster, 1937).
2. About 50 percent of stutterers fail to predict the majority of words they will stutter on. The ability to predict does not seem to increase with age (Silverman and Williams, 1972). (Only school-aged children were sampled.)
3. The stutterer's expectation of stuttering decreases with repeated readings of the same material (Brutten, 1957; 1963a).
4. Stutterers show a decrease in alpha activity before saying a feared word as compared with a nonfeared word or a nonspeech task, regardless of whether they stutter on the word (Peters et al., 1976).

Theory

Most stutterers have some advance warning that a word they have decided to say will prove difficult. Some stutterers have a less accurate early warning system than others and fail to predict correctly very often. Others are remarkably accurate. A sizable minority of stutterers have no advance knowledge of stuttering at all.

One theory advanced in the earliest years of the profession was that the expectation of stuttering created the problem in a kind of self-fulfilling prophecy. If the stutterers could only stop expecting to stutter, they would stop doing so. This idea fails badly as a theory because it is so difficult to test. Furthermore, the data show that only some stutterers have some ability to predict, so expectation of stuttering can never do more than contribute to the problem. This is probably true, however. Given some sense that they are about to have trouble getting through a word, most young stutterers will do something to cope with the problem they think they are going to have, and what they do—pushing airflow with greater force, forcing the word out, using a timer or starter, avoiding the word and substituting another one, or any of the countless avoidance behaviors—adds more extraneous behavior and effort to the process of speech production. In this sense, expectation of stuttering creates stuttering behavior. But of course for many stutterers some of the time and for a few stutterers all of the time, there is no advance warning, and for these, stuttering behaviors are clearly not the result of expectation and the avoidance behavior it prompts.

The learning theory interpretations of stuttering suggested early on that the stutterer expects to stutter because the experiences he has had with the disorder make him knowledgeable about his problem, and there is a kind of probabilistic prediction, based on an assessment, made in some cases with little awareness, of the various environmental cues that have been associated with stuttering in the past. Surveying these cues, the stutterer gains a sense of the probability that he will stutter, and if the probability exceeds some threshold, which would be expected to vary from person to person, the expectation of stuttering occurs.

This interpretation of expectancy—that it is based on the stutterer's experience with the disorder—generates the prediction that stutterers who have been stuttering for a longer period of time and therefore have had more experience with the disorder, will be more accurate predictors. Silverman and Williams (1972) did not find this, although the fact that they sampled only schoolchildren suggests that they may have overlooked those stutterers whose experiences with the disorder were greatest, the confirmed adult stutterers. Furthermore, their failure to observe an anticipated outcome does not constitute evidence in opposition to the idea that generated the predicted outcome. It may still be that expectancy is a result of personal experience.

Peters' (1976) study establishes that there really is some neurological event that happens when the stutterer expects to stutter, but of course it doesn't tell us very much about the nature of the event.

To my knowledge, motor control theories have not attempted to deal with this aspect of stuttering, but those who believe that stuttering is caused either by poor vocal tract coordination or excessive muscle activity within the vocal tract (which may be the same thing) would doubtless suggest that the stutterer's expectation of stuttering comes from an awareness of growing tension in the vocal tract. Although the muscles are on the whole small, one can be aware of tension in them. This awareness might be expected to vary for a number of reasons. The tension levels required for disruption might vary from individual to individual, the ability to sense this particular kind of tension or tension in these particular areas might vary from individual to individual, and some individuals may learn to deny or ignore these signals, either for emotional reasons or because awareness of vocal tract activity may interfere somewhat with effective communication.

Prediction based on a sensation of tension (which, by the way, stutterers often report) might not always be an accurate sign of stuttering because different words place different demands on coordination according to the movements required to produce the word, which themselves vary in speed and timing depending on the word's position in the sentence, context, and a number of other factors. So it is not surprising that some stutterers cannot predict very well. What is surprising is that some stutterers can predict with perfect accuracy. These may be stutterers who have clearly elevated vocal tract tension levels, who can sense these levels and have learned to pay close attention to them, and who recognize which word and phrase characteristics are likely to make greater demands on coordination.

Brutten's (1963a) finding that expectancy adapts just as overt stuttering does fits well with either a learning theory or a motor control theory of stuttering. The learning theorist would say that expectancy adapts because the stutterer knows enough about his disorder to recognize that repetitive material elicits less stuttering. The motor control theorist would suggest that repeated practice actually reduces vocal tract tension, which stutterers can sense, and from which they can make a more or less accurate prediction.

REFERENCES

ABBS, J. H., and SMITH, K. U., Laterality differences in the auditory feedback control of speech, *Journal of Speech and Hearing Research*, 13 (1970), 298–303.

ADAMCZYK, B., Use of instruments for the production of artificial feedback in the treatment of stuttering, *Folia Phoniatrica*, 11 (1959), 216–18.

ADAMS, M. R., Vocal tract dynamics in fluency and stuttering: a review and interpretation of past research, in *Vocal Tract Dynamics and Dysfluency*, eds. L. M. Webster and L. C. Furst. First Annual Hayes Martin Conference on Vocal Tract Dynamics. Speech and Hearing Institute, New York City, 1975.

ADAMS, M. R., and MOORE, W. H., Jr., The effects of auditory masking on the anxiety level, frequency of disfluency, and selected vocal characteristics of stutterers, *Journal of Speech and Hearing Research*, 15 (1972), 572–78.

ADAMS, M. R., LEWIS, J. I., and BESOZZI, T. E., The effect of reduced reading rate on stuttering frequency, *Journal of Speech and Hearing Research*, 16 (1973), 572–78.

ADAMS, M. R., and HUTCHINSON, J., The effects of three levels of auditory masking on selected vocal characteristics and the frequency of disfluency of adult stutterers, *Journal of Speech and Hearing Research*, 17 (1974), 682–88.

ADAMS, M. R., and RAMIG, P., Vocal characteristics of stutterers and normal speakers during choral reading, *Journal of Speech and Hearing Research*, 23 (1980), 457–65.

ANDREWS, G., CRAIG, A., FEYER, A–M., HODDINOTT, S., HOWIE, P., and NEILSON, M., Stuttering: a review of research findings and theories circa 1982, *Journal of Speech and Hearing Disorders*, 48 (1983), 226–46.

ARMSON, J., Recent research on the motor control of normal movements. Unpublished manuscript, Temple University, Philadelphia, 1986.

BACHRACH, D. L., Sex differences in reactions to delayed auditory feedback, *Perceptual and Motor Skills*, 19 (1964), 81–82.

BACKUS, O., Incidence of stuttering among the deaf, *Annals of Otology, Rhinology, and Laryngology*, 47 (1938), 632–35.

BARBER, V. A., Studies in the psychology of stuttering: chorus reading as a distraction in stuttering, *Journal of Speech Disorders*, 4 (1939), 371–83.

BARBER, V. A., Rhythm as a distraction in stuttering, *Journal of Speech Disorders*, 5 (1940), 29–42.

BARDRICK, R. A., and SHEEHAN, J. G., Emotional loadings as a source of conflict in stuttering, *American Psychologist*, 11 (1956), 391 (abst.).

BARON, M., The effect of eyelid conditioning of a speech variable in stutterers and nonstutterers. Ph.D. dissertation, University of Iowa, Iowa City, 1949.

BEECH, H. R., and FRANSELLA, F., *Research and Experiment in Stuttering*. New York: Pergamon, 1968.

BELMORE, N., KEWLEY-PORT, D., MOBLEY, R., and GOODMAN, V., The development of auditory feedback monitoring: delayed auditory feedback studies on the vocalizations of children aged six months to nineteen months, *Journal of Speech and Hearing Research*, 16 (1973), 709–20.

BERWICK, N., Stuttering in response to photographs of listeners. M.A. thesis, University of Iowa, Iowa City, 1939.

BLANKENSHIP, J., Stuttering in normal speech, *Journal of Speech and Hearing Research*, 7 (1964), 65–86.

BLOODSTEIN, O., Hypothetic conditions under which stuttering is reduced or absent, *Journal of Speech and Hearing Disorders*, 15 (1950), 142–53.

BLOODSTEIN, O., and GANTWERK, B. F., Grammatical function in relation to stuttering in young children, *Journal of Speech and Hearing Research*, 10 (1967), 786–89.

BLOODSTEIN, O., and SHOGAN, R. L., Some clinical notes on forced stuttering, *Journal of Speech and Hearing Disorders*, 37 (1972), 177–86.

BOHR, J. W. F., The effects of electronic and other external control methods on stuttering: a review of some research techniques and suggestions for future research, *Journal of the South African Logopedic Society*, 10 (1963), 4–13.

BOOMER, D. S., Review of F. Goldman-Eisler, Psycholinguistics experiments in spontaneous speech, *Lingua*, 25 (1970), 152–64.

BORDEN, G., An interpretation of research on feedback interruption in speech, *Brain and Language*, 7 (1979), 307–19.

BROEN, P. A., and SIEGEL, G. M., Variations in normal speech disfluencies, *Language and Speech*, 15 (1972), 219–31.

BROWN, S. F., Stuttering with relation to word accent and word position, *Journal of Abnormal and Social Psychology*, 32 (1938), 112–20.

BROWN, S. F., and MOREN, A., The frequency of stuttering in relation to word length during oral reading, *Journal of Speech Disorders*, 7 (1942), 153–59.

BRUCE, M. C., and ADAMS, M. R., Effects of two types of motor practice on stuttering, *Journal of Speech and Hearing Research*, 21 (1978), 421–28.

BRUTTEN, E. J., A colorimetric anxiety measure of stuttering and expectancy adaptation. Ph.D. dissertation, University of Illinois, Urbana, 1957.

BRUTTEN, E. J., Fluency and disfluency: an investigation of expectancy adaptation, ASHA: *Journal of the American Speech and Hearing Association*, 6 (1963a), 781.

BRUTTEN, E. J., Palmar sweat investigation of disfluency and expectancy adaptation, *Journal of Speech and Hearing Research*, 6 (1963b), 40–48.

BRUTTEN, E. J., and SHOEMAKER, D. J., *The Modification of Stuttering.* Englewood Cliffs, N.J.: Prentice-Hall, 1967.

BUXTON, L. F., An investigation of sex and age differences in speech behavior under delayed auditory feedback. Ph.D. dissertation, Ohio State University, Columbus, 1969.

CHASE, R. A., SUTTON, S., and RAPIN, I., Sensory feedback influences on motor performance, *Journal of Auditory Research*, 1 (1961), 212–23.

CHERRY, E., *On Human Communication.* New York: John Wiley, 1957.

CHERRY, E., and SAYERS, B., Experiments upon total inhibition of stammering by external control and some clinical results, *Journal of Psychomotor Research*, 1 (1956), 233–46.

CHERRY, E., SAYERS, B., and MARLAND, P., Some experiments on the total suppression of stammering and a report on some clinical trials, *Bulletin of the British Psychological Society*, 30 (1956), 43–44.

CONDON, W. S., and OGSTON, W. D., Soundfilm analysis of normal and pathological behavioral patterns, *Journal of Nervous and Mental Disease*, 143 (1966), 338–47.

CONTURE, E., The influence of rhythmic stimulation on certain vocal characteristics of stutterers. Convention address, New York State Speech and Hearing Association, 1974a.

CONTURE, E., Some effects of noise on the speaking behavior of stutterers, *Journal of Speech and Hearing Research*, 17 (1974b), 714–23.

CONTURE, E. G., McCALL, G., and BREWER, D. W., Laryngeal behavior during stuttering, *Journal of Speech and Hearing Research*, 20 (1977), 661–68.

CONTURE, E. G., and METZ, D. E., The influence of rhythmic stimulation on certain vocal characteristics of stutterers. Convention address, New York State Speech and Hearing Association, 1982.

CONWAY, J., and QUARRINGTON, B., Positional effects in the stuttering of contextually organized verbal material, *Journal of Abnormal and Social Psychology*, 47 (1963), 299–303.

DANCER, J. E., An investigation of stuttering adaptation and recovery under conditions of massed and spaced practice. M.A. thesis, Southern Illinois University, Carbondale, 1966.

DENES, P. B., and PINSON, E., *The Speech Chain.* Oradell, N.J.: Bell Laboratories, 1963.

DIXON, C. C., Stuttering adaptation in relation to assumed level of anxiety. M.A. thesis, University of Iowa, Iowa City, 1947.

DUCHAN, J., OLIVA, J., and LINDNER, R., Performative acts defined by synchrony among intonational verbal and nonverbal systems in a one-and-a-half-year-old child, *Sign Language Studies*, 22 (1979), 75–88.

EISENSON, J., and HOROWITZ, E., The influence of propositionality on stuttering, *Journal of Speech Disorders*, 10 (1945), 193–97.

FAIRBANKS, G., Some correlates of sound difficulty in stuttering, *Quarterly Journal of Speech*, 23 (1937), 67–69.

FLETCHER, J. M., *The Problem of Stuttering.* New York: Longmans, 1928.

FROESCHELS, E., Pathology and therapy of stuttering, *The Nervous Child*, 2 (1943), 148–61.

FRANK, A., and BLOODSTEIN, O., Frequency of stuttering following repeated unison readings, *Journal of Speech and Hearing Research*, 14 (1971), 519–24.

FRANSELLA, F., Rhythm as a distractor in the modification of stuttering, *Behavior Research and Therapy*, 5 (1967), 253–55.

FRANSELLA, F., and BEECH, H. R., An experimental analysis of the effect of rhythm on the speech of stutterers, *Behavior Research and Therapy*, 3 (1965), 195–201.

FROESCHELS, E., New viewpoints on stuttering, *Folia Phoniatrica*, 13 (1961), 187–201.

GARBER, S., and MARTIN, R., Effects of noise on increased vocal intensity and stuttering, *Journal of Speech and Hearing Research*, 20 (1977), 233–40.

GAY, T., Effect of speaking rate on vowel formant movements, *Journal of the Acoustical Society of America*, 63 (1978), 223–30.

GOLDFARB, W., and BRAUNSTEIN, P., Reactions to Delayed Auditory Feedback in Schizophrenic Children, in *Psychotherapy of Communication*, ed. P.H. Hock and J. Zubin. New York: Grune & Stratton, 1958.

GOLDMAN-EISLER, F., The predictability of words in context, and the length of pauses in speech, *Language and Speech*, 1 (1958), 226–31.

GOLDIAMOND, I., Stuttering and fluency as manipulable operant response classes, in *Research in Behavior Modification*, eds. L. Krasner and L. Ullman. New York: Holt, Rinehart & Winston, 1965.

GOLDIAMOND, I., ATKINSON, C. J., and BILGER, R. C., Stabilization of behavior and prolonged exposure to delayed auditory feedback, *Science*, 137 (1962), 437–38.

GRAY, B. B., and BRUTTEN, G. J., The relationship between anxiety, fatigue, and spontaneous recovery in stuttering, *Behavior Research and Therapy*, 2 (1965), 251–59.

GREENBERG, J. B., The effect of a metronome on the speech of young stutterers, *Behavior Therapy*, 1 (1970), 240–44.

GROSS, M. S., and NATHANSON, S. N., A study of the use of a DAF shaping procedure for adult stutterers. Convention address, American Speech and Hearing Association, 1966.

HAHN, E., A study of the relationship between stuttering occurrence and grammatical factors in oral reading, *Journal of Speech Disorders*, 7 (1942), 329–55.

HAM, R., and STEER, M. D., Certain effects of alterations in auditory feedback, *Folia Phoniatrica*, 19 (1967), 53–62.

HARMS, M. A., and MALONE, J. Y., The relationship of hearing acuity to stammering, *Journal of Speech Disorders*, 4 (1939), 363–70.

HAROLDSON, S. K., MARTIN, R. R., and STARR, C. D., Time-out as a punishment for stuttering, *Journal of Speech and Hearing Research*, 11 (1968), 560–66.

HEALEY, E. C., and ADAMS, M. R., Speech timing skills of normally fluent and stuttering children and adults, *Journal of Fluency Disorders*, 6 (1981), 233–46.

HEALEY, E. C., MALLARD, A. R., and ADAMS, M. R., Factors contributing to the reduction of stuttering during singing, *Journal of Speech and Hearing Research*, 19 (1976), 475–80.

HEJNA, R. F., A study of the loci of stuttering in spontaneous speech. *Dissertation Abstracts*, 15 (1955), 1674–75.

HUNNICUTT, S., Intelligibility versus redundancy—conditions of dependency, *Language and Speech*, 28 (1985), 47–56.

JAYARAM, M., Distribution of stuttering in sentences: relationships to sentence length and clause position, *Journal of Speech and Hearing Research*, 27, 1984, 338–41.

JOHNSON, W., and BROWN, S. F., Stuttering in relation to various speech sounds, *Quarterly Journal of Speech*, 21 (1935), 481–96.

JOHNSON, W., and KNOTT, J. R., Certain objective cues related to the precipitation of the moment of stuttering, *Journal of Speech Disorders*, 2 (1937), 17–19.

JOHNSON, W., and ROSEN, L., Effects of certain changes in speech patterns upon the frequency of stuttering, *Journal of Speech Disorders*, 2 (1937), 101–4.

KERN, A., Der Einfluss des Horens auf das Stottern, *Archive für Psychiatrie und Nervenkrankheiten*, 97 (1932), 429–49.

KLEMM, M., in *Psychopathology and the Problems of Stuttering*, ed. H. Freund, Springfield, Ill.: Charles C Thomas. 1966.

KNOTT, J. R., JOHNSON, W., and WEBSTER, M., Studies in the psychology of stuttering I. A quantitative evaluation of expectation of stuttering in relation to the occurrence of stuttering, *Journal of Speech Disorders*, 2 (1937), 20–22.

LADEFOGED, P., SILVERSTINE, R., and PAPCUN, G., Interruptibility of speech, *Journal of the Acoustical Society of America*, 54 (1973), 1105–08.

LANYON, R. I., Speech: relation of nonfluency to information value, *Science*, 164 (1970), 451–52.

LEE, B. S., Artificial stuttering, *Journal of Speech and Hearing Disorders*, 16 (1951), 53–55.

LEUTENEGGER, R. R., Adaptation and recovery in the oral reading of stutterers, *Journal of Speech Disorders*, 22 (1957), 276–87.

LOTZMAN, V., Zur anwendung variierter verzogerungszeiten bei balbuties, *Folia Phoniatrica*, 13 (1961), 276–312.

MacKAY, D. G., Metamorphosis of a critical interval: age-linked changes in the delay in auditory feedback that produces maximal disruption of speech, *Journal of the Acoustical Society of America*, 19 (1968), 811–21.

MAHAFFEY, R. B., and STROMSTA, C., Effects of peak-clipped and center-clipped delayed sidetone, *ASHA: Journal of the American Speech and Hearing Association*, 7 (1965), 413–14.

MAHL, C, Disturbances and silences in the patient's speech in psychotherapy, *Journal of Abnormal Social Psychology*, 53 (1956), 1–15.

MARAIST, J. A., and HUTTON, C., Effects of auditory masking upon the speech of stutterers, *Journal of Speech and Hearing Disorders*, 22 (1957), 385–89.

MARTIN, R., Rhythmic (hierarchical) versus serial structure in speech and other behavior, *Psychological Review*, 79 (1979), 487–509.

MARTIN, R., SIEGEL, G., JOHNSON, L., and HAROLDSON, S., Sidetone amplification, noise, and stuttering, *Journal of Speech and Hearing Research*, 27, 1984, 518–27.

McCLAY, H., and OSGOOD, E. I., Hesitation phenomena in spontaneous English speech, *Word*, 15 (1959), 19–44.

MEYER, V., and MAIR, J. M., A new technique to control stammering: a preliminary report, *Behaviour Research and Therapy*, 1 (1963), 251–54.

MILISEN, R., Frequency of stuttering with anticipation of stuttering controlled, *Journal of Speech Disorders*, 3 (1938), 207–14.

MILLER, G. A., Speech and Language, in *Handbook of Experimental Psychology*, ed. S. S. Stevens, New York: John Wiley, 1951.

MINIFIE, F., HIXON, T., and WILLIAMS, F., *Normal Aspects of Speech, Language, and Hearing*. Englewood Cliffs, N.J.: Prentice-Hall, 1973.

MURRAY, F. P., An investigation of variably induced white noise upon moments of stuttering, *Journal of Communication Disorders*, 2 (1969), 109–14.

NADOLECZNY, M., Stuttering as a manifestation of a spastic coordination neurosis, *Archiv für Psychiatrie und Nervenkrankheiten*, 82 (1927), 235–46.

NEELEY, J. N., A study of the speech behavior stutterers and nonstutterers under normal and delayed auditory feedback, *Journal of Speech and Hearing Disorders Monograph Supplement*, No. 7 (1961).

NETSELL, R., and DANIEL, B., Neural and mechanical response time for speech production, *Journal of Speech and Hearing Research*, 17 (1974), 608–18.

NEWMAN, P., A study of adaptation and recovery of the stuttering response in self-formulated speech, *Journal of Speech and Hearing Disorders*, 19 (1954), 312–21.

PETERS, R. W., LOVE, L., OTTO, D., WOOD, T., and BENIGNUS, V., Cerebral processing of speech and nonspeech signals by stutterers, *Proceedings, 16th International Congress of Logopedics and Phoniatrics*, Interlaken, 1974, ed. E. Loebell, Basel: S. Karger, 1976.

QUARRINGTON, B., CONWAY, J., and SIEGEL, N., An experimental study of some properties of stuttered words, *Journal of Speech and Hearing Research*, 5 (1962), 387–94.

QUINN, P. T., Stuttering: some observations on speaking when alone, *Journal of the Australian College of Speech Therapists*, 21 (1971), 92–94.

RAMIG, P., and ADAMS, M. R., Rate reduction strategies used by stutterers and nonstutterers during high- and low-pitched speech, *Journal of Fluency Disorders*, 5 (1980), 27–41.

RAWNSLEY, Q. F., and HARRIS, J. D., Comparative analysis of normal speech and speech with delayed sidetone by means of sound spectrographs, Bureau of Medical Research Project #NM003–04.56.03, 1954.

RONSON, I., Word frequency and stuttering: the relationship to sentence structure, *Journal of Speech and Hearing Research*, 19 (1976), 813–19.

ROUSEY, C., Stuttering severity during prolonged spontaneous speech, *Journal of Speech and Hearing Research*, 1 (1958), 40–47.

SCHLESINGER, I. M., MELKMAN, R., and LEVY, R., Word length and frequency as determinants of stuttering, *Psychonomic Science*, 6 (1966), 255–56.

SERGEANT, R. L., Concurrent repetition of a continuous flow of words, *Journal of Speech and Hearing Research*, 4 (1961), 373–80.

SHANE, M. L. S., Effect on Stuttering of Alteration in Auditory Feedback, in *Stuttering in Children and Adults*, ed. W. Johnson, Minneapolis: University of Minnesota Press, 1955.

SHEEHAN, J. G., The modification of stuttering through nonreinforcement, *Journal of Abnormal and Social Psychology*, 46 (1951), 51–63.

SHEEHAN, J., *Stuttering: Research and Therapy*. New York: Harper & Row, 1970.

SIEGENTHALER, B. M., and BRUBAKER, R. S., Suggested research in delayed auditory feedback, *Pennsylvania Speech Annual*, 14 (1957), 24–31.

SILVERMAN, E-M., Word position and grammatical function in relation to preschoolers' speech disfluency, *Perceptual and Motor Skills*, 39 (1974), 267–72.

SILVERMAN, F. H., Course of nonstutterers' disfluency adaptation during 5 consecutive oral readings of the same material, *Journal of Speech and Hearing Research*, 13 (1970a), 382–86.

SILVERMAN, F. H., A note on the degree of adaptation by stutterers and nonstutterers during oral reading, *Journal of Speech and Hearing Research*, 13 (1970b), 173–77.

SILVERMAN, F. H., The effect of rhythmic auditory stimulation on the disfluency of nonstutterers, *Journal of Speech and Hearing Research*, 14 (1971), 350–55.

SILVERMAN, F. H., Disfluency and word length, *Journal of Speech and Hearing Research*, 15 (1972), 788–91.

SILVERMAN, F. H., and WILLIAMS, D. E., Loci of disfluencies in the speech of nonstutterers during oral reading, *Journal of Speech and Hearing Research*, 10 (1967), 790–94.

SILVERMAN, F. H., and WILLIAMS, D. E., The adaptation effect for six types of speech disfluency, *Journal of Speech and Hearing Research*, 14 (1971), 525–30.

SILVERMAN, F. H., and WILLIAMS, D. E., Prediction of stuttering by school age stutterers, *Journal of Speech and Hearing Research*, 15 (1972), 189–93.

SODERBERG, G., The relations of stuttering to word length and word frequency, *Journal of Speech and Hearing Research*, 9 (1966), 584–89.

SODERBERG, G., Linguistic factors in stuttering, *Journal of Speech and Hearing Research*, 10 (1967), 801–10.

SODERBERG, G., Delayed auditory feedback and stuttering, *Journal of Speech and Hearing Disorders*, 33 (1968), 260–67.

STARK, R. A., and PIERCE, B. R., Effects of delayed auditory feedback upon a speech related task in stutterers, *Journal of Speech and Hearing Research*, 13 (1970), 245–53.

STARKWEATHER, C. W., Recent research on stuttering and vocalization: clinical and theoretical implications. Short course, American Speech and Hearing Association, 1978.

STARKWEATHER, C. W., Speech fluency and its development in normal children, in *Speech and Language: Advances in Basic Research and Practice*, New York: Academic Press, 1981.

STARKWEATHER, C. W., Stuttering and laryngeal behavior: a review. American Speech and Hearing Association, Monograph No. 21, 1982.

STARKWEATHER, C. W., and GORDON, P., Stuttering: the language connection. Short course, American Speech and Hearing Association, Cincinnati, 1983.

STEPHEN, S., and HAGGARD, M., Acoustic properties of masking/delayed feedback on the fluency of stutterers and controls, *Journal of Speech and Hearing Research*, 23 (1980), 527–38.

STROMSTA, C., The effects of altering the fundamental frequency of masking on the speech performance of stutterers. Technical Report, National Institute of Health Project # B–1331, Bethesda, Md., 1958.

STROMSTA, C., The effect of altering the frequency of auditory masking on the speech performance of stutterers. Technical Report, Public Service Grant # B–1331, Ohio State University, 1967.

SUTTON, S., and CHASE, R., White noise and stuttering, *Journal of Speech and Hearing Research*, 4 (1961), 72.

TAYLOR, I. K., The properties of stuttered words, *Journal of Verbal Learning and Verbal Behavior*, 5 (1966), 112–18.

TIFFANY, W. R., The effects of syllable structure on diadochokinetic and reading rates, *Journal of Speech and Hearing Research*, 23 (1980), 894–908.

TIMMONS, B. A., Sex as a factor influencing sensitivity to DAF, *Perceptual and Motor Skills*, 32 (1971), 824–26.

TORNICK, G., and BLOODSTEIN, O., Stuttering and sentence length, *Journal of Speech and Hearing Research*, 19 (1976), 651–54.

UMEDA, N., Vowel duration in American English, *Journal of the Acoustical Society of America*, 58 (1975), 434–45.

UMEDA, N., Consonant duration in American English, *Journal of the Acoustical Society of America*, 61 (1977), 846–58.

VANDANTZIG, M., Syllable-tapping: a new method for the help of stammerers, *Journal of Speech Disorders*, 5 (1940), 127–32.

VAN RIPER, C., *The Nature of Stuttering*, 2nd ed. Englewood Cliffs, N.J.: Prentice-Hall, 1982.

WALL, M., The location of stuttering in the spontaneous speech of young child stutterers. Ph.D. dissertation, City University of New York, 1977.

WALL, M., STARKWEATHER, C., and CAIRNS, H., Syntactic influences on stuttering in young child stutterers, *Journal of Fluency Disorders*, 6 (1981), 283–98.

WALLE, G., *Prevention of Stuttering*, (film). Memphis, Tenn.: Speech Foundation of America, 1975.

WEBSTER, R. L., and DORMAN, M. F., Decreases in stuttering frequency as a function of continuous and contingent forms of auditory masking, *Journal of Speech and Hearing Research*, 13 (1970), 82–86.

WINGATE, M. E., Sound and pattern in "artificial" fluency, *Journal of Speech and Hearing Research*, 12 (1969), 677–86.

WINGATE, M. E., Effect on stuttering of changes in audition. *Journal of Speech and Hearing Research*, 13 (1970), 861–73.

WINGATE, M. E., *Stuttering: Theory and Treatment*. New York: Irvington, 1976.

WISCHNER, G. J., An experimental approach to expectancy and anxiety in stuttering behavior, *Journal of Speech and Hearing Disorders*, 17 (1952), 139–54.

WITT, M., Statistische erhebungen über den Einfluss des Singens und Flustern auf Stottern, *Vox*, 5 (1925), 41–43.

WONG, C. Y., and BLOODSTEIN, O., Effect of adjacency on the distribution of new stutterings in two successive readings, *Journal of Speech and Hearing Research*, 20 (1977), 35–39.

ZERNERI, E., Attempts to use delayed speech feedback in stuttering therapy, *Journal Francais d' Oto-Rhino-Laryngologie et Chirurgie Maxillo-Faciale*, 15 (1966), 415–18.

ZIMMERMANN, G., Stuttering: a disorder of movement, *Journal of Speech and Hearing Research*, 23 (1980), 122–36.

Differences Between Stutterers and Nonstutterers

INTRODUCTION

This chapter introduces a new approach. So far, I have been discussing information that describes stuttering. Now information that explains it or can be used to explain it will be presented. Not that this text will provide an explanation, but rather that the theory presented will be explanatory rather than descriptive. I will, in other words, begin now to confront that most difficult of questions: Why do people stutter?

Information bearing on the answer to this question comes from diverse experiments, and I have divided them somewhat arbitrarily into two large categories—general comparisons between stutterers and nonstutterers, which is the subject of this chapter, and comparisons of the communicative (speech, language, or hearing) performance of stutterers, which is the subject of the next chapter.

GENERAL PHYSIOLOGICAL DIFFERENCES

Findings

1. Stutterers have more diseases of the respiratory system than nonstutterers (Berry, 1938).
2. Stutterers are more likely to have pathological nystagmoid reflexes than nonstutterers (Schilling, 1959; Baldan, 1965; Bruno, Camarda, and Curi, 1965).
3. Stuttering is more common in twins than in uniparous individuals (Nelson, Hunter, and Walter, 1945; Graf, 1955).
4. Despite much research, the biochemistry of stutterers seems to be the same as that of nonstutterers. These studies have been mostly con-

cerned with low calcium levels and parathyroid insufficiency (Hill, 1954).

Theory

Are stutterers different from nonstutterers in some general physiological way? For some years during the 1940s and 1950s, when the theorists were impressed by the spasmodic, involuntary nature of stuttering behaviors, a great search went on to find the cause of stutterers' supposed predisposition to spasm. There was, at the same time, a widespread belief that people with diabetes did not stutter. This belief arose because a respected authority on the subject of stuttering stated that he had never encountered a diabetic who stuttered. Other clinicians seconded this idea, and it began to be accepted as a fact. But of course it was not a fact but the absence of one; and as is usually the case with "information" of this sort, it had a brief life, terminated by one and then a flood of announcements to the contrary. But it contributed for a while to the feeling that there must be some constitutional difference between stutterers and nonstutterers.

The idea that stutterers' muscles might be more reactive than nonstutterers' led to a search for evidence of low calcium levels and parathyroid insufficiency. Despite much searching, nothing was established. This too is a nonfact, but the search has been wide and intensive enough to conclude at least that there is no evidence to support the idea that stutterers have lower then normal calcium levels or parathyroid insufficiency.

Finding 2 is probably a consequence of finding 1. Because stutterers are more likely to have upper respiratory infections (URIs), one would expect to find a higher incidence of middle ear infections as well, causing the tendency for them to show pathological nystagmoid reflexes. However, the more important question remains: Why are stutterers more likely to have respiratory infections? There are three possible types of explanations: (1) URIs somehow cause children to be more likely to acquire stuttering; (2) stuttering somehow causes children to be more likely to acquire URIs; or (3) the probabilities of a child's acquiring stuttering and a cold are both somehow increased by a third factor.

The first type of explanation is the more powerful theoretical notion: that the respiratory infection actually causes the person to acquire stuttering or, since so many children with colds do not become stutterers, causes the person to be more likely to acquire stuttering. However, although the idea is theoretically powerful, it doesn't fit well with other information about stuttering, that is, young stutterers' parents do not invariably report that their children had colds when stuttering began. And the behaviors of stuttering don't seem directly related to edema, or any other aspect of URIs. As a result, we are likely to reject the most powerful explanation. One weak possibility should be mentioned: during URIs, the airway is often partially occluded, and this may change the aerodynamic properties of the airway enough so that children who are already at risk for stuttering are somehow nudged over a threshold into the disorder. Such a combination of circumstances would of course happen only rarely, yet perhaps often enough to produce a statistical effect.

The second explanation—that stuttering somehow causes or contributes to URIs—is also weak. Perhaps the stress of early stuttering predisposes children to infection, or perhaps the additional tension in the vocal tract musculature which is a common feature of established stuttering weakens the tissues a little and makes them more likely to be infected.

The third explanation, which is the least interesting from a theoretical point of view, is probably the most likely: that some third factor increases the probability of both respiratory infection and stuttering. For example, in a household under stress, as might be produced by illness or marital discord, there are likely to be both high levels of emotion, with many concomitant effects on speech such as poor turn-taking, rapid speech rates, inattention, and also less than perfect parenting, at least from time to time. Or, even more likely, during periods of stress, family members may hug and kiss each other more often, transmitting infection in the process. Events such as these might increase the probabilities of stuttering and URIs at the same time.

Finding 3—that stuttering is more common in twins—is also difficult to explain with any precision. One obvious explanation is that the genetic predisposition to bear twins is related to a genetic predisposition to stutter. One piece of evidence confirms such an explanation. Berry (1938) examined the families of twins who stuttered and found an incidence of stuttering of 2.9 percent among the singleton siblings of stuttering twins, an incidence that is somewhat higher than the incidence in the general population. There are several reasons, however, why this idea should be treated with some caution. The main reason for caution is that one can never be certain what a difference in incidence may be attributable to. The singleton siblings of twins may undergo considerable stress, lack of attention in comparison to their more interesting brothers or sisters, or their environment may be different in some other important way. Maybe their parents talk less to them, or at a faster rate.

As for the finding itself, that twins are more likely to stutter, there are many differences in the environments of twins that could contribute to stuttering. Higher levels of parental interest and concern for twins could make the parents of twins more likely to react negatively to disfluent speech. Higher levels of parental anxiety in coping with the care of twin infants could lead to emotional dynamics, including feelings of rejection of the twins or resentment of their demands, that could contribute to an emotionally unhealthy environment.

The slower development of twins, specifically in the acquisition of speech and language skills, could also play a role in making the incidence of stuttering higher in this population. The parents may respond to this delay with increased concern, which the children may begin to share. A concern over speech and language might cause some children to learn to talk with tension and struggle. It has already been noted that girls are more likely to recover from stuttering than boys, and this fact has been explained with the idea that girls develop speech and language skills faster than boys. Similarly, if twins develop speech and language skills more slowly than uniparous children, they may be less likely to recover from stuttering. This possibility could be investigated by a study comparing the recovery rates of twin stutterers with those of nontwin stutterers.

Twins, of course, have a higher risk of many disorders. These disorders are related for the most part to the additional difficulties twins experience during birth and shortly thereafter. It is possible that the higher incidence of stuttering seen in twins is actually a result of the inclusion in the sampled twin pairs of children whose brains were injured, perhaps minimally, perhaps even without the knowledge of the parents or physician.

This discussion has not done much to answer the question of why some children become stutterers, but it has provided a few hints. It has hinted that perhaps the final answer will have something to do with speech and language development; it has suggested once again the possibility of a genetic predisposition to stutter; and it has suggested that the reactions of parents to their children may play a role. These suggestions are hardly specific, but perhaps more specific ideas will develop as more information about stuttering is described.

CENTRAL NERVOUS SYSTEM DIFFERENCES AND EFFECTS

Information on the differences between stutterers and nonstutterers that may be attributed to central nervous system (CNS) function falls into two groups: differences related to the lateralization of brain function and differences related to motor control. Both areas have generated considerable research activity. A third area—differences in sensory functioning—might have been placed here but is instead discussed (excepting those related to laterality) in the next chapter under differences in communicative performance, specifically audition.

Lateralization

Findings

Handedness

1. When groups of stutterers are compared with groups of nonstutterers, a larger percentage of left-handed individuals is found in the group of stutterers (Bryngelson and Rutherford, 1937; Bryngelson, 1939; Johnson, 1942).

General Perceptual Laterality

2. Stutterers perceive a phi phenomenon stimulus as inconsistently moving from right to left, which is the way nonstutterers with mixed dominance see it (Jasper, 1932).
3. Stutterers have higher right ear thresholds for pure tones than nonstutterers (Hugo, 1972).

Dichotic Listening

4. Stutterers are more likely to have higher left ear scores than normals and show smaller differences between left and right ears in dichotic listening tasks (Curry and Gregory, 1967; Perrin, 1970; Quinn, 1971). Some researchers have failed to find this effect (Dorman and Porter, 1975). Quinn (1971) suggests that differences are more pronounced when semantically significant stimuli are used.
5. Thirty percent of stutterers compared with 79 percent of nonstutterers have a right ear advantage (REA) for verbal and a left ear advantage (LEA) for nonverbal stimuli in a unilateral DAF key-tapping task. Twenty percent of stutterers, but no nonstutterers, had an REA for both verbal and nonverbal stimuli (Tsunoda and Moriyama, 1972).

Visual Hemifield

6. Most normal speakers perceive words more accurately when they are presented to the right visual hemifield. Most stutterers show no difference (Moore, 1976).

Reaction Time (RT)

7. Stutterers show a significant group × field interaction in a tachistoscopically presented, visual hemifield, linguistic stimulus, RT task (Hand and Haynes, 1981).
8. Stutterers' voice RTs to auditory stimuli are slower than nonstutterers', but there is no difference between left and right ears for either stutterers or controls (Cross and Shadden, 1977).
9. Normal speakers have a LEA of neural response time for a nonspeech task (bilateral lip closure in response to a tone) which most stutterers lack (MacFarlane, 1976).

Electroencephalogram (EEG) Findings

10. Most nonstutterers show a longer percentage of time in alpha negative activity in the left hemisphere preceding oral reading. Most stutterers show a longer time in the right hemisphere (Moore and Lang, 1978).
11. Of normal speakers, 80 percent show a larger contingent negative variation (CNV) in the left hemisphere than in the right. Only 22 per-

cent of stutterers showed this effect when electrodes were placed over the inferior frontal areas (Zimmerman and Knott, 1974).

Tracking

12. In a monaural auditory tracking task, where a tone of varying pitch is presented to one ear while a similar tone in the other ear is controlled by the jaw or tongue, most nonstutterers showed an REA, doing better when the tone they controlled was in the right ear. Only 57 percent of stutterers showed this REA (Sussman and MacNeilage, 1975). The study was not replicated by Neilson, Quinn, and Neilson (1976).

Theory

The idea that stutterers are less well lateralized than nonstutterers has one of the longest histories of any line of investigation in our field. It began not long after the turn of the century, and it continues today. The first publications were concerned with the idea that stuttering developed as a consequence of training children to shift from natural left-handedness to right-handed use (Ballard, 1912; Wallin, 1924), but this was vigorously disputed (Parson, 1924). Soon after, attempts were made to survey stutterers and nonstutterers to see if there was a different distribution of handedness. Widely variable results were reported, but most studies reported that there was a higher percentage of outright left-handers and ambidextrous individuals among the stutterers than among the nonstutterers. The concept of handedness was challenged, however, as being more a matter of degree than of category, leading to the development of a dextrality quotient. Few if any differences were found when stutterers were compared with nonstutterers using this quotient.

Techniques for measuring lateral dominance that were more comprehensive than handedness, including preferred use of the feet, eyes, and so on, were devised and more testing was done. The results continued to be contradictory and uncertain until a thorough and carefully controlled study by Spadino (1941) compared seventy young stutterers with an equal number of young nonstutterers and found no differences between the two groups. This laid to rest the idea that being left-handed or ambidextrous, or being forced to shift from inherent left-handedness to right-handed usage, caused stuttering. But this one study, although well executed, should not have completely discounted the many previous studies that had found higher percentages of left-handers and ambidextrous among stutterers than among nonstutterers. It seems unlikely that all of these results were attributable to poor method. And anyway the idea that stutterers might be different in the way their brains were organized was not going to die.

Orton and Travis (1929) had noted that the motor control of speech depended on coordinated neural signals to the speech muscles. Because most of the structures of speech were located at the midline and innervated by nerves from both sides of the brain, it was necessary that one side be "dominant" over the other to ensure that neural signals arrived at the paired musculature at the same time. Previous investigations indicating that stutterers were more likely to be left-handed or ambidextrous provided some weak support for this idea. Perhaps the most important contribution of the Orton-Travis theory, however, was in focusing for the first time on the lack of motor control that stutterers had over their speech mechanism. The dominance question seemed ultimately not to lead very far. To prove the case, laterality differences other than a lack of motor control needed to be found, and a number of studies were designed to investigate the perceptual side of laterality.

A few studies (Jasper, 1932; Hugo, 1972) found differences between stutterers and nonstutterers in the perception of visual and auditory stimuli suggestive of a different pattern of brain organization, one with less clearly established dominance. But these studies did little to explain how such a difference could be related to stuttering. The method of Western science, which is to accumulate small pieces of information and construct from these a full theory or idea, has the drawback of occasionally producing pieces that don't fit into the total theoretical picture very easily. In some few cases these pieces that don't fit turn out to be very important later, and so we don't want to forget them, just to set them aside in a separate pile, waiting for some new piece to come along that will make it clear how they fit. But most of the pieces in such a pile remain anomalous. When the full picture finally becomes clear, these pieces are recognized as anomalies of one sort or another, and discarded. Many of the studies in the laterality area of stuttering research are in this sort of pile of anomalous data, waiting for some other piece of information to explain their relation to the total picture.

After the Orton-Travis theory had all but disappeared from the minds of clinicians and researchers, a similar idea emerged. Perhaps stutterers, regardless of their handedness, might lack hemispheric dominance for speech and language. A number of small *N,* anecdotal studies were reported suggesting that this might be the case. But there was no way, short of the somewhat dangerous Wada test (Jones, 1966), to demonstrate which hemisphere was dominant for language in an individual. The dichotic listening tests, in which competing stimuli are presented simultaneously to the two ears, suggested a solution. Although both ears send information to both hemispheres, the distribution of acoustic nerve fibers is asymmetrical. As a result, the right ear supplies more information to the left hemisphere, and the left ear more to the right. When stimuli are presented simultaneously and at the same level above threshold to both ears, there is an equally asymmetrical distribution of information. If linguistic stimuli are used, most individuals show an REA because in most individuals the left-hemisphere processes language stimuli. Individuals who do not show such an effect probably have language dominance in the right hemisphere, or in both hemispheres.

A number of dichotic listening studies comparing stutterers and non-stutterers have been carried out. Typically, the distribution of subjects who show an REA is different in the group of stutterers than in the group of nonstutterers, but typically also, there is a strong minority report. There are usually stutterers in the group, and not just one or two anomalies but a notable minority, who show the REA. Similarly, there are usually nonstutterers in the other group who do not show the REA. This is information, to be sure, but it is not information that has great theoretical power.

Other tests for language dominance have been devised and used to compare stutterers and nonstutterers. The RT paradigm, in which the experimenter measures the time interval between presentation of a signal and performance of a motor task, was originally used for different purposes (see pp. 221–225), but it clearly had the potential for comparing one ear, eye, or hand with the other. No difference was found between the two ears, for stutterers or for nonstutterers, as should have been expected. The differential distribution of nerve fibers to the two hemispheres gives an advantage to the contralateral hemisphere in the amount of information it receives, but it gives no such advantage in the speed with which the information is transmitted from the ear to the brain.

In the case of the eye, however, the experimental situation can be arranged so that information is presented to only one of the two hemispheres. Of course, once the information is presented to one of the hemispheres it is quickly (within an estimated 17 msec) shared with the other hemisphere, provided the brain being tested is healthy. But a test with RT, which depends for correct performance only on which hemisphere receives information first, can still be used to test one hemisphere against the other. When a linguistic stimulus is used, the visual hemifield, RT paradigm becomes a test of language dominance. Hand and Haynes (1981) performed such a test and found results similar to those found previously for handedness and for dichotic listening: as a group the stutterers' left hemispheres were slower in responding to linguistic stimuli than the left hemispheres of the matched nonstutterers, but there were some stutterers whose left hemispheres seemed dominant for language, and there were nonstutterers who seemed to lack left-hemisphere dominance for language.

MacFarlane (1976) performed an experiment with similar results evaluating a motor response to a nonlinguistic stimulus. A tone was presented to each of the two ears, and in reaction to the tone, the subjects pressed their lips together, activating a switch located in a squeezable device held between the lips. Thus the speech system was tested but without having to have the subjects talk. The nonlinguistic stimulus was apparently processed more readily in the right hemisphere by most of the nonstutterers, but

among the stutterers not so many subjects showed this advantage. The results indicated that for some stutterers, but not for all, the pattern of brain
organization is different from that in most, but not all, of nonstutterers.

The EEG method assesses brain activity. One aspect of brain activity
is the presence or absence of a characteristically rhythmic pattern of brain
activity known as the alpha wave. This rhythmic activity is typically present
when the brain is relatively inactive and disappears when it is engaged. Just
before a person begins to speak, the alpha wave disappears, indicating presumably that the brain is formulating language. The inference, although
logical, is rather far from the observation. The EEG observation only tells
us that the brain is relatively busy, not what it is doing. Indeed we have no
way of observing brain function that is more direct or reliable than hearing
what people tell us about their thoughts. The results of the EEG studies are
similar to the other methods for assessing language dominance. A stutterer
is more likely to show the pattern that we assume indicates language dominance in the right or in neither of the two hemispheres, while the nonstutterer is more likely to show the pattern that we assume indicates language dominance in the left. The difference in distribution is most clearly
shown in the Zimmermann and Knott (1972) study.

Pursuit auditory tracking is considered to reflect something more specific than simply dominance for language. Speech motor control is assumed
to rely on the presence of certain patterns of CNS organization, which link
the motor structure for speech with the sensory apparatus for hearing
speech, the ear. The pursuit auditory tracking task measures the person's
ability to make immediate adjustments of the speech mechanism in response to ongoing changes in the acoustic signal. The ability to perform
well in this kind of task depends partly on the speed of reaction to the
changing signal (i.e., it is partly an RT task) and partly on the ability to
discriminate changes in the auditory signal as they occur. Here too the results have shown that some stutterers perform as if they lacked the patterns
of organization that most nonstutterers have, but again the minority report
is strong, and as a result, it is difficult to relate the information obtained
to a more general picture of stuttering.

Dominance for language or for speech motor control, as determined
by these tests, is clearly not what causes, or even closely related to what
causes, stuttering to develop in some individuals. There are too many exceptions. Still, the trend is there. What could it mean as far as the nature
of stuttering is concerned?

Several possibilities need to be explored. It may be that whatever
causes stuttering to develop in some children also causes language dominance in some cases to develop in the right rather than in the left hemisphere. Perhaps the presence of stuttering itself, or the presence of some
unknown factor which results in stuttering, causes dominance for language
to develop in the opposite hemisphere in some cases. Or perhaps stuttering

can develop in children for a variety of causes, of which one is right-hemisphere dominance for language. We know so little about brain function and development that almost any interpretation of these facts is as likely as any other.

Although we think of the brain as being in control of behavior, it is a mistake to assume that any difference in brain anatomy and physiology must be causative of a behavioral difference. The brain, like other parts of the body, develops in response to other physiological events and, to an uncertain degree, to environmental events. Thus brain differences in stutterers could conceivably be a result of the disorder rather than a cause of it. The experience of being a stutterer could conceivably alter brain physiology.

Information in this area is premature. We don't know enough to decide what it means and we have to put it aside in that shrinking pile of interesting and hard-to-explain pieces of information. Someday it may fit. Or it may be discarded as unrelated to stuttering except by some odd coincidence.

Motor Differences

Findings

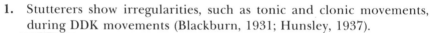

1. Stutterers show irregularities, such as tonic and clonic movements, during DDK movements (Blackburn, 1931; Hunsley, 1937).
2. Adult stutterers have slower DDK rates than nonstutterers while performing nonspeech movements of jaw, eyebrow, and hand (Chworowsky, 1951).
3. Stutterers have slower DDK for CV syllables representing lip, alveolar, and velar articulations (Rickenberg, 1956).
4. Stutterers make more errors than nonstutterers in imitating sequences of rhythmic finger-tapping and in repeating the exact timing of spoken material (Zaleski, 1965; Cooper and Allen, 1977).
5. "Stuttering" has been observed in a few nonspeech activities requiring precise sequential coordination, such as the playing of musical instruments (Froeschels, 1943; Van Riper, 1952) and penmanship (Scripture, 1909; Fagan, 1932; Roman, 1959), but these reports are anecdotal and rare.
6. The vocal RTs of stutterers are slower than those of nonstutterers when they respond to an auditory stimulus by producing an isolated vowel (Adams and Hayden, 1976), when they respond to a visual stimulus by producing a wide variety of syllables (Starkweather, Hirschman, and Tannenbaum, 1976), or when they respond by producing both isolated vowels and isolated consonants in response to a visual stim-

ulus presented independently to the left and right hemispheres (Adler, 1977). And stutterers are slower than nonstutterers in neural response time for nonspeech bilabial closure electromyograph (EMG) potential for both auditory and visual stimuli, particularly when stimulation is via the left ear (MacFarlane, 1976).

7. Stutterers are slower than nonstutterers in adjusting their vocal mechanisms from voiced to voiceless, voiceless to voiced, and from voiced to voiced sounds (Kerr, 1976).

8. Stutterers have slower RTs than nonstutterers, even when nonspeech activities are involved (Dinnan, McGuiness, and Perrin, 1970; Cross and Luper, 1979; Hand and Haynes, 1981; Starkweather, Franklin, and Smigo, 1984), although the difference for nonspeech activities is typically less than the differences for speech activities.

9. There is a high correlation between speech and nonspeech RTs in both stutterers and nonstutterers (Luper and Cross, 1978.)

10. The differences between stutterers and nonstutterers in reaction times is greater in children than in adults (Luper and Cross, 1978).

11. Stutterers have higher levels of EMG "tension" in masseter than nonstutterers, but tension level is not correlated with stuttering severity (Kolotkin et al., 1979).

12. When speech is motorically simplified so that there are fewer gestures per unit of time, as in whispered or lipped speech, the frequency of stuttering decreases (Perkins et al., 1976).

13. Zimmermann (1980) has suggested that stuttering is a disorder of movement. He suggests that the inputs to motoneuron pools are altered by a combination of constitutional and environmental effects to raise the ongoing background tension level of muscles in the speech mechanism and the tension levels associated with transient inputs to muscles for specific movements.

Theory

Investigation into the motoric abilities of stutterers has a long history. In the earliest days of research in speech pathology, DDK tests of motor skill were a standard part of any diagnostic battery. In this test, clients are asked to move some part of their speech mechanisms, such as a tonguetip, back and forth or up and down repeatedly and as quickly as possible. The number of such movements is counted and timed, and the rate of movement is calculated. Since it was the standard test of motor skill, it was naturally used to test many stutterers, and they were found to be slower than nonstutterers in these tests and in addition to perform them with irregularities that were not unlike stuttering itself—hesitation and jerkiness. These two facts—slower performance and uncoordinated performance—suggest several interpretations.

Early interpretations centered around the idea that anxiety impaired motor skill, but few independent tests of anxiety showed a relation between anxiety level and motor performance. Another interpretation is that the motor performance of stutterers is reduced because of a generally higher level of muscle activity or tension. The presence of anxiety (or any form of autonomic arousal) would increase this tension. The more recent idea is that muscular tension is often present in the absence of excessive levels of arousal. A chronically tense musculature stiffens the movable speech structures, and this slows movements. Chronic muscle tension would also introduce a tendency to tremulous or shaky movement that could result in errors of timing and coordination.

In later years, the RT paradigm was borrowed from experimental psychology as a simpler and more direct test of motor skill. The DDK test was, after all, a little strange. We do not talk by performing the same movements repeatedly. It is probably more difficult to repeat the same movements over and over again than it is to perform the more varied movements involved in talking. It is certainly not representative of speech movements.

In the RT arrangement, the repetitiveness of DDK is removed, and only one movement is required. The elapsed time from the presentation of the stimulus to the beginning of the movement is measured. There is the possibility of close control over what anatomical structures are tested and also the possibility of testing different sensory inputs separately. Ideally, the reaction time paradigm is seen as a brief moment from the sequence of typical speech gestures. During ordinary talking each speech gesture is initiated at a particular time to be coordinated with other speech gestures and to result in an acoustic product that contributes to the overall intelligibility of the message. What signals the beginning of a movement is uncertain. Perhaps it is other movements we respond to, having learned a chain of movements, or perhaps it is some aspect of the auditory signal.

The effect of delayed auditory feedback (DAF) suggests that we do not finish syllables until we hear ourselves reaching a certain point in the syllable. Or perhaps we initiate movements according to a sense of the rhythm of the language. It may be that in adults the timing and rhythm of speech movements is so well learned and habituated that stimuli of any sort play a minor role in signaling the initiation of movements, but at least in children, whose speech habits are less well learned, stimuli of some sort must play a role. So the RT paradigm is used to test the person's ability to initiate movement rapidly.

Nevertheless, the RT paradigm, like DDK, is not perfectly representative of speech movements. We do not usually perform the movements of speech in isolation. Also—and this seems a crucial failure of the RT paradigm—it has not yet been found to be correlated with any aspects of speech production. If RT really tests speech motor production, it should be correlated with speech rate, disfluency, or some similar variable in normal speakers. There have not been many attempts to find such a relation, so the relevance of reaction time may yet be established.

In RT too, the movements of stutterers are slower than those of non-stutterers. The first few studies were motivated by interest in the vocal mechanism and showed that this particular set of structures moved more slowly. Soon, however, it was apparent that it was not just the vocal mechanism but the upper articulators as well that were slower. Furthermore, the differences between stutterers and nonstutterers are present for visual as well as acoustic stimuli, suggesting that it is not an auditory disfunction that is responsible for the result. However, it should be noted that differences seem to be greater for auditory than for visual presentation, suggesting that there is another variable, in addition to a motoric difference, that determines RT performance, a variable that is sensory specific.

Motor explanations of stuttering, such as chronic tension, raise a number of questions. One of them is: If the musculature of stutterers is chronically tense, and if this chronic tension is responsible for stuttering behaviors, then why is it that stutterers speak without stuttering so much of the time? There are several answers to this question. One is that the chronic tension may vary in level from moment to moment as a result of changing levels of arousal. This is a suggestion that Zimmermann (1980) has made, one which predicts that stuttering will be more likely during high arousal, a fact already established. The second answer is that demands for performance may vary as a result of changing requirements during the speech act. This is a suggestion that Starkweather (1981) has made, noting that the rate of speech accelerates and decelerates slightly according to syntactic and phonological structure. Stuttering tends to occur at those locations where a change in rate is predictable.

These two answers are not mutually exclusive. In fact, it is certain that both linguistic and situational demands for rapid, coordinated, well-timed speech movements vary from moment to moment, and if the motor abilities of stutterers to meet these demands are chronically impaired, performance will be determined by a summation of the two sets of demands. In such a case the prediction of stuttering will be difficult, at least for the outside observer. The stutterer may have a sense, either physiological or probabilistic, of the summation of these demands and be able to predict the occurrence of stuttering more easily than the outside observer.

Both the RT and the DDK tests of motor performance suffer from being speeded tests. The person is instructed to move as quickly as possible. This introduces the possibility that some subjects, more competitive perhaps, or motivated in some other way, will perform better, even though their motor skills are no different. Conversely, the additional pressure to perform and to perform quickly may have different effects on some subjects than on others. It isn't unreasonable to suppose that stutterers might be more likely to deteriorate in performance of a motor task under conditions of time pressure. Their speech often reflects such a tendency. If this is so, then reaction time or DDK differences between stutterers and nonstutterers might not be a result of different levels of motor skill or coordination but of different levels of test anxiety.

An important question is: Do people stutter because their motor skill is less than that of nonstutterers, or is their motor performance less than that of nonstutterers because they are in some sense "stuttering" during the test? The DDK and RT tests of performance with nonspeech structures are designed to resolve this issue. Nonspeech motor performance cannot be influenced by stuttering because stuttering is something that one does during speech. Can a person stutter when doing something other than talking? The answer to this question depends partly on what one means by "stuttering." If "stuttering" means moving (not just speech movements) with hesitation, repetition, and jerkiness, then the answer appears to be "yes," but the difference is greater for speech than for nonspeech movements.

It comes as no surprise that stutterers are less able than nonstutterers to move their speech mechanisms quickly or to control these movements. The problem in this line of investigation has always been, as in many other lines, a problem of separating the cause from the effect. There are two ways to approach this problem. One is to test the motoric ability of the speech mechanism as it performs movements other than speaking. The other is to test the motoric ability of movements by other parts of the body. Both of these strategies have been used, and both of them have helped investigators discover differences between stutterers and nonstutterers. Furthermore, significant correlations between speech and nonspeech reaction times have been observed.

However, it has proved easier to find differences when the speech mechanism itself was tested, whether by RT measures or by DDK measures, than when nonspeech structures, such as the hand, were tested. This combination of effects suggests an interesting interpretation. Perhaps there is a general motor difference between stutterers and nonstutterers, which predisposes some children to be disfluent. Some of these children recover from this predisposition and go on to become fluent speakers. Others, however, learn to approach speech as a tense and difficult activity requiring force and struggle. The additional muscle tension created in the speech mechanism by this learned attitude slows motor performance in the speech mechanisms even further. Some such dual explanation seems required to explain the presence of small but significant differences in nonspeech motor performance between stutterers and nonstutterers and larger differences in speech motor performance.

Another prediction from this explanation is that the speech and nonspeech performances will be correlated. If the slower speech performance is based on a more general motoric difference, even though there may be a learned component that makes the speech differences greater than the nonspeech differences, then there should be a correlation between non-speech and speech performance. Those stutterers who have a greater impairment of the general motor system should be, for the most part, the ones who end up with a greater impairment of the speech motor system. Such a correlation has been found in one study (Luper and Cross, 1978) but not in a replication (Starkweather, Franklin, and Smigo, 1984).

Another prediction that can be derived from the predisposition plus learning explanation (suggested by the greater speech than nonspeech differences) is that stutterers who have had more experience with the disorder, who have been stuttering longer, will have more of a deficit in motor skill of the speech musculature than those who have been stuttering for a shorter time. The opposite of this was found by Luper and Cross (1978). Stuttering children differ from nonstuttering children more than stuttering adults differ from nonstuttering adults. Apparently the motor difference tends to improve with age. But, of course, it could be the general motor impairment that improves with age, not the specific speech impairment. It may be that the general motor impairment is a more important determiner of performance than the specific one. Answers to this question could be found by speech versus nonspeech RT tests in both children and adults.

The idea that stuttering behaviors are a result of increased muscle tension also predicts that greater levels of muscle tension will be associated with greater severity of stuttering behavior. Kolotkin, Manschreck, and O'Brien (1979) measured EMG tension levels in the masseter muscles of stutterers and nonstutterers and confirmed the higher levels in stutterers that other investigators had found, but failed to find a significant correlation between tension levels and severity of stuttering behaviors. Of course, one failure of prediction does not ruin a theory, and some other investigator may find such a relation. The possibility exists, and is indeed suggested by a number of other findings, that the severity of stuttering is determined by different factors than its mere presence. One explanation, suggested in other sections of this book, is that severity has not been measured very well in most studies. Another explanation is that the severity of stuttering is determined more by environmental factors associated with stuttering's development, while the presence or absence of stuttering is determined more by genetic factors.

Any theory of stuttering needs to account for fluency-enhancement effects. Perkins and colleagues (1976) pointed out that many of the fluency-enhancing conditions create circumstances in which there are fewer speech movements per unit of time. This simplification of the motor act of speaking can occur because one whole system is restricted in its movement, as the vocal mechanism is during whispered speech, or it can occur because fewer movements are required over all, as in slowed speech. This explanation accounts somewhat less well for the fluency-enhancing effect of rhythmically paced speech which doesn't seem obviously simplified, and seems not to depend on slowed rate. The explanation offered for this effect is that the speaker's motoric task is also simplified in paced speech because decisions about the timing of speech gestures are externally controlled. This explanation may be true, but it is less verifiable than others. We will probably never be able to observe these "decisions" being made.

In summary, tests of motor performance have shown repeatedly that stutterers exhibit poorer performance than nonstutterers, and explanations of stuttering based on chronically tense muscle systems seem compatible with most of the observations. But it is not certain whether stutterers' motoric deficiencies are a cause or a result of the disorder.

PSYCHOBEHAVIORAL DIFFERENCES

Findings

1. Stutterers are late in passing speech milestones, perform less well on language tests, and show three times as much articulation disorder as nonstutterers (Andrews et al., 1983).
2. Stutterers score 0.5 SD lower on "intelligence" tests (Andrews et al., 1983).
3. Stutterers are less adept than nonstutterers in cognitive tasks related to speech sounds (Wingate, 1967, 1971) and in "sound-mindedness" (Perozzi, 1970).
4. Stutterers are less able than nonstutterers to match auditory-temporal patterns with corresponding visual-spatial patterns (Cohen and Hansen, 1975).
5. Stutterers perform less well than nonstutterers on tests of central auditory function (Andrews et al., 1983).

Theory

Taken together, these findings suggest that stutterers' CNSs do not function as well as those of nonstutterers, at least not in areas of function related to speech and language. Three kinds of interpretations need to be considered: (1) people who stutter are deficient in these areas, and the deficit causes stuttering to develop or diminishes the chances of its recovery, (i.e., diminished CNS performance causes stuttering); (2) people who stutter develop habits of reticence from an early age, which prevent them from developing certain cognitive and language skills, which diminish their performance on tests that assess, or even just rely on, these skills, (i.e., stuttering causes diminished CNS performance); and (3) some factor, common to the development of these cognitive functions and to the development of fluency, causes both diminished CNS performance and stuttering.

The first possibility is the most powerful theoretically, that the disorder of stuttering develops as a consequence of diminished CNS performance. It is not difficult to imagine how this might be so. Children between three and five years of age who have such CNS deficits might well be expected to speak with more than the usual hesitation and uncertainty. This might manifest itself in certain children (not necessarily in all children) in the excessively repetitive speech that typifies incipient stuttering. The explanation fits well with observations that stuttering is related to language development (see pp. 251–255). Then, if the communicative environment surrounding the child is too demanding, additional habits of struggle, tension, and forcing could develop, resulting in a full-fledged stuttering problem.

This explanation makes the prediction that the CNS deficits already identified in adults who stutter should be equally present in children who stutter. The first two facts noted above are true of children. The rest have been established by testing adults. It also suggests that the *motoric* differences between people who stutter and people who don't may develop as a consequence of the disorder and should not be present in children who stutter. This is apparently not the case. That is, motoric differences seem to be present in children who stutter (Cross and Luper, 1979; Caruso and Conture, 1982).

However, these findings were obtained from a test population of children including individuals who had been stuttering for a period of time. Some of them may not have been just incipient stutterers but children who had already begun to develop habits of struggle and forcing because of environmental demands for fluent speech that they could not meet. To be an adequate test of this question, children who show no sign of struggle and tension but who nonetheless have excessively repetitious speech should be tested for motoric differences. The one finding that is difficult to refute in asserting a cognitive linguistic cause of stuttering is the observation by Cross and Luper (1979) that the motoric differences between children who stutter and those who don't become less with increasing age. However, the observation has been challenged (Reich et al., 1981).

Another approach to this question can be derived by not assuming that the origins of stuttering must lie with either motoric or linguistic factors. Clearly, it is possible that both the motor and the CNS differences are present in children who stutter. That is, there could be a pattern of deficiency, including both motor and cognitive-linguistic components, which is present in young children and results in their speaking with hesitation, uncertainty, and excessive repetitiveness. Indeed, where CNS deficits are known to exist, that is, in the brain-injured population, combinations of motor and cognitive-linguistic deficits are more the norm than the exception. Further, it might be expected that these two components would not necessarily be present in the same proportion. Some children would show more of a motoric and less of a cognitive-linguistic deficit, while for others the reverse pattern would be present.

Interesting as these theoretical notions are, we must be aware that there are two other explanations of the cognitive-linguistic differences of stutterers, explanations which are also possible but suggest a less interesting relation between the observed differences and the causes of the disorder. The first of these explanations is that the observed cognitive-linguistic differences are attributable to the disorder itself. That is, they are not one of the causes of stuttering but one of the effects. Stuttering children clearly have a different set of experiences than nonstutterers as they develop speech and language. They gradually become aware that their speech is different; they learn to use excessive amounts of effort when they talk; and often they learn to avoid speaking. These attitudes may hinder the development of cognitive skills that depend on language.

Differences in Attitudes

Findings

1. There is a cultural stereotype of the male stutterer as nervous, shy, and withdrawn, and the stereotype is independent of the stutterer's age and of the listener's experience with stutterers (Woods and Williams, 1976). This is not to say that the stutterer is nervous, shy, and withdrawn but rather that most stutterers probably expect to encounter the stereotypical attitudes among their listeners, and this expectation may influence their behavior.
2. In Britain, and doubtless in the United States and in many other societies, stuttering is considered something to laugh at (Brook, 1957).
3. The female who stutters is stereotyped more negatively than the male who stutters. The stuttering female is seen as more different from nonstuttering females than the stuttering male is from nonstuttering males. The stereotype of the stuttering female is naive, lacking influence, insecure, boring, unsociable, and masculine (Silverman, 1982).
4. The attitudes of stuttering women are different from those of nonstuttering women and from those of stuttering men (Silverman, 1980).
5. Black and white stutterers show different trends with regard to the predominance of different stuttering behavioral subtypes (more covert behaviors and more accessory features among the Blacks), presumably because of different cultural attitudes toward stuttering and speech (Leith and Mims, 1975).
6. Listeners who count more stutterings in a speech sample tend to have a more tolerant attitude toward the disorder than those who count less (Emerick, 1960).
7. The parents of stuttering children are no less tolerant of disfluency than the parents of nonstuttering children (Berlin, 1960).
8. The mothers of stutterers may be more overtly accepting but covertly rejecting than the mothers of nonstutterers (Kinstler, 1961).

9. Adults talk more rapidly and interrupt more often when talking to children who stutter (Meyers and Freeman, 1985).

Theory

The attitudes people have toward a category of people determine how they will react to those people. These reactions may in turn influence the behaviors of that category. People interacting with stutterers and believing that they are nervous, shy, and withdrawn may react in a predictable way. Children may be cruel. Parents may be protective. Some stutterers encountering these reactions may acquire an attitude of helplessness; others may become aggressive. Children whose parents, out of a sense of protectiveness, ignore their child's stuttering, may come to believe that the behaviors are not as evident as they really are. In this way, the stereotypical views of stuttering found within any culture may influence the development of the disorder.

But there is another important element. The person who stutters, being a member of the culture, is also aware of the cultural stereotype. He consequently knows or suspects what reactions might be occurring unspoken in the people he talks to. This knowledge of the reactions of others may not always be accurate, but regardless of its accuracy it is sure to influence the behavior of the stutterer. Knowing, or thinking you know, that people are inwardly laughing at you or contemptuous of you will have a powerful influence on your behavior. In this way too, the cultural stereotypes of stuttering may influence the form the disorder takes.

Still another mechanism related to culture is the reactions of parents to their children who stutter. If the culture finds stuttering repulsive or amusing, parents will naturally react with concern or even alarm when they believe or suspect that their child is beginning to develop stuttering. The parents' concern will influence their behavior, and this may in turn influence the development of the child's disorder. Meyers and Freeman (1985) have shown that adults talk more rapidly to children who stutter and interrupt them more often than they do children who do not stutter. These different ways of talking to stuttering children may reflect the sense of discomfort that most people feel when talking to a stutterer, and which is probably traceable to the cultural stereotype of the stutterer as nervous, shy, and withdrawn. Regardless of its origin, these unusual ways of speaking that adults display when talking to a child who stutters are surely strong candidates for influencing the child's speech.

The role of cultural stereotypes in shaping stuttering behavior is clearly not very well understood. A further exploration of the attitudes held toward stuttering by different cultural groups, and a close look at the correlative behaviors displayed by stutterers in the same culture, would be helpful in understanding the kind of role that cultural stereotyping plays in the development of this disorder.

REFERENCES

ADAMS, M. R., A clinical strategy for differentiating the normally nonfluent child and the incipient stutterer, *Journal of Fluency Disorders*, 2 (1977), 141–48.

ADAMS, M. R., and HAYDEN, P., The ability of stutterers and nonstutterers to initiate and terminate phonation during production of an isolated vowel, *Journal of Speech and Hearing Research*, 19 (1976), 290–96.

ADLER, J., Hemispheric differences in vocal and articulatory reaction times to linguistic and nonlinguistic visual stimuli in stutterers and nonstutterers. M.A. thesis, Temple University, Philadelphia, 1977.

ANDREWS, G., CRAIG, A., FEYER, A–M., HODDINOTT, S., HOWIE, P., and NEILSON, M., Stuttering: a review of research findings and theories circa 1982, *Journal of Speech and Hearing Disorders*, 48 (1983), 226–46.

BALDAN, O., Study of the vestibular function in a group of stutterers: electronystagmographic researches, *De Therapia Vocis et Loquellae*, 1 (1965), 349–51.

BALLARD, P., Sinistrality and speech, *Journal of Experimental Psychology*, 1 (1912), 298–316.

BERLIN, C. I., Parents' diagnoses of stuttering, *Journal of Speech and Hearing Research*, 3 (1960), 372–79.

BERRY, M. F., Developmental history of stuttering children, *Journal of Pediatrics*, 12 (1938), 209–17.

BLACKBURN, B., A study of the diaphragm, tongue, lips, and jaw in stutterers and normal speakers, *Psychology Monographs*, 41 (1931), 1–13.

BROOK, F., *Stammering and its Treatment*. London: Pitman, 1957.

BRUNO, G., CAMARDA, V., and CURI, L., Contribution to the study of organic causal factors in the pathogenesis of stuttering, *Bolletino delle Malattie dell' Orecchio, della Gola, del Naso*, 83 (1965), 753–58.

BRYNGELSON, B., A study of the laterality of stutterers and normal speakers, *Journal of Speech Disorders*, 4 (1939), 231–34.

BRYNGELSON, B., and RUTHERFORD, B., A comparative study of laterality of stutterers and non-stutterers, *Journal of Speech Disorders*, 2 (1937), 15–16.

CARUSO, A., and CONTURE, E., Speech physiology associated with young stutterers' (dys) fluency: preliminary observations. Convention address, American Speech and Hearing Association, 1982.

CHWOROWSKY, C., A comparative study of the diadochokinetic rates of stutterers and nonstutterers in speech related and nonspeech related movements. M.A. thesis, University of Wisconsin, Madison, 1951. Abstracts of theses, *Speech Monographs*, 19 (1952), 192.

COHEN, M. S., and HANSEN, M. L., Intersensory processing efficiency of fluent speakers and stutterers, *British Journal of Disorders of Communication*, 10 (1975), 11–22.

COOPER, M. H., and ALLEN, G. D., Timing control accuracy in normal speakers and stutterers, *Journal of Speech and Hearing Research*, 20 (1977), 55–71.

CROSS, D. E., and SHADDEN, B., Stimulus ear presentation and voice reaction time for stutterers and nonstutterers. Convention address, American Speech and Hearing Association, 1977.

CROSS, D. E., and LUPER, H. L., Voice reaction time of stuttering and nonstuttering children and adults, *Journal of Fluency Disorders*, 4 (1979), 59–77.

CURRY, F. K. W., and GREGORY, H. H., A comparison of stutterers and nonstutterers on three dichotic listening tasks. Convention address, American Speech and Hearing Association, 1967.

DINNAN, J. A., McGUINNESS, E., and PERRIN, L., Auditory feedback: stutterers v. nonstutterers, *Journal of Learning Disorders*, 3 (1970), 209–13.

DORMAN, M. F., and PORTER, R. J., Jr., Hemispheric lateralization for speech perception in stutterers, *Cortex*, 11 (1975), 181–85.

EMERICK, L., Extensional definition and attitude toward stuttering, *Journal of Speech and Hearing Research*, 3 (1960), 181–86.

FAGAN, L. B., Graphic stuttering, *Psychology Monographs*, 43 (1932), 67–71.

FROESCHELS, E., Pathology and therapy of stuttering, *The Nervous Child*, 2 (1943), 148–61.

GRAF, O. I., Incidence of stuttering among twins, *Stuttering in Children and Adults*, ed. W. Johnson, Minneapolis: University of Minnesota Press, 1955.

HAND, R., and HAYNES, W. O., Hemispheric and reaction time differences in stutterers and nonstutterers. Convention address, American Speech and Hearing Association, 1981.

HILL, H., An experimental study of disorganization of speech and manual responses in normal subjects, *Journal of Speech and Hearing Research,* 19 (1954), 295–305.

HUGO, R., 'n kommunikatiegefundeerde ondersoek na bepaalde waarnemingsverskynesis bei disfemie, *Journal of South African Speech and Hearing Association,* 19 (1972), 39–51.

HUNSLEY, Y. L., Disintegration in the speech musculature of stutterers during the production of a nonvocal temporal pattern, *Psychology Monographs,* 49 (1937), 32–49.

JASPER, H. H., A laboratory study of diagnostic indices of bilateral neuromuscular organization in stutterers and normal speakers, *Psychology Monographs,* 43 (1932), 172–74.

JOHNSON, W., A study of the onset and development of stuttering, *Journal of Speech Disorders,* 7 (1942), 251–57.

JONES, R. K., Observations on stammering after localized cerebral injury, *Journal of Neurology, Neurosurgery, and Psychiatry,* 29 (1966), 192–95.

KERR, S. H., Phonatory adjustment times in stutterers and nonstutterers. Convention address, American Speech and Hearing Association, 1976.

KINSTLER, D. B., Covert and overt maternal rejection in stuttering, *Journal of Speech and Hearing Disorders,* 26 (1961), 145–55.

KOLOTKIN, M., MANSCHRECK, T., and O'BRIEN, D., Electromyographic tension levels in stutterers and normal speakers, *Perceptual and Motor Skills,* 49 (1979), 109–10.

LEITH, W., and MIMS, H., Cultural influences in the development and treatment of stuttering: a preliminary report on the black stutterer, *Journal of Speech and Hearing Disorders,* 40 (1975), 459–66.

LUPER, H. L., and CROSS, D. E., Relation between finger reaction time and voice reaction time in stuttering and nonstuttering children and adults. Convention address, American Speech and Hearing Association, 1978.

MACFARLANE, S. C., Neural response time of stutterers and nonstutterers for certain oral motor tasks as a function of auditory stimulation. Convention address, American Speech and Hearing Association, 1976.

MEYERS, S. C., and FREEMAN, F. J., Mother and child speech rates as a variable in stuttering and disfluency, *Journal of Speech and Hearing Research,* 28 (1985), 436–44.

MOORE, W. H., Jr., Bilateral tachistoscopic word perception of stutterers and normal subjects, *Brain and Language,* 3 (1976), 434–42.

MOORE, W. H., Jr., and LANG, M. K., Alpha asymmetry over the right and left hemispheres of stutterers and control subjects preceding massed oral readings: a preliminary investigation, *Perceptual and Motor Skills,* 44 (1977), 223–30.

NEILSON, P., QUINN, P., and NEILSON, M., Auditory tracking measures of hemispheric asymmetry in normals and stutterers, *Australian Journal of Human Communication Disorders,* 4 (1976), 121–26.

NELSON, S. E., HUNTER, N., and WALTER, M., Stuttering in twin types, *Journal of Speech Disorders,* 10 (1945), 335–43.

ORTON, S., and TRAVIS, L., Studies in stuttering: studies of action currents in stutterers, *Archives of Neurology and Psychiatry,* 21 (1929) 61–68.

PARSON, B. S., *Lefthandedness.* New York: Macmillan, 1924.

PERKINS, W. H., RUDAS, J., JOHNSON, L., and BELL, J., Stuttering: discoordination of phonation with articulation and respiration, *Journal of Speech and Hearing Research,* 19 (1976), 509–22.

PEROZZI, J. A., Phonetic skill (sound-mindedness) of stuttering children, *Journal of Communication Disorders,* 3 (1970), 207–10.

PERRIN, K. L., An examination of ear preference for speech and nonspeech stimuli in a stuttering population, *Dissertation Abstracts* (1970), 1213.

QUINN, P. T., Stuttering: some observations on speaking when alone, *Journal of the Australian College of Speech Therapists,* 21 (1971), 92–94.

REICH, A., TILL, J., GOLSMITH, H., and PRINS, D., Laryngeal and manual reaction times of stuttering and nonstuttering adults, *Journal of Speech and Hearing Research,* 24 (1981), 192–96.

RICKENBERG, H. E., Diadochokinesis in stutterers and nonstutterers, *Journal of the Medical Society of New Jersey,* 53 (1956), 324–26.

ROMAN, K. G., Handwriting and speech, *Logos,* 2 (1959), 29–39.

SCHILLING, A., Electronystagmographic findings as indication of central coordination defect in stutterers, *Archiv fur Ohren- Nasen- Kehlkopfheilkunde vereinigt mit Zeitschrift fur Hals- Nasen- und Ohrenheilkunde,* 175 (1959), 457–61.

SCRIPTURE, E. W., Penmanship stuttering, *Journal of the American Medical Association,* 52 (1909), 1480–81.

SILVERMAN, E-M., Communication attitudes of women who stutter, *Journal of Speech and Hearing Disorders,* 45 (1980), 533–39.

SILVERMAN, E-M., Speech-language clinicians' and university students' impressions of women and girls who stutter, *Journal of Fluency Disorders,* 7 (1982), 469–78.

SPADINO, E., *Writing and Laterality Characteristics of Stuttering Children.* New York: Teachers College, Columbia University Press, 1941.

STARKWEATHER, C. W., Speech fluency and its development in normal children, in *Speech and Language: Advances in Basic Research and Practice,* (vol. 4), ed. N. Lass. New York: Academic Press, 1981.

STARKWEATHER, C. W., HIRSHMAN, P., and TANNENBAUM, R., Latency of vocalization: stutterers v. nonstutterers, *Journal of Speech and Hearing Research* 19 (1976), 481–92.

STARKWEATHER, C. W., FRANKLIN, S., and SMIGO, T., Voice and finger reaction times: differences and correlations, *Journal of Speech and Hearing Research,* 27 (1984), 193–96.

SUSSMAN, H., and MACNEILAGE, P., Hemispheric specialization for speech production and perception in stutterers, *Neuropsychologia,* 13 (1975), 19–26.

TSUNODA, T., and MORIYAMA, H., Specific pattern of cerebral dominance for various sounds in adult stutterers, *Journal of Auditory Research,* 12 (1972), 216–27.

VAN RIPER, C., Report of stuttering on a musical instrument, *Journal of Speech and Hearing Disorders,* 17 (1952), 433–34.

WALLIN, J., Studies of mental defects and handicaps, *Miami University Bulletin,* series 22, No. 5 (1924).

WINGATE, M. E., Slurvian skill of stutterers, *Journal of Speech and Hearing Research* 10 (1967), 844–48.

WINGATE, M. E., Phonetic ability in stuttering. *Journal of Speech and Hearing Research,* 14 (1971), 189–94.

WOODS, C. L., and WILLIAMS, D. E., Traits attributed to stuttering and normally fluent males, *Journal of Speech and Hearing Research,* 19 (1976), 267–78.

ZALESKI, T., Rhythmic skills in stuttering children, *De Therapia Vocis et Loquellae,* 1 (1965), 371–72.

ZIMMERMANN, G., Stuttering: a disorder of movement, *Journal of Speech and Hearing Research,* 23 (1980), 122–36.

ZIMMERMANN, G., and KNOTT, J. D., Slow potentials of the brain related to speech processing in normal speakers and stutterers, *Electroencephalography and Clinical Neurophysiology,* 37 (1974), 599–607.

Stuttering
and Communicative
Processes

TOPICS COVERED IN THIS CHAPTER

- *Experimental findings on stuttering and vocalization*
- *Theoretical implications of the literature on stuttering and vocalization*
- *Experimental findings on stuttering and audition*
- *Theory:*
  Stuttering
  Audition
- *Experimental findings on stuttering and touch/pressure during speech*
- *Theory:*
  Feedback theory
  Oral sensory deprivation
  Intraoral air pressure changes
- *Experimental findings on rate and timing in stuttering*
- *Theory of rate and timing in stutterers:*
  Voice onset time, segment duration, and formant frequencies in stutterers
  Fluency enhancement and speech rate
- *Experimental findings on stuttering and language*
- *Theory of the relation of stuttering to language performance:*
  Stuttering and language formulation
  Stuttering and language skill
  Stuttering and language disorders

INTRODUCTION

This chapter deals with differences in speech, language, or hearing between stutterers and nonstutterers. Information of this kind can be used in two different types of theory construction. The first type is descriptive theory. Stuttering is itself a way of talking, and some of the findings in this chapter simply help to describe the disorder more completely. Like the bricks of a building, each piece of information plays a part in supporting the complete edifice. The theory, in this case, explains how a particular fact fits in, what part of the building it is located in, and what other bricks it supports or is supported by. The second type is explanatory theory, of which a good deal has already been seen in this book. But in this chapter the problem of explanation is somewhat more difficult than usual. Here we deal with differences in communicative behavior between stutterers and nonstutterers, and some of the differences are present as part of the disorder. Often this is obvious, but in a few cases, it is not so clear, and a finding appears to have explanatory power, but a more careful interpretation will show that it has only descriptive power.

STUTTERING AND VOCALIZATION

Findings

1. Stuttering is ameliorated under conditions that involve a change in vocal functioning (Wingate, 1970), such as whispering or pitch change, but there are also changes other than vocalization in the conditions that enhance fluency (Starkweather, 1982).
2. Stuttering occurs less often on reading material that involves fewer

off-on vocal adjustments (Adams and Reis, 1971), but this finding has been questioned in several ways (Young, 1975; Hutchinson and Brown, 1978; Starkweather, 1982). On the other hand, stuttering is more likely to occur following silence and when the second sound of the word is voiced (Wall, Starkweather, and Harris, 1981), but this result may have been due to effects on stuttering caused by syntactic variations.

3. Out-loud rehearsal of memorized sentences is more effective in reducing the frequency of stuttering than silent, whispered, lipped, or no rehearsal (Brenner, Perkins, and Soderberg, 1972).

4. The decrease in fluency that occurs during choral speech is only partially attributable to changes in vocalization (Ingham and Carroll, 1977; Adams and Ramig, 1980).

5. Changes in vocalization cannot account for all of the decrease in stuttering that occurs during singing (Healey, Mallard, and Adams, 1976).

6. The masking effect occurs, and is in fact more pronounced, when stutterers speak with normal vocal intensity (Garber and Martin, 1977).

7. The laryngeal events accompanying part-word repetitions are different than those accompanying prolongations (Conture, McCall, and Brewer, 1977).

8. Stutterers have abnormal (nonreciprocal) laryngeal muscle (adductor-abductor) activity and a higher level of laryngeal activity during stuttering (Freeman and Ushijima, 1975, 1978; Shapiro, 1980), and other laryngeal anomalies such as phonatory breaks and tremoring (Chevrie-Mueller, 1963). Laryngeal stuttering behaviors seem similar to supralaryngeal (oral articulatory) stuttering behaviors (Starkweather, 1982).

9. Stutterers have slower reaction times to voiced than to whispered /a/, although nonstutterers do not show any difference (Venkatigiri, 1981)

10. The voice initiation times of stutterers improve under conditions of metronomic pacing and masking noise (Hayden, Adams, and Jordahl, 1982).

11. The intervocalic interval (VOT) associated with voiceless stop consonants is longer in the "fluent" speech of stutterers than in nonstutterers, both in nonsense syllable production (Agnello and Wingate, 1972), and in contextual material, although the differential effects on VOT of place of consonant articulation are the same for stutterers as for nonstutterers (Hillman and Gilbert, 1977). This seems to be because the stutterers are slower in moving their laryngeal and oral articulatory structures (Starkweather and Myers, 1978).

12. There is wide individual variation in the locus of disruption in stuttering; some are more laryngeal than others (Ford and Luper, 1975).

13. It may be that there are nonvocal (periods of absent phonation) and vocal (excessive repetitions and prolongations) subtypes of stuttering (Quarrington and Douglass, 1960).

Theory

The first seven of the findings listed above fit into one part of the puzzle, the remaining six into another. I'll discuss findings 1 through 7 first. Wingate (1970) reviewed fluency-enhancing conditions and concluded that they had in common a change in the way the voice was used. Each of the fluency-enhancing conditions—whispering, singing, metronomic pacing, slowed speech, high- or low-pitched speech, choral speech—involves a change in the way the person talks. Wingate suggested that what the conditions had in common was a change in the manner of vocalization, but it is not just the vocalization of the speaker that changes.

When speech is altered by changing one aspect of it, other aspects of it change also. In singing, speech is slower, louder, and more rhythmic. Also, familiar words are produced, and the vowels are greatly lengthened relative to the consonants. When the pitch of the voice is raised or lowered, the rate of airflow is also changed and the voice is louder or softer, and the rate of syllable production is reduced. And so on. Any single deviation from the usual manner of talking results in many other deviations. The speech mechanism, although it contains a number of different parts that perform different functions, is physiologically tied together by muscle origins and insertions and acts as a complete unit. It should be thought of as an organ of the body, serving one purpose. When we ask it to do something different from the usual, the whole mechanism responds to perform the required task. It is difficult, if not impossible, to single out one function.

Wingate's idea was a simple and sensible interpretation of the facts as he saw them. From that interpretation, there was an obvious implication. If stutterers spoke fluently when they changed their pattern of vocalization, it might be that their stuttering occurred because of aberrant vocal, particularly laryngeal, behavior. There were a few inferential leaps in the subsequent literature (one of which jumped entirely over the respiratory system), and this idea came to be known as the vocalization hypothesis. It excited many people, perhaps because it suggested, finally, a relatively simple explanation for the problem of stuttering. Simple explanations are always appealing, but not always correct. In spite of the unwarranted inferences, however, the vocalization hypothesis produced some important research.

Adams and Reis (1971) sought to test the vocalization hypothesis. They reasoned that what would be difficult for stutterers in the act of vocalizing was the rapid adjustments that were required to turn the voice off and on during continuous speech. In the production of a sound like /p/ in the phrase "Can you see Peter?" the glottis is widened very briefly after the word "see" to diminish vocal fold vibration and then closed again for the vowel in "Peter." In continuous speech, there are many of these rapid adjustments, and considering the slower reaction times of stutterers, and the fact that they speak more fluently when they slow down, perhaps the speed of these rapid adjustments is too much for them.

To test this idea, Adams and Reis constructed a passage that contained only voiced sounds. It required relatively few vocal adjustments. They gave this passage and another one that had not been altered to a group of stutterers to read five times in a row in a typical adaptation sequence. As expected, the stutterers tended to stutter more on the normal passage than on the one that contained fewer vocal adjustments. The authors concluded that stuttering behavior could be reduced if the number of off-on vocal adjustments were reduced. However, there were several problems. In constructing a passage without vocal adjustments, an experimenter might use unusual words and unusual sentence constructions. Of course, if this were true, it would unbalance the two passages with regard to syntax and vocabulary, which are variables known to influence the frequency of stuttering. The odd sentences and words would tend to produce more stuttering, and the suspected fluency-enhancing effect of fewer vocal adjustments would not be seen. So in constructing the passage they were careful to use simple words and simple sentences.

Unfortunately, this attempt may have biased the passage in the opposite direction, making it easier for the stutterers to say, and producing the result they did in fact obtain. In other words, in trying to avoid a type I error, the researchers increased the possibility of a type II error. There is no substitute for actual control, balancing the passages for vocabulary and syntax, and indeed other aspects of speech and language that might influence the frequency of stuttering. The problem is that if too many elements have to be controlled, it may be impossible to create the passage. The different aspects of language—phonology, syntax, semantics, and pragmatics—are interdependent, and, like the different parts of the speech mechanism, it is difficult to change one without changing the other.

A number of other challenges of Adams and Reis' experiment were made. Young (1975) questioned the method used to measure the adaptation effect, and Hutchinson and Brown (1978) wondered why an adaptation sequence was used at all. For these reasons, neither the Adams and Reis study, nor the replication of it that they did a few years later (1974), constitute good evidence for the vocalization hypothesis.

Brenner, Perkins, and Soderberg (1972) made another attempt to test the vocalization hypothesis. They asked stutterers to rehearse sentences before saying them. The rehearsals were of different kinds—whispered, mouthed movements without voice, and silent reading. In a control condition, there was no rehearsal at all. Here too there was an attempt to isolate different parts of the speech mechanism and test them independently. They found that the out-loud rehearsal was the only one that produced a significant reduction in the frequency of stuttering on the final, test reading, and they concluded that the use of the voice was necessary to achieve the rehearsal effect.

The test would have been more complete had there been a condition in which voice was produced without articulatory movements, a kind of humming condition in which the melody and stress patterns of the sentences were practiced but not the articulatory movements. This kind of condition, compared to the articulatory movement without voice (whispered) condition would have been a reasonable test of the hypothesis. Because this condition was omitted, a conclusion in support of the vocalization hypothesis was premature. Another explanation of the results, just as tenable, was that all parts of the speech mechanism needed to be practiced in combination, and that any change, not just a change in vocal functioning, rendered the rehearsal ineffective. There were other problems—whispering does not produce an absence of vocal function but alterations of it, nor does mouthing, or possibly even silent reading. All parts of the mechanism tend to work together.

Other tests of the vocalization hypothesis began to show another pattern of conclusions. Ingham and Carrol (1977) identified a number of variables that changed during choral speech that were not directly related to vocalization. Adams and Ramig (1980) showed that the rate of speech changed, indeed it tended to speed up, during choral speech.

Healey, Mallard, and Adams (1976) discovered that familiarity with the lyrics, and by implication a number of other variables, played a role in the fluency-enhancing effect of singing.

Garber and Martin (1977) compared the effects of masking when the subjects' voices were loud and when, through instruction, subjects kept their voices soft. Garber and Martin found that it was not the increased loudness of the voice that enhanced fluency, because fluency enhancement was strongest when the softer voice was used. They did not assess the rate of speech, which might also have been a factor.

Conture, McCall, and Brewer (1977) looked directly at stutterers' larynges with an endoscope. They found that laryngeal behavior during stuttered speech was, like laryngeal behavior during fluent speech, coordinated with events going on in other parts of the vocal tract. Even during stuttering, when a listener might be inclined to judge the speech as uncoordinated, there were correlations between the events occurring at the larynx and events occurring in other parts of the vocal tract. This latter conclusion, that stuttering itself is highly coordinated, has been confirmed (Borden, Baer, and Kenney, 1985).

Taken together, this information means that the vocalization hypothesis—the idea that stuttering was a disorder that occurred because of a faulty voice-producing mechanism—was too simple an answer. The mechanism, and the process of talking, were too complicated and interdependent for adequate tests of the functioning of individual aspects. Furthermore, fluency enhancement seemed to occur for reasons other than changes in vocalization. Indeed, it appeared that a number of changes, including changes in vocalization, could produce fluency-enhancing effects. The need to search for words and formulate sentences seems to put a strain on fluency, hence the more fluently produced familiar lyrics of a song. The role of audition, which I will examine more closely in the next section, was also implicated; at least talking when one couldn't hear oneself seemed to enhance fluency independent of vocal function. And changes in rate also seemed to have an effect.

Finding 8 has been very important in the evolution of stuttering theory. Freeman and Ushijima (1975, 1978) inserted hooked wire electrodes directly into the intrinsic muscles of the larynx in four stutterers and then asked them to produce a number of different kinds of speech tasks, some under fluency-enhancing conditions. The signals picked up by the electrodes were amplified and recorded. This technique, electromyography, records the levels of activity of individual muscles over a period of time. The experimenters then compared the EMG signals produced when the subjects spoke fluent words with those produced when they stuttered the same words. An equally small group of nonstutterers was also examined in the same way. The method was highly invasive and technically difficult, so the small size of the sample is understandable. Even so, caution should be used in interpreting the results from such a small number of observations.

They found that the muscle activity during the stuttered tokens was abnormal in several ways. First, the muscles were simply too active. There was much more muscle activity in the stuttered than in the nonstuttered words. Second, the muscle activity in the stuttered tokens was likely to be misplaced with regard to the timing of the speech gesture itself, usually occurring earlier than in the nonstuttered tokens. Third, the muscle activity of antagonistic muscles was not reciprocal. Antagonistic muscles, muscles that work in opposition to each other, are typically coordinated in that one is relaxed while the other is flexing, and vice versa. In the stuttered tokens this reciprocity of muscle activity was often not seen, both muscles of an antagonistic pair flexing simultaneously, working against each other. In the nonstutterers, muscle activity was more normal. However, it should be noted that in some of the stuttered tokens of the stutterers, muscle activity was not abnormal, and in some of the fluently produced tokens of both groups, some heightened, misplaced, and nonreciprocal muscle activity was observed. There was a notable minority report.

The experimenters were properly cautious in their interpretation of these results. The data showed only that during stuttered words muscle activity was overreactive, uncoordinated, and mistimed, as one would have expected. This is not to say that the results of this experiment were unimportant. Far from it. For the first time there was physiological evidence that the overreactions, mistimings, and miscoordinations of stuttered speech went deeper than the behavior and were present at the level of the muscle itself.

There was a tendency, however, for these results to be misinterpreted. The Freeman and Ushijima observations were interpreted to mean that stuttering was a muscular disorder, a malfunction at the level of the muscles. This may be true, but the Freeman and Ushijima observations do not prove it, although they are the observations one would expect if stuttering were a disorder of muscle activity. In other words, nothing in their observations could lead one to conclude that the abnormal muscle events they saw were a cause of stuttering. They could just as easily be a result of stuttering, or a manifestation of stuttering, at a physiological level.

The results were also misinterpreted to mean that stuttering was somehow a problem of the vocal mechanism. This misinterpretation was quickly put to rest, however, by the observations of Shapiro. Shapiro (1980) replicated the Freeman and Ushijima procedure, and in addition examined the muscle activity of a few of the facial muscles as well as the laryngeal muscles. He found the same patterns that Freeman and Ushijima had, but he found them in the facial as well as the laryngeal muscles. Clearly, stuttering was not restricted to the laryngeal mechanism.

Shapiro also noted the significance of the minority report in the Freeman and Ushijima observations. Many of the words that had been spoken fluently, as judged by trained listeners, showed patterns of muscle activity that looked just like the patterns observed for the stuttered words. Other words that sounded fluent did not show these abnormal patterns. It was evident that stuttering could occur on a physiological, muscular level without producing any perceptual deviation in the acoustic signal of speech. Stuttering could be present but not be observed, at least not without EMG equipment.

This finding of "subclinical" or "physiological" stuttering in the absence of overt stuttering behavior was very important. It meant that many of the experiments done in the past on the perceptually "fluent" speech of stutterers may have been contaminated. Experimenters who thought they were looking at fluently produced words in stuttering subjects were looking at words, some of which were fluent and some of which were stuttered at the physiological level. The study of stutterers' fluent speech had long been an interesting topic, and many previous observations were cast into doubt by Shapiro's description of subclinical stuttering.

A number of studies were done to follow up the observations of Freeman and Ushijima and Shapiro. Most of these are discussed elsewhere, because the implications of Freeman and Ushijima's and Shapiro's observations went well beyond the question of vocalization. Findings 9 and 10, however, resulted from studies done to test the implication that stuttering was primarily a disorder of laryngeal malfunction. Venkatigiri (1981) recalled the finding, reported just a few years before Freeman and Ushijima's and Shapiro's observations, that stutterers had slower reaction times for movements of the speech mechanism. If stuttering were a disorder of the voice-producing mechanism, then the reaction time of movements used to produce voiced speech sounds should differ from the reaction times of voiceless speech sounds. This experimenter then asked a group of stutterers to respond to an external stimulus as quickly as possible by saying /a/ in one condition. In the other condition, they responded by whispering the same vowel. Because the whispered response does not involve as much vocal activity (it does involve some), the reaction times should differ for the two tasks. A control group of matched nonstutterers was also given the same task. The results confirmed the hypothesis. The reaction times of the stutterers were slower for the voiced than for the whispered vowel, and this difference was not present in the responses of the nonstutterers.

Here, and in many similar experiments, the possibility of physiological stuttering needs to be considered. Of course, Venkatigiri did not include in the data any reaction times that occurred on responses on which the stutterers stuttered. Probably there were none of these anyway, because stutterers don't usually stutter on a task as simple as saying /a/. However, the possibility still exists that abnormally high, mistimed, and nonreciprocal muscle activity was present in some of the responses. The presence of this increased muscle activity would tend to slow the reaction time by stiffening the entire mechanism and damping its movements. Furthermore, these abnormal muscle events would be more likely to occur on the vocalized /a/ than on the whispered /a/, just as stuttering is more likely to occur on words spoken out loud than on whispered words.

Hayden, Adams, and Jordahl (1982) made a similar observation. Just as Venkatigiri had looked at reaction time during whisper, they looked at reaction time during metronomic pacing and masking noise, two other conditions known to enhance fluency. And they found the same thing: faster reaction times under fluency-enhancing conditions. Here too the differences observed could be attributed to abnormal muscle activity present in the apparently fluent words.

Finding 11, which was produced before Shapiro's identification of subclinical stuttering, has nonetheless to fall to the same axe. First Agnello and Wingate (1972), then Hillman and Gilbert (1977), looked at the VOT interval in stutterers and compared its duration with that of nonstutterers. VOT is the duration of the relatively silent period between the burst portion of a voiceless stop consonant and the onset of voicing. The motive for these investigations was to look for evidence that stutterers mistimed the movements of speech even when they were not stuttering, to see if there was not some more general timing deficit. Indeed, these experimenters found longer VOTs in the fluent speech of stutterers than in the fluent speech of nonstutterers, but of course the value of the observation is undercut by the possibility that the words on which the observation was made may not have been totally fluent. They may have sounded fluent, but there may nonetheless have been abnormal muscle activity present, and this abnormal muscle activity would have slowed the movements of speech and lengthened the duration of the VOT.

Finally, any consideration of the theory that stuttering is a disorder of voice production should take note of the observations of Ford and Luper (1975) and the hypothesis of Quarrington and Douglass (1960) that stutterers vary in the type of stuttering that they show. Ford and Luper looked at a number of physiological measures of stutterers' speech while they stuttered. Each showed a different physiological pattern. Some seemed to have most difficulty coordinating the movements of the larynx; others showed excessive tension and uncoordination in the movements of the upper articulators; still others seemed to have the most difficulty coordinating the outflow of air with the movements of the mouth and larynx.

Quarrington and Douglass had theorized in 1960 that some stutterers seem to be overt, stuttering in a way that is audible to listeners, while others are more likely not to stutter overtly but to perform other less noticable behaviors. Some stutterers expend a lot of effort to hide stuttering; others either don't, won't, or can't. Those whose stuttering is more overt will naturally have more muscular tension involved in the production of voice and articulation. Those who hide their stuttering better may have more of the subclinical type. Given this possibility, studies with small N's focusing on one anatomical area should be interpreted with caution.

STUTTERING AND AUDITION

Findings

1. Stuttering is found only rarely among the congenitally deaf and often disappears with the onset of adventitious deafness (Backus, 1938; Harms and Malone, 1939; Wingate, 1970).

2. Stutterers read more slowly than nonstutterers when they read with one ear masked (Stromsta, 1966).

3. Stutterers are less able than nonstutterers to localize sound (Rousey, Goetzinger, and Dirks, 1959; Asp, 1965).

4. Stutterers differ from nonstutterers in the interear phase relationship of bone-conducted sidetone (Stromsta, 1972).

5. Normal male speakers experience a blockage of phonation, pitch alterations, and vocal quality changes while continuously sustaining a vowel in falsetto when sidetone is distorted by reducing energy in the upper partials relative to the energy in the fundamental (nonlinear distortion) (Vannier et al., 1954; Stromsta, 1959).

6. Stutterers have a lower threshold of auditory discomfort than nonstutterers (MacCullough and Eaton, 1971).

7. Stutterers have slower galvanic skin responses (GSR) to auditory stimuli (Dinnan, McGuinness, and Perrin, 1970).

Theory

There is a long history of interest in the area of audition in stutterers. Surely the most interesting of the facts in this area is the first one. There simply are not many stutterers who have severe bilateral hearing loss. There are a few, however, and of these there are fewer yet, but still some, who are congenitally, completely, bilaterally deaf. You don't have to be able to hear to be a stutterer, but it helps. Hearing clearly seems to play a role in the disorder. But it is not easy to discern what that role is. The absence of hearing in a prelinguistic infant greatly changes the course of speech and language development, and stuttering typically begins during the preschool years. A child who was predisposed to stutter, but who was also bilaterally deaf, would have a very different course of speech development than one whose hearing was fully functional. So the fact that there are not many deaf stutterers may result from the unusual development of speech, and consequently of stuttering, in these children.

Similarly, when an adult or older child loses the ability to hear in both ears, there is a change in speech behavior. Gradually, there is a drifting away from the phonological system of the language and a corresponding deterioration of speech performance. Here too, it may not be deafness per se, but the speech changes that accompany deafness that are responsible for the effect of deafness on stuttering. Stutterers who lose their hearing will gradually begin to talk differently than they did before the loss.

Nevertheless, it is true that hearing is an important, but not mandatory, condition for stuttering to develop. The most obvious and straightforward explanation of this fact is that as children begin to develop stuttering, they react more and more to the aberrant sound of their own speech and try hard, too hard perhaps, to avoid or escape from the repetitions and prolongations in their speech. It would be difficult to develop such an avoidant attitude toward stuttering without being able to hear oneself and others.

However, the reactions of listeners would probably be discernible in nonverbal behavior, and some children might learn, even in the absence of usable hearing, to react to their stuttering with struggle, tension, and avoidance. Several other facts, described in other sections, also fit with this explanation: stutterers are usually more fluent under masking noise, particularly when they speak in a softer voice (Garber and Martin, 1977); and stutterers are more fluent when they whisper (Wingate, 1970). If one had acquired a fearful, avoidant, or otherwise negative attitude toward the sound of one's own speech, it might be expected that the symptoms produced by such an attitude would be reduced when the sound was reduced.

However, other explanations should also be noted. A likely one is simply that deaf speech is timed differently; it is often higher in pitch, with aberrant vocal quality. The vowels are likely to be longer than in the speech of the hearing. All of these differences, which are similar to the effects of masking noise on nondeaf speakers, are known to produce speech that is either fluent or less severely stuttered. So it may simply be that deaf individuals are not likely to stutter because they talk differently.

A third explanation, and one that is theoretically more interesting, although probably less likely to be true, is that stuttering is somehow caused by an aberration of the hearing mechanism, an aberration that cannot be present if the hearing mechanism is not fully functional. It is this possibility, that stutterers hear themselves differently than nonstutterers, that has given rise to most of the research in this area.

Findings 2 through 4 have to do with differences between the two ears in stutterers or with a possible difference in stutterers in the way information from the two ears is integrated by the brain. Stromsta has been one of the most active proponents of this idea. His first observation—that stutterers show a difference, when compared to nonstutterers, in the phase relationship between the two ears of bone-conducted feedback during speech—suggested that the signals sent to the brain by the two ears were perhaps arriving at different times. It also suggested that the brain was consequently receiving information difficult to interpret about the speech that was simultaneously being produced. The resulting uncertainty about what the mouth was doing at any given moment might result in hesitation and uncertainty in speech behavior. It is generally believed now that feedback plays a relatively minor role in speech production in adults (Borden, 1979), but this does not take much away from the theory because, first, stuttering usually begins in the very young child when feedback is still important in speech production, and, second, a distortion of feedback can have a dramatic effect on speech even though under ordinary circumstances it is not much used. The observation of differences in the bone-conducted sidetone of stutterers was later successfully replicated, although the replication was also carried out by Stromsta (1972).

Two tests of the theory have been made. One, by Stromsta (1972), had stutterers read with masking on one ear. The masking of one ear should have removed the disparity between the two signals and produced an alleviation of stuttering. But instead the stutterers were observed to read more slowly. This is interesting in its own right, and uncertain of interpretation, but it failed to confirm the theory.

Another test, however, by Asp (1965), did confirm the theory. He reasoned that if stutterers hear differently than nonstutterers in a way that affects the relative timing of signals between the two ears, then this difference should affect their ability to localize sounds, because the localization of sound depends on the phase relationship of an arriving signal between the two ears. The study showed that, indeed, stutterers do not localize sound as well as nonstutterers. Of course there may be other explanations. It would be useful for someone to replicate Asp's experiment.

Another test of the theory was less well related to the theory in question. A team of researchers (Vannier et al., 1954) asked stutterers to produce a soft falsetto tone and sustain it while the researchers altered the quality of the signal fed back to the stutterers' ears. They distorted the signal by reducing harmonic energy. The result of this distortion is a sound that is similar to a low-quality loudspeaker; it might be described as tinny. When this kind of a signal was fed back to the subjects as they produced a soft falsetto tone, the tone tended to waver and drop out. The result seems less than compelling. Sustaining falsetto softly is producing a voice that is on the verge of disappearing anyway. That it should be affected by a change in feedback of any kind seems unremarkable. The experiment would have been more compelling had other types of feedback and perhaps other kinds of sound production tasks also been done for comparative purposes.

Findings 6 and 7 are unrelated to the interear phase theory but have to do with audition. MacCullough and Eaton (1971) observed that stutterers report discomfort at a lower level of intensity than nonstutterers do. It is not clear how this observation fits into the general picture of the audition of stutterers. Dinnan, McGuinness, and Perrin (1970) set out to test the idea that stutterers might have a different auditory feedback system, but found instead that they simply responded more slowly. The observation may have something to do with the auditory feedback systems of stutterers, or it may be related to the reaction time literature. It should be noted, however, that the GSR that Dinnan and colleagues used did not involve movement, so that its relation to the reaction time literature is unclear.

TOUCH AND PRESSURE SENSATION DURING SPEECH

Findings

1. Pressure on parts of the speech musculature may completely inhibit stuttering in some stutterers (Fujita, 1955), but in others, pressure may set off tremors (Van Riper, 1971).
2. Oral sensory deprivation increases the frequency and severity of stuttering (Hutchinson and Ringel, 1975).
3. Intraoral air pressure, airflow durations, and airflow rates are higher during oral sensory deprivation in normal speakers, but with little effect on speech quality (Hutchinson and Putnam, 1974).

Theory

This small body of information developed during a period of interest in the idea that stuttering was a disorder of feedback. The feedback theory developed from the effects of DAF on normal speakers and on stutterers, and from the apparent relation between stuttering and audition. If audition was, or might be, related to stuttering, it was logical to pursue a relation between stuttering and other forms of feedback. Touch, pressure, and motion sense seemed like good candidates.

The early information on touch and pressure was largely anecdotal, and it still has not been clearly demonstrated that stuttering can be either enhanced or diminished by pressure on parts of the speech musculature during speech. Assuming that such a phenomenon is real, there is a possibility that the effect is based on learning. That is, the stutterer, having had much experience with certain sounds and the touch and pressure sensations associated with them, may react to the stimulus of pressure with a tremor-like response. Similarly, other sensations of touch or pressure, associated by virtue of the stutterer's experience with fluent speech rather than stuttering, may have an ameliorative effect. To establish that touch and pressure are related to stuttering in a way that is theoretically important, it would be necessary not only to document the effect, but to show how it is related or unrelated to the stuttering patterns of the subjects involved.

Hutchinson and Ringel (1975) approached the problem systematically. If stuttering was related to touch, pressure, or movement, its symptoms should respond to the removal of these sensations through anesthesia. Consequently, they anesthetized the mouths of a number of stutterers and recorded their speech. Stuttering was significantly increased by the procedure. This seemed to suggest with some clarity that stuttering did not result from a faulty or hypersensitive sense of touch, pressure, or proprioception. Indeed, it would appear that information derived from these feedback systems was, if anything, helping the stutterers speak as fluently as they normally did.

These results could be said to complement the findings, noted earlier, that stuttering is aleviated under conditions of masking noise. If speech is monitored in some way by information from both auditory and cutaneous-muscular sensations, the removal of auditory feedback throws more of the monitoring burden on the cutaneous and muscular sensations and enhances fluency. On the other hand, a reduction of the cutaneous and muscular sensations throws more of a burden on the auditory system and diminishes fluency. It could also be, however, that the bilateral and complete anesthetization of the mouth raised the subjects' anxiety level, which is a common effect.

Another explanation comes from the experiment by Hutchinson and Putnam (1974) in which they measured aspects of airflow and air pressure within the mouths of normal speakers during oral sensory deprivation. The higher air pressure, more rapid air flow, and longer durations all suggest that speaking with an anesthetized mouth requires considerable effort. Articulatory contacts are made more firmly and probably held for a longer period of time, during which air pressure builds up to higher levels, and then, when it is released it flows with greater velocity. Speech with an anesthetized mouth is slow and labored, much like stuttering itself. Given this information, it is not surprising that stutterers showed more frequent and more severe stuttering when deprived of oral sensation. This condition reduces fluency in nonstutterers as well.

RATE AND TIMING

Van Riper (1982) first suggested that stuttering was a disorder of timing. Clearly the time dimension of speech is altered by stuttering. The repetitions, blockages, and secondary extraneous behaviors slow the rate of information flow. The velocity of movement of stutterers has not been specifically measured, to my knowledge, but I would guess that it varies from faster than normal during certain types of stuttering, such as part-word repetitions, to slower than normal during blockages and other labored articulations. This too suggests that stuttering is a disorder of timing.

A third possibility is that stuttering arises because stutterers are deficient in their ability to time the articulatory events of speech. Allen (1975) has speculated that speech is timed by reference to a kind of central clock. If this theory is correct, one might further theorize that stutterers lack such a clock or that their clocks function improperly. Martin (1979) has related timing to speech rhythm. This might suggest that a rhythmic deficiency is present in stutters, an idea that is currently under test. Kelso and Tuller (1983) and Fowler (1978) have suggested that the timing of speech movements is constrained and enhanced by the physical properties of the vocal tract, functioning like a mass-spring system. From this point of view, the aberrations of timing present in the speech of stutterers might arise because the vocal tracts of stutterers have resonant frequencies that are different, perhaps too springy because of heightened background muscle tonus (Zimmermann, 1980).

Findings

1. The voice onset time or intervocalic interval (VOT) associated with voiceless stop consonants is longer in the "fluent" speech of stutterers than in the speech of nonstutterers, both in nonsense syllable production (Agnello and Wingate, 1972) and in contextual speech, although in contextual speech at least the differential effects on VOT of place of consonant production is the same for stutterers as for nonstutterers (Hillman and Gilbert, 1977). (This finding was discussed earlier under vocalization.)
2. The "fluent" speech of stutterers shows longer durations of consonants in VCV syllables and of vowels in CVC syllables than the speech

of nonstutterers. There is also a greater variance of duration in the stutterers. The differential effects on duration of adjacent phonemes (manner), however, is the same for stutterers as for nonstutterers (DiSimoni, 1974).

3. In their "fluent" speech, stutterers may move their speech mechanisms at a slower speed than nonstutterers (Starkweather and Myers, 1978; Zimmermann, 1980).

4. Although they speak more slowly to begin with, stutterers, both adults and children, modify their speech rate in the same way as nonstutterers when asked to speak more slowly (Healey and Adams, 1981).

5. The formant frequencies of stutterers' "fluent" speech show a tendency to produce more centralized vowels, indicating a tendency to speak with restricted movements, both spatially and temporally, than nonstutterers (Klich and May, 1982).

6. When stutterers speak under fluency-enhancing conditions, they show longer duration of phonation (time between pauses) and slower speech rate (Andrews et al., 1982).

7. When naive listeners are asked to rate the "naturalness" of stutterers' speech, their ratings are correlated −.81 with the rate at which the stutterers produce words and −.81 with the frequency of stuttering (Martin, Haroldson, and Triden, 1984). The naturalness of a sample of speech can be predicted from the rate at which the speech is produced as accurately as it can be from the frequency of stuttering. It seems a fair conclusion that listeners find slow speech as unnatural as stuttered speech.

Theory

Findings 1 through 5 fit one part of the picture, while findings 6 and 7 fit another part. The first five findings are based on analyses of the speech of stutterers when judged by listeners to be free of stuttering. As we have seen, acoustic judgments of fluency do not entirely eliminate abnormalities that may still be present at the muscular level. Although this problem diminishes the importance of some of these studies, it does not render them all entirely worthless.

The first finding has already been discussed in the section on vocalization. From the point of view of timing, the slower VOTs of stutterers suggest simply that stutterers talk more slowly, even when they are not stuttering. This fact is not of great value, however, when the possibility of physiological stuttering is considered. Because the samples on which the measurements of VOT were made could have contained words produced with underlying muscle activity that was abnormally high and improperly timed, it may be that the observation of longer VOTs in stutterers was simply a reflection of these underlying abnormalities.

The same point can be made with regard to the second finding.

DiSimoni (1974) took samples of specific sound combinations within a sentence frame from stutterers and nonstutterers. Any productions that were stuttered, as judged acoustically, were discarded. He then made spectrograms and measured the durations of specific consonants and vowels. The segments produced by the stutterers tended to be longer, consistent with a slower rate of speech production. In this case, however, the case for contamination by physiological stuttering is made somewhat stronger by DiSimoni's additional observations of greater variability of segment durations in the stutterers, which would be expected if the samples contained stuttering behavior.

The third finding falls in the same group. In these two studies, sections of spontaneous speech produced by stutterers but judged by listeners to be free of stuttering were analyzed to determine the duration of the segments. The stutterers produced longer segments, consistent with a slower rate of speech. However, the possibility of underlying physiological stuttering cannot be discounted, and the effects may be attributable to it. So, although the speech of stutterers may be slower than the speech of nonstutterers, the reduced rate may be simply a result of stuttering and not the result of some underlying deficit in timing or motor control.

Healey and Adams (1981) asked both stutterers and nonstutterers to speak at a slower rate and verified that they had done so. They then measured the duration of pauses and the rate of syllable production. Both groups of subjects used either one or the other or both strategies to reduce the rate of their speech. This is one of the rare studies that is interesting for what it did not find. If stuttering were a result of a deficit of timing, it might be expected that stutterers would show a different pattern of rate reduction than nonstutterers, perhaps pausing longer but still producing syllables rapidly, or vice versa. But such was not the case. This does not, of course, provide any evidence against a timing theory of stuttering, just the absence of a result that might have been expected.

Klich and May's analysis (1982) of the formant frequencies of stutterers' "fluent" speech noted a tendency for the average formant frequencies to be shifted in a central direction, suggesting that stutterers talked with speech movements that were less extensive and briefer. This pattern is consistent with the possibility that, despite the judgments of acoustical fluency, aberrations of muscle activity of the type associated with stuttering may nonetheless have been present. It suggests also that there may be an underlying increased level of muscle tonus, stiffening the entire speech mechanism and restricting its movement.

Andrews and his colleagues (1982) analyzed the speech of stutterers under the most powerful of the fluency-enhancing conditions. They wanted to see if there were any common influences of the conditions, other than the tendency for stuttering to be reduced. They found that the conditions increased the duration of phonation, that is, the time spent talking between pauses, and that the stutterers' rate was slowed. Of these the first is probably a by-product of fluency enhancement. Stutterers talk in longer utterances when stuttering is relieved because it is the stuttering that shortens their phonation time in the first place. However, the second of these observations, that the rate is slowed, is important because when stuttering is removed rate typically increases. If the rate of nonstuttered speech is slowed by fluency-enhancing conditions, it may be that what causes stuttering in the first place is a rate that is too fast for the person's motor control skills. I believe this interpretation is important because it fits so well with the facts of stuttering development and beneficial effects on stuttering of slowed speech rate.

Finding 7 simply says about stuttering what we have already observed about normal fluency: that the rate at which syllables are produced is an important part of the picture. When listeners are asked to judge the speech of stutterers who have been through therapy programs that make use of reduced rate, they judge as more natural the subjects who speak at a faster rate. It is natural to speak quickly, and slow speech sounds unnatural or tends to accompany other aspects of speech that sound unnatural.

STUTTERING AND LANGUAGE

In the earlier descriptive sections findings were presented that related language and stuttering. These descriptive findings showed that stuttering in adults and children was located with regard to language variables—at clause boundaries, on less frequently used words, and so on. In this section, findings are presented that relate stuttering to language acquisition in children, and the theory that can be built on these facts explains the cause and development of stuttering rather than describing its location.

Findings

1. Young stutterers stutter more at clause boundaries (Bloodstein, 1974; Wall, 1977; Wall, Starkweather, and Cairns, 1981).
2. Nonstuttering children show more disfluency when producing modeled sentences of greater syntactic complexity (Haynes and Hood, 1978).
3. Nonstuttering three- and four-year-olds show more disfluencies with increased syntactic complexity in elicited imitation tasks (Pearl and Bernthal, 1980).
4. Nonstuttering five-year-olds show more disfluencies with increased syntactic complexity in a sentence modeling task but not in an elicited imitation task (Gordon, 1982).
5. Nonstuttering boys with high verbal ability use more and longer ut-

terances and more complex language but still have fewer and shorter pauses than boys of low verbal ability (Jones, 1974).

6. Highly disfluent but nonstuttering preschool children use less complex language than highly fluent children of the same age (Muma, 1971).

7. Young stutterers seem to use less complex language than nonstutterers of the same age (Wall, 1977).

8. Stuttering children are often delayed in developing reading skills (Schindler, 1955). Others have failed to find this result (Conture and van Naersson, 1977).

9. Nonstuttering children become more disfluent, and their disfluencies include relatively more part-word repetitions, as the linguistic complexity of reading material increases (Cecconi, Hood, and Tucker, 1977).

10. Language-delayed children are more disfluent than normals if, and only if, they have been in therapy (Merits-Patterson and Reed, 1977).

11. Stuttering children are significantly, but not pathologically, delayed in language development (Kline and Starkweather, 1979).

Theory

The findings in this section fall into two groups. Findings 1 through 4 and 9 demonstrate the relation between disfluency and language formulation. First, in children, as in adults, stuttering is located at clause boundaries. Bloodstein (1974) first suggested this as one of the characteristics of early stuttering, but the suggestion was based on clinical accounts. Subsequently, a careful syntactic analysis of the corpora of a group of young stuttering children documented clearly that there was a powerful tendency for stuttering, even in the very young stutterer, to be located with regard to syntax, specifically at major clause boundaries (Wall, 1977; Wall, Starkweather, and Cairns, 1982). It is not clear, however, if stuttering occurs at clause boundaries *because* of any linguistic activity that may be occurring there. There are differences in the motoric production of speech that occurs at these same locations—requirements for greater precision of articulation and intelligibility (Hunnicutt, 1985) and, at the same time, requirements for greater velocities of movement (Umeda, 1975).

Haynes and Hood (1978) asked children who were not stutterers to produce sentences based on a model. In this task, a sentence is produced for the child along with a picture that the sentence provides. Then a second picture with the same structure but different content is presented, and the child is asked to produce a sentence describing it. The resulting production has the same syntactic structure but different forms than the modelled sentences. Using this procedure, Haynes and Hood (1978) showed that when nonstuttering children produced more complex sentences, they were more likely to be disfluent than when they produced less complex sentences. It was not immediately apparent, however, whether the effect was attributable to difficulty in receiving the more complex sentence, in its greater length, its faster rate of production, or to other factors.

A second study by Pearl and Bernthal (1980) with a younger age group demonstrated a similar effect using an elicited imitation task. The results, discussed earlier, are illustrated in Figure 4–8. Once more, the greater syntactic complexity produced the most disfluency, but again it was not possible to be certain that the tendency for more complex sentences to produce more disfluency was a result of sentence formulation or some other aspect of the production of complex sentences, such as faster articulatory rate.

Gordon (1982) compared modeling and elicited imitation tasks in young nonstuttering children, and found that the tendency for complexity to produce disfluency was greater in the modeling than in the elicited imitation task (see Figure 4–9), and this seemed to show decisively that the reason more complex sentences were produced more disfluently was because they were more difficult to formulate. Other aspects of speech production were controlled. This was an important finding because it linked, for the first time, the effort of language formulation with the effort of speech production. When the linguistic task becomes difficult, the motor speech production task can suffer. There is, in other words, a trading relationship between language and speech, and if there is a trading relationship the possibility of interference is strong. Interference, in this case, refers to the fact that demands on the child for language formulation, when high enough, may detract from motor speech performance. Language fluency (see pp. 11–13) is related to speech fluency.

The second group, findings 5 through 11, shows that there is a relation between stuttering (and disfluency) and general verbal or language skill. Children who are not so skilled at language are likely to be less fluent speakers than those who are more skilled, and conversely, children who are less fluent are likely to be less verbally skilled.

Jones' (1974) and Muma's (1971) findings illustrate this relation as well as any. A speaker will pause more often and for longer durations when producing material that is linguistically more difficult (Goldman-Eisler, 1961). Despite this, Jones (1974) found that children who were highly skilled with words and language, and who consequently used sentences that were longer and more complex than those used by children who were not so skilled, nevertheless paused less often and for briefer durations. Similarly, Muma (1971) found that when children were divided into highly fluent and highly nonfluent groups, their language skills as reflected in the length and complexity of their sentences were different. Clearly, verbal skill shows itself not only in the length and complexity of sentences, but also in the ease with which those sentences are formulated and produced. This is not to say, necessarily, that children with high language skills are motorically superior as well. The duration of pauses and the frequency of pauses is clearly related to language formulation, but it may also be related to motoric skill (Amster, 1984). It is simply not possible at present to distinguish motoric and linguistic fluency.

Wall (1977), in an informal analysis, observed that the sentences of children who stuttered were less complex than those of children who did not stutter. Similarly, Kline and Starkweather (1979) found that young stutterers had a significantly shorter mean length of utterance than matched nonstutterers. In the Kline and Starkweather study, the receptive skills of the stuttering children were also found to be significantly less well developed than those of their matched peers. The results of this study are shown in Figure 9–1. Furthermore, there was a small but significant correlation between the expressive and receptive measures. These findings also suggest that stutterers have somewhat lower language abilities than nonstutterers. They do not, however, show that the lesser language abilities of stutterers are related to the etiology of stuttering.

It is possible that stutterers do not develop language as rapidly as nonstutterers because they stutter. Stutterers are often reticent at this age, and this reticence may produce language performance that suggests a lower level of development. The poorer test performance could be simply a reflection of the children using shorter and simpler sentences because they have learned through experience with stuttering that sentences like these are less likely to be stuttered. Or it could be that being a stutterer restricts the use of speech to the point where language is not learned as rapidly. Several

FIGURE 9-1   The language skills of young stutterers and nonstutterers.

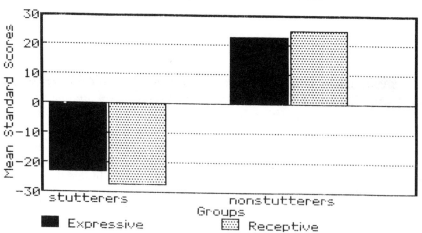

facts argue against such a superficial relationship, however. First, the low receptive scores observed by Kline and Starkweather (1979) argue against the idea that simple reticence produced the low expressive scores. Similarly the observation of Schindler (1955) that stutterers are delayed in their reading suggests that language skills themselves, and not just the performance of them, may be involved, although it is not clear to what extent performance plays a role in the development of reading skills. In addition, of course, Conture and van Naersson (1977) failed to replicate Schindler's finding.

Finding 10 is one of the most interesting, and one of the most worrisome, pieces of information in the area of language and stuttering. Merits-Patterson and Reed (1977) compared the speech of children who were on the waiting list for language therapy with that of children who were actually in language therapy and found a higher incidence of stuttering in the latter group. The implication is clear that language therapy, not the presence of a language disorder, tends to increase the chances that a child will stutter. Perhaps children with language disorders are prone to stuttering to begin with, but therapy for the language disorder is likely to bring it out. This suggests first of all that the therapy introduces a kind of pressure on the child to perform, which in turn causes the child to stutter.

The implication is clear that children in therapy for language disorders should be closely monitored for fluency, and when stuttering begins to appear, therapy plans should be altered drastically to reduce pressure for performance. A second implication is that language performance and speech production are related in much the same way as described above and in the sections on normal fluency. This is not to suggest that stuttering develops because of a language disorder, but rather that the production of speech and the formulation of language place a simultaneous demand on the young person. If the demands in either of these two dimensions are excessive, performance in the other dimension may be reduced.

From this review of language and stuttering three major points emerge: (1) disfluency and stuttering occur at points where language is being formulated; (2) children who stutter are less skilled verbally than children who don't; and (3) children with delayed language development sometimes begin to stutter when they encounter the more demanding environment of the language clinic. Together these facts, viewed most conservatively, suggest that the production of fluent speech and the use of language put simultaneous demands on the same system. If stuttering is present so that the child is already devoting much energy to the motoric acts of speaking, language performance will be diminished. If the child's language is delayed so that additional energy must be devoted to language production to meet the increased expectations of significant adults, motor speech production may suffer in consequence.

REFERENCES

ADAMS, M. R., and REIS, R., The influence of the onset of phonation on the frequency of stuttering, *Journal of Speech and Hearing Research,* 14 (1971), 639–44.

ADAMS, M. R., and REIS, R., The influence of the onset of phonation in the frequency of stuttering: a replication and re-evaluation, *Journal of Speech and Hearing Research,* 17 (1974), 752–54.

ADAMS, M. R., and RAMIG, P., Vocal characteristics of stutterers and normal speakers during choral reading, *Journal of Speech and Hearing Research,* 23 (1980), 457–65.

AGNELLO, J. G., and WINGATE, M. E., Some acoustic aspects of stuttered speech, *Journal of the Acoustical Society of America,* 52 (1972), 159.

ALLEN, G., Speech rhythm: its relation to performance universals and articulatory timing, *Journal of Phonetics,* 3 (1975), 75–86.

AMSTER, B., The rate of speech in normal preschool children. Ph.D. dissertation, Temple University, Philadelphia, 1984.

ANDREWS, G., HOWIE, P., DOZSA, M., and GUITAR, B., Stuttering: speech pattern characteristics under fluency inducing conditions, *Journal of Speech and Hearing Research,* 25 (1982), 208–16.

ASP, C., An investigation of the localization of interaural stimuli by clicks and the reading times of stutterers and nonstutterers under monaural sidetone conditions, *De Therapia Vocis et Loquellae,* 1 (1965), 353–56.

BACKUS, O., Incidence of stuttering among the deaf, *Annals of Otology, Rhinology and Laryngology,* 47 (1938), 632–35.

BLOODSTEIN, O., The rules of early stuttering, *Journal of Speech and Hearing Disorders,* 39 (1974), 79–94.

BORDEN, G., An interpretation of research on feedback interruption in speech, *Brain and Language,* 7 (1979), 307–19.

BORDON, G., BAER, T., and KENNEY, M., Onset of voicing in stuttered and fluent utterances, *Journal of Speech and Hearing Research,* 28 (1985), 363–72.

BRENNER, N. C., PERKINS, W. H., and SODERBERG, G. A., The effect of rehearsal on frequency of stuttering, *Journal of Speech and Hearing Research,* 15 (1972), 483–86.

CECCONI, C., HOOD, S., and TUCKER, R., Influence of reading level difficulty on the disfluencies of normal children, *Journal of Speech and Hearing Research,* 20 (1977), 475–84.

CHEVRIE-MUELLER, C., A study of laryngeal function in stutterers by the glottographic method, in *Proceedings of the Seventh Congrès de la Société Francaise de Médecine de la Voix et de la Parole,* Paris, 1963.

CONTURE, E. G., MCCALL, G., and BREWER, D. W., Laryngeal behavior during stuttering, *Journal of Speech and Hearing Research,* 20 (1977), 661–68.

CONTURE, E., and VAN NAERSSON, E., Reading abilities of school age stutterers, *Journal of Fluency Disorders,* 2 (1977), 295–300.

DINNAN, J., MCGUINNESS, E., and PERRIN, L., Auditory feedback: stutterers v. nonstutterers, *Journal of Learning Disorders,* 3 (1970), 209–13.

DISIMONI, F., Preliminary study of certain timing relationships in the speech of stutterers, *Journal of the Acoustical Society of America,* 56 (1974), 695–96.

FORD, S. C., and LUPER, H. L., Aerodynamic, phonatory, and labial EMG patterns during fluent and stuttered speech. Convention address, American Speech and Hearing Association, 1975.

FOWLER, C., Timing control in speech production, *Dissertation Abstracts International,* 38 (1978), 3927–28.

FREEMAN, F., and USHIJIMA, T., Laryngeal activity accompanying the moment of stuttering: a preliminary report of EMG investigation, *Journal of Fluency Disorders,* 1 (1975), 36–45.

FREEMAN, F., and USHIJIMA, T., Laryngeal muscle activity during stuttering, *Journal of Speech and Hearing Research,* 21 (1978), 538–62.

FUJITA, K., Tremor control as a factor in stuttering, *Japanese Journal of Otology,* 58 (1955), 287–91.

GARBER, S. F., and MARTIN, R. R., Effects of noise on increased vocal intensity and stuttering, *Journal of Speech and Hearing Research,* 20 (1977), 233–40.

GOLDMAN-EISLER, F., The distribution of pause durations in speech, *Language and Speech,* 4 (1961), 18–26.

GORDON, P., The effects of syntactic complexity on the occurrence of disfluencies in five-year-old children. Poster session, American Speech and Hearing Association, 1982.

HARMS, M., and MALONE, J. Y., The relationship of hearing acuity to stammering, *Journal of Speech Disorders,* 4 (1939), 363–70.

HAYDEN, P., ADAMS, M. R., and JORDAHL, N., The effects of pacing and masking on stutterers' and nonstutterers' speech initiation times, *Journal of Fluency Disorders,* 7 (1982), 9–19.

HAYNES, W., and HOOD, S., Disfluency changes in children as a function of the systematic modification of linguistic complexity, *Journal of Communication Disorders,* 11 (1978), 79–93.

HEALEY, E. C., MALLARD, A. R., and ADAMS, M. R., Factors contributing to the reduction of stuttering during singing, *Journal of Speech and Hearing Research,* 19 (1976), 475–80.

HEALEY, C., and ADAMS, M., Rate reduction strategies used by normally fluent and stuttering children and adults, *Journal of Fluency Disorders,* 6 (1981), 1–14.

HILLMAN, R. E., and GILBERT, H. R., Voice onset time for voiceless stop consonants in the fluent reading of stutterers and nonstutterers, *Journal of the Acoustical Society of America,* 61 (1977), 610–11.

HUNNICUTT, S., Intelligibility v. redundancy: conditions of dependency, *Language and Speech,* 28 (1985), 47–56.

HUTCHINSON, J., and PUTNAM, A., Aerodynamic aspect of sensory deprived speech, *Journal of the Acoustical Society of America,* 56 (1974), 1612–17.

HUTCHINSON, J., and RINGEL, R., The effect of oral sensory deprivation on stuttering behavior, *Journal of Communication Disorders,* 8 (1975), 249–58.

HUTCHINSON, J. M., and BROWN, D., The Adams and Reis observations revisited, *Journal of Fluency Disorders,* 3 (1978), 149–54.

INGHAM, R. J., and CARROLL, P. J., Listener judgment of differences in stutterers' nonstuttered speech during chorus and nonchorus conditions, *Journal of Speech and Hearing Research,* 20 (1977), 293–302.

JONES, Elaborated speech and hesitation phenomena, *Language and Speech,* 17 (1974), 199–203.

KELSO, S., and TULLER, B., Compensatory articulation under conditions of reduced afferent information: a dynamic formulation, *Journal of Speech and Hearing Research,* 26 (1983), 217–24.

KLICH, R., and MAY, G., Spectrographic study of vowels in stutterers' fluent speech, *Journal of Speech and Hearing Research,* 25 (1982), 364–70.

KLINE, M., and STARKWEATHER, C., Receptive and expressive language performance in young stutterers. Convention address, American Speech and Hearing Association, 1979.

MACCULLOUGH, M., and EATON, R., A note on reduced auditory pain threshold in 44 stuttering children, *British Journal of Disorders of Communication,* 6 (1971), 148–53.

MARTIN, J., Rhythmic (hierarchical) versus serial structure in speech and other behavior, *Psychology Revue,* 79 (1979), 487–509.

MARTIN, R., HAROLDSON, S., and TRIDEN, K., Stuttering and speech naturalness, *Journal of Speech and Hearing Disorders,* 49 (1984), 53–58.

MERITS-PATTERSON, R., and REED, C., Disfluencies in the speech of language-disordered children, *Journal of Speech and Hearing Research,* 46 (1981), 55–58.

MUMA, J., Syntax of preschool fluent and disfluent speech: a transformational analysis, *Journal of Speech and Hearing Research,* 14 (1971), 428–41.

PEARL, S., and BERNTHAL, J., The effect of grammatical complexity upon disfluency behavior of nonstuttering preschool children, *Journal of Fluency Disorders,* 5 (1980), 55–68.

QUARRINGTON, B., and DOUGLASS, E., Audibility avoidance in nonvocalized stutterers, *Journal of Speech and Hearing Disorders,* 25 (1960), 358–65.

ROUSEY, C., GOETZINGER, C., and DIRKS, D. Sound localization of normal, stuttering, neurotic, and hemiplegic subjects, *American Medical Association Archives of General Psychiatry,* 1 (1959), 640–45.

SCHINDLER, M., A study of educational adjustments of stuttering and nonstuttering children, in *Stuttering in Children and Adults,* eds. W. Johnson and R. Leutenegger. Minneapolis: University of Minnesota Press, 1955.

SHAPIRO, A., An electromyographic analysis of the fluent and dysfluent utterance of several types of stutterers, *Journal of Fluency Disorders*, 5 (1980), 203–31.

STARKWEATHER, C. W., Stuttering and laryngeal behavior: a review. American Speech and Hearing Association Monograph No. 21, 1982.

STARKWEATHER, C. W., and MYERS, M., The duration of subsegments within the intervocalic intervals of stutterers and nonstutterers. *Journal of Fluency Disorders*, 4 (1979), 205–14.

STROMSTA, C., Experimental blockage of phonation by distorted sidetone, *Journal of Speech and Hearing Research*, 2 (1959), 286–301.

STROMSTA, C., Interaural phase disparity of stutterers and nonstutterers, *Journal of Speech and Hearing Research*, 15 (1972), 771–80.

UMEDA, N., Vowel duration in American English, *Journal of the Acoustical Society of America*, 58 (1975), 434–45.

VANNIER, J., SAUMONT, R., LABARRAQUE, L., and HUSSON, R., Production experimental des blocages synaptiques recurrentials par des stimulations auditives homorhythmiques avec dephasages reglables, *Revue de laryngologies*, Supplement 1, Bordeau, 1954.

VAN RIPER, C., *Speech Correction: Principles and Methods*, 5th ed. Englewood Cliffs, N.J.: Prentice-Hall, 1971.

VENKATIGIRI, H. S., Reaction time for voiced and whispered /a/ in stutterers and nonstutterers, *Journal of Fluency Disorders*, 6 (1981), 265–71.

WALL, M., The location of stuttering in the spontaneous speech of young child stutterers, Ph.D. dissertation, City University of New York, New York, 1977.

WALL, M., STARKWEATHER, C., and CAIRNS, H., Syntactic influences on stuttering in young child stutterers, *Journal of Fluency Disorders*, 6 (1981), 283–98.

WALL, M., STARKWEATHER, C., and HARRIS, K., The influence of voicing adjustments on the location of stuttering in the spontaneous speech of young child stutterers, *Journal of Fluency Disorders*, 6 (1981), 299–310.

WINGATE, M. E., Effect on stuttering of changes in audition, *Journal of Speech and Hearing Research*, 13 (1970), 861–73.

YOUNG, M., Letter to the editor, *Journal of Speech and Hearing Research*, 18 (1975), 600–602.

ZIMMERMANN, G., Stuttering: a disorder of movement, *Journal of Speech and Hearing Research*, 23 (1980), 122–36.

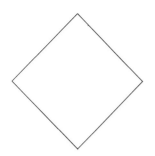

Author Index

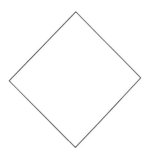

Subject Index